19 Update in Intensive Care and Emergency Medicine

Edited by J.-L. Vincent

W. J. Sibbald J.-L. Vincent (Eds.)

Clinical Trials for the Treatment of Sepsis

With 61 Figures and 74 Tables

Springer-Verlag
Berlin Heidelberg New York
London Paris Tokyo
Hong Kong Barcelona
Budapest

Series Editor

Prof. Dr. Jean-Louis Vincent
Clinical Director, Department of Intensive Care
Erasme University Hospital
Route de Lennik 808, 1070 Brussels, Belgium

Volume Editors

Prof. Dr. W.J. Sibbald
Department of Critical Care, Victoria Hospital
375 South Street, N6A 4G5 London, Ontario, Canada

and

Prof. Dr. Jean-Louis Vincent

ISBN-13:978-3-642-79226-7 e-ISBN-13:978-3-642-79224-3
DOI: 10.1007/978-3-642-79224-3

Softcover reprint of the hardcover 1st edition 1995

SPIN: 10478360 19/3130-5 4 3 2 1 0 – Printed on acid-free paper

Preface

Sepsis and Innovative Treatment: The Odyssey

R. C. Bone

The Odyssey by Homer, dates back to the 8th century, B.C. [1]. It is a great epic adventure of Odysseus's dramatic journey from Troy back home to Ithaca. Odysseus survives the ordeals of this journey and returns with new powers and insights. The study of the pathogenesis and treatment of sepsis has also been an odyssey. I feel we will return from this odyssey with new insights and treatments. However, as with Odysseus, this will occur only after considerable struggle.

In the 1980s we had a rather simplistic view of sepsis. It was a highly lethal complication caused by infection and often characterized by shock and multi-organ failure. Our knowledge of the inflammatory responses associated with sepsis was embryonic compared to today. The inflammatory response was often treatment with mega-dose corticosteroids along with fluid resuscitation, vasopressors and antibiotics. Because of the paucity of multi-center controlled trials documenting the risk/benefit ratio of the treatment of sepsis with corticosteroids, two large multi-center controlled trials were organized to evaluate the role of corticosteroids in sepsis [2, 3]. Because animal models showed benefits of corticosteroids only with pre-treatment or early treatment, a definition of sepsis was used that did not require positive culture documentation or septic shock to be included in the studied population. The sepsis syndrome was used as a definition and is as follows:

> Sepsis syndrome consists of sepsis which is clinical evidence of infection, tachypnea, tachycardia and hyperthermia or hypothermia plus evidence of altered organ perfusion including one or more of the following:
>
> 1) acute changes in mental status;
> 2) $PaO_2/FiO_2 \leq 280$ without other pulmonary or cardiovascular diseases as the cause;
> 3) increased lactate, and
> 4) oliguria [4].

The sepsis syndrome had a predictable mortality rate, incidence of shock, incidence of bacteremia, and subsequent development of multi-organ failure. This definition or a modification of it has been used for all subsequent large sepsis trials.

Our hope of finding a "magic bullet" to treat sepsis has been frustrating. Part of this frustration emanates from our incomplete understanding of sepsis and the conduct of clinical trials. However, like Odysseus, we now recognize that we are now on an incredible journey with a destination yet to be determined. What are the bright spots?

1) Our knowledge of the pathogenesis of sepsis has made incredible advances in the past two decades;
2) Our knowledge of the epidemiology of sepsis has advanced;
3) Our appreciation of the complexity of the inflammatory response and its beneficial and detrimental aspects are now appreciated more completely; and
4) Our design and conduct of clinical trials have achieved greater scrutiny.

These advances have been achieved because of dedicated investigators that have carefully documented the results of their trials, a pharmaceutical industry that has fostered the support and leadership possible to conduct such trials, and the Federal Drug Administration (FDA) which has worked diligently with investigators and the pharmaceutical industry to learn from our past clinical trials.

I believe we are now on an analytic review of our sepsis trials that may allow us to enter a new stage in the understanding of sepsis. This Round Table Conference on Clinical Trials for the Treatment of Sepsis is such a much-needed scrutiny. I regret that I was unable to attend the Conference in Brussels on March 12–14, 1994, because of a hypernephroma that hopefully was cured by a nephrectomy. Indeed, I was encountering my own odyssey. I appreciate the invitation from Drs Vincent and Sibbald to write a preface to this Round Table Conference. I feel we are on the brink of a new understanding and possible new treatments for sepsis. Our odyssey with sepsis has just begun!

References

1. The Homeric Epics. The New Encyclopaedia Britannica Macropaedia (1985) Encyclopaedia Britannica, Chicago, Vol. 20, pp 695–698
2. Bone RC, Fisher CJ Jr, Clemmer TP, Slotman GJ, Metz CA, Balk RA, and the Methylprednisolone Severe Sepsis Study Group (1987) A controlled clinical trial of high-dose methylprednisolone in the treatment of severe sepsis and septic shock. N Engl J Med 317:653–658
3. Hinshaw L and The Veterans Administration Systemic Sepsis Cooperative Study Group (1987) Effect of high-dose glucocorticoid therapy on mortality in patients with clinical signs of systemic sepsis. N Engl J Med 317:659–665
4. Bone RC (1991) Let's agree on terminology: Definitions of sepsis. Crit Care Med 19:973–976

Table of Contents

Monitoring Illness Severity

Clinical Management of Sepsis

Investigational Therapy of Sepsis

Designing the Optimum Clinical Trial for the Treatment of Sepsis

List of Contributors

Baumgartner J. D.
Dept. of Medicine,
Morges Hospital, Morges,
Switzerland

Bernard G. R.
Dept. of Intensive Care, Vanderbilt
University, T-1219 MCN, Nashville
TN 37232-2650, USA

Bloos F.
Dept. of Anesthesiology,
Friedrich-Schiller University
Hospital, Bachstrasse 18,
07740 Jena, Germany

Bone R. C.
Dept. of Medicine, The Medical
College of Ohio, 3000 Arlington
Avenue, Toledo OH 42699-0008,
USA

Brazzi L.
Dept. of Anesthesiology, Milan
Hospital, Via Francesco Sforza 35,
20122 Milan, Italy

Brunet F.
Dept. of Intensive Care, Cochin
Port-Royal Hospital, 27 rue du
Faubourg St Jacques, 75014 Paris,
France

Calandra T.
Medical Research, The Picower
Institute, 350 Community Drive,
Manhasset NY 11030, USA

Calvano S. E.
Dept. of Surgery, New-York
Hospital-Cornell Medical Center,
68th street, New York NY 10021,
USA

Carlet J.
Dept. of Intensive Care, St Joseph
Hospital, rue Pierre Larousse 7,
75743 Paris Cedex 15, France

Cerra F. B.
Dept. of Surgery, University of
Minnesota, 406 Harvard Street
South East, Minneapolis MN 55455,
USA

Christman J. W.
Dept. of Intensive Care, Vanderbilt
University, T-1219 MCN, Nashville
TN 37232-2650, USA

Cohen J.
Dept. of Infectious Diseases,
Hammersmith Hospital, Du Cane
Road, London W12 0NN,
United Kingdom

Cook D. J.
Dept. of Medicine, St Joseph
Hospital, 50 Charlton Avenue East,
Hamilton ONT L8N 46A, Canada

Cronin L.
Dept. of Clinical Epidemiology and
Biostatistic Minister, Mac Master
Hospital, Hamilton ONT L8N 46A,
Canada

Damas P.
Dept. of Anesthesiology, Liège
University Hospital B35, Domaine
du Sart Tilman, 4000 Liège,
Belgium

Deby-Dupont G.
Dept. of Anesthesiology, Liège University Hospital B35, Domaine du Sart Tilman, 4000 Liège, Belgium

Dhainaut J. F.
Dept. of Intensive Care, Cochin Port-Royal Hospital, 27 rue du Faubourg St Jacques, 75014 Paris, France

Doig G. S.
Dept. of Epidemiology, University of Western Ontario, London ONT N6A 5C1, Canada

Draper E. A.
APACHE Medical Systems, Inc., 1901 Pennsylvania avenue, suite 900, Washington D. C. 20006, USA

Eidelman, L. A
Dept. of Anesthesiology and Critical Care, Hadassah-Hebrew University Medical Center, P. O. Box 12000, Jerusalem 91120, Israel

Fink M. P.
Dept. of Surgery, Beth Israel Hospital, 330 Brookline Avenue, Boston MA 02215, USA

Fisher C. J.
Dept. of Critical Care, The Cleveland Clinic Foundation, 9500 Euclid avenue, Cleveland MA 02215, USA

Gasche Y.
Dept. of Intensive Care, University Hospital, Geneva 1211, Switzerland

Gattinoni L.
Dept. of Anesthesiology, Milan Hospital, Via Francesco Sforza 35, 20122 Milan, Italy

Harrell F. E.
Dept. of Biometry, Duke University Medical Center, P. O. Box 3363, Durham NC, USA

Holden E.
Dept. of Intensive Care, Vanderbilt University, T-1219 MCN, Nashville TN 37232-2650, USA

Knaus W. A.
Dept. of Anesthesiology, George Washington Medical Center, 2300 K Street, Washington D. C. 20037, USA

Lamy M.
Dept. of Anesthesiology, Liège University Hospital B35, Domaine du Sart Tilman, 4000 Liège, Belgium

Le Gall J. R.
Dept. of Intensive Care, St Louis Hospital, avenue Claude Vellefaux 1, 75010 Paris, France

Lemeshow S.
School of Public Health, University of Massachusetts, Morrille Science Center, Amherst MA 01003, USA

Lowry S. F.
Dept. of Surgery, New-York Hospital-Cornell Medical Center, 68th street, New York NY 10021, USA

Lynn W. A.
Dept. of Infectious Diseases, Hammersmith Hospital, Du Cane Road, London W12 0NN, United Kingdom

Marshall J. C.
Dept. of Surgery, Toronto General Hospital, 200 Elizabeth Street, Toronto ONT M5G 2C4, Canada

Meunier F.
EORTC Data Center, avenue E. Mounier 83, 1200 Brussels, Belgium

Mira J. P.
Dept. of Intensive Care, Cochin Port-Royal Hospital, 27 rue du Faubourg St Jacques, 75014 Paris, France

Morisaki H.
Dept. of Critical Care, Victoria Hospital, 375 South Street, London ONT N6A 4G5, Canada

Nyman D. J.
Dept. of Anesthesiology and Critical Care, Hadassah-Hebrew University Medical Center, P.O. Box 12000, Jerusalem 91120, Israel

Pelosi P.
Dept. of Anesthesiology, Milan Hospital, Via Francesco Sforza 35, 20122 Milan, Italy

Pittet D.
Dept. of Intensive Care, University Hospital, Geneva 1211, Switzerland

Reinhart K.
Dept. of Anesthesiology, Friedrich-Schiller University Hospital, Bachstrasse 18, 07740 Jena, Germany

Rochon J.
Dept. of Epidemiology, University of Western Ontario, London ONT N6A 5C1, Canada

Sibbald W. J.
Dept. of Critical Care, Victoria Hospital, 375 South Street, London ONT N6A 4G5, Canada

Spies C.
Dept. of Anesthesiology, Friedrich-Schiller University Hospital, Bachstrasse 18, 07740 Jena, Germany

Sprung C. L.
Dept. of Anesthesiology and Critical Care, Hadassah-Hebrew University Medical Center, P.O. Box 12000, Jerusalem 91120, Israel

Suter P. M.
Dept. of Intensive Care, University Hospital, Geneva 1211, Switzerland

Sylvester R. J.
EORTC Data Center, avenue E. Mounier 83, 1200 Brussels, Belgium

Thijs L. G.
Dept. of Internal Medicine, Free University Hospital, De Boelelaan 1117, 1081 HV Amsterdam, The Netherlands

van der Poll T.
Dept. of Surgery, New-York Hospital-Cornell Medical Center, 68th street, New York NY 10021, USA

Vincent J. L.
Dept. of Intensive Care, Erasme University Hospital, route de Lennik 808, 1070 Brussels, Belgium

Wagner D. P.
Dept. of Intensive Care, George Washington Medical Center, 2300 K Street, Washington DC 20037, USA

Common Abbreviations

ALI	Acute lung injury
ARDS	Acute respiratory distress syndrome
ATP	Adenosine triphosphate
AIDS	Acquired immuno-deficiency syndrome
COP	Colloid osmotic pressure
CPAP	Continuous positive airway pressure
DIC	Disseminated intravascular coagulation
DNA	Desoxyribonucleic acid
DO_2	Oxygen delivery
G-CSF	Granulocyte-colony stimulating factor
GI	Gastrointestinal
GSH	Glutathione
ICU	Intensive care unit
IL	Interleukin
IV	Intravenous
IVIG	Intravenous immunoglobulin G
IL-1ra	Interleukin-1 receptor antagonist
LPS	Lipopolysaccharide
MODS	Multiple organ dysfunction syndrome
MOF	Multiple organ failure
NADPH	Nicotinamide adenine dinucleotide phosphate
NAC	N-acetylcysteine
NMR	Nuclear magnetic resonance
PAF	Platelet activating factor
PCr	Phosphocreatine
PDH	Pyruvate dehydrogenase
PEEP	Positive end-expiratory pressure
pHi	Gastric intramucosal pH
REE	Resting energy expenditure

ROC	Receiver-operator-characteristics
ROS	Reactive oxygen species
SIRS	Systemic inflammatory response syndrome
SOD	Superoxide dismutase
TNF	Tumor necrosis factor
TPN	Total parenteral nutrition
VO_2	Oxygen consumption/uptake

Clinical Trials in the Treatment of Sepsis: An Evidence-Based Approach

D. J. Cook

Using the Literature to Solve Patient Problems

The purpose of this Round Table Conference on Clinical Trials for the Treatment of Sepsis is to summarize the current, most valid literature in the field.

The biomedical literature is expanding at a compound rate of 6–7% per year; it doubles every 10 to 15 years [1]. Keeping abreast of the latest medical developments in sepsis is a daunting prospect for clinicians. Today, more than ever, practitioners require the ability to efficiently assess the validity and applicability of published evidence, and the ability to incorporate this assessment into patient care [2, 3]. When any promising therapeutic option is available to clinicians, they are burdened with the dilemma of deciding who, if anyone, should receive this therapy. To make these difficult treatment decisions involves proficiently selecting, critiquing, synthesizing and applying relevant information from the critical care literature. It also involves identifying all available options and possible outcomes, weighing the benefits against the risks and costs, and factoring in logistic, economic, legal and possibly social considerations [4]. If every intensivist attempted to do this for every diagnostic or therapeutic decision, the result would be exhaustion!

Clearly, shortcuts are needed. Physicians are now beginning to use the medical literature more effectively to guide clinical therapy. A profusion of articles instructing clinicians on how to access [5], evaluate [6], and interpret [7] the medical literature exist. Another solution to the complexity of day to day decision making in the ICU is replacing preference-based practice with practice based on current, comprehensive summaries and evidence-based clinical recommendations [8].

We hope that the proceedings of this conference, in which we critically appraise and summarize the relevant literature on the management of sepsis, will help to serve this goal, and direct future research in this field.

Organization of the Conference

The conference was divided into five sessions. Session I is "The Epidemiology of Sepsis", in which an overview of the distribution and determinants of sepsis has been provided. Session II focused on "Monitoring the Treatment of Sepsis". Endotoxins and inflammatory mediators, measures of total body and organ-specific oxygen availability, multiple organ dysfunction and illness severity scores will be discussed in light of their descriptive and prognostic utility in the septic state. In Session III, entitled "The Clinical Management of Sepsis", widely used therapeutic interventions were critically examined, with reference to the quality of evidence supporting their use in daily practice. In these chapters, we will refer readers to the level of evidence provided by the current literature on the use of antibiotics, intravenous fluids, transfusion therapy, vasoactive drugs and nutrition. Session IV is on the "Investigational Therapy of Sepsis". In this session, newer experimental modalities have been highlighted, including anti-endotoxin therapy, non-steroidal anti-inflammatory drugs and steroids, anti-TNF, interleukin antibodies, platelet activating factor antagonists, granulocyte-colony stimulating factors, pentoxifylline, prostaglandins, N-acetylcysteine and bradykinin antagonists. Because many of these agents have not been evaluated in randomized clinical trials in humans, the strenght of inference that can be drawn from these studies will be tempered by the fact that the evidence may be biologic but not clinical. Though they may yield important information about modifying the pathophysiology of sepsis, many of these studies are hypothesis-generating, and must still be rigorously evaluated in clinical trials before they are adopted into daily practice. Session V in this conference is entitled, "Designing the Ideal Clinical Trial for the Treatment of Sepsis". In these addresses, the principles of clinical epidemiology and biostatistics were used to highlight crucial issues in the design and conduct of trials in sepsis. Strategies which were addressed included choosing the design, specifying the population, intervention and outcomes, avoiding bias and minimizing random error, and considering statistical and economic issues. Practical problems about trial monitoring and the ethics of experimentation in animals and humans were also addressed.

Clinical Judgement and Evidence in Therapeutic Decision-Making

What rules of evidence ought to apply when expert committees meet to generate recommendations for the clinical management of patients with sepsis? Should only the thoroughly validated results of randomized clinical trials be admissible to avoid or minimize the application of useless or harmful therapy? Or, to maximize the potential benefits to patients, should a synthesis of the experience of seasoned clinicians form the basis for such recommendations?

Ample precedent exists for the latter approach even when attempts are made to replace it [9]. However, for the following reasons, the non-experimental evidence that represents the recalled experiences of clinicians will tend to overestimate efficacy:

1. Even in critically ill patients with marked physiologic derangements, some symptoms (e.g. transient ischemic attacks) or signs (e.g. increased intracranial pressure) and extreme laboratory test results, when they are reassessed a short time later, tend to return toward the more usual, normal result [10]. Because of this universal tendency for regression toward the mean, which may be part of the natural history of a condition, any treatment (regardless of it efficacy) that is initiated in the interim will appear efficacious, even when it might not be.
2. Routine clinical practice is never "blind"; clinicians always know when active treatment is under way. As a result, the desire of clinicians for success can cause an overestimate of the efficacy of an intervention (recall bias). The overestimate may in part be a consequence of bias in interpretation of diagnostic tests which indicate whether patients have developed an adverse outcome (such as the radiographic diagnosis of ARDS). In rare situations when critically ill patients are conscious and aware of their treatment in a clinical trial, their desire for a successful outcome, and the well-known placebo effect [11] may also tend to overestimate the benefit of treatment.
3. Favorable treatment responses are more likely to be recognized and remembered by clinicians when their patients comply with treatments. There are already 6 documented instances in which compliant patients in the placebo groups of randomized trials exhibited far more favorable outcomes (including survival) than their non-compliant companions [12–17]. Because high compliance is therefore a marker for better outcomes, even when treatment is useless, our uncontrolled clinical experiences often will cause us to conclude that compliant patients (i.e. most ICU patients) must have been receiving efficacious therapy.

For the preceding reasons, treatment based upon uncontrolled clinical experience risks precipitating the widespread application of treatments that are useless or even harmful. These same treatments are much less likely to be judged efficacious in double-blind, randomized trials than in uncontrolled case series of unblinded, "open" comparisons with contemporaneous or historical series of patients; hence the maxim: "Therapeutic reports with controls tend to have no enthusiasm, and reports with enthusiasm tend to have no controls."

The foregoing discussion should not be misinterpreted as constituting a mandate for discarding the large body of uncontrolled observations by clinicians who have managed patients with sepsis. For some treatments of sepsis, randomized control trials have not yet been carried out (nor because of overwhelming evidence of efficacy from cohort studies, are they likely to be conducted), and the only information base for generating some of the recommendations comes from systematic clinical observations.

However, it is clear that it is important, whenever possible, to base firm recommendations (and especially those involving risk to patients) on the results of rigorously controlled investigations and scientific overviews, and to be much more circumspect when recommendations rest only on the results of data from subexperimental studies, non-human studies and uncontrolled clinical observations. This philosophy and approach to practice is often referred to as evidence-based medicine [13].

Levels of Evidence and Grades of Recommendations

In this conference, we use a set of guidelines called, "Levels of Evidence and Grades of Recommendations". These guidelines for interpreting the literature were fruitfully adopted by the participants of the First [14] and Second [15] American College of Chest Physicians Antithrombotic Consensus Conferences. The result was a series of evidence-based clinical recommendations supported by summaries of the best available evidence for all treatments of thrombotic disorders. The definition of levels of evidence and grades of recommendations were also adopted by the Canadian Cardiovascular Society Task Force on the Use of Thrombolytic Therapy; the Canadian Cardiovascular Society Consensus Conference on the Management of the Postmyocardial Infarction Patient [16]; The Ontario Oncology Group, and is now being used to formulate recommendations of the US Preventive Health Services Task Force (David Sackett, personal communication, Washington 1992).

These guidelines are simple, and useful in evaluating the validity of primary clinical trials. The guidelines we are using in this conference are also relevant in evaluating the validity of scientific review articles. If a comprehensive and unbiased overview of methodologically rigorous studies is available, it follows that this should be used in developing treatment policies. An overview that incorporates a quantitative summary of the data is called a meta-analysis, and, in resolving issues of therapeutic effectiveness, represents the highest form of evidence for deciding on the strength of inference supporting a treatment recommendation [17]. Scientific overviews, when optimally conducted, include all the relevant trials of high quality (Level I or II evidence), chosen in an explicit, unbiased fashion.

The participants in this conference, when summarizing what was known about the causes, clinical course, and management of sepsis, began by specifying the level of evidence that was used in each case, according a classification described below. This framework can be applied to primary research (individual studies) and synthetic research (scientific overviews or meta-analyses).

Primary Research: Individual Studies

Level I: Randomized Trials with Low False-Positive (α) and Low False-Negative (β) Errors (High Power)

By "low false-positive (α) error" is meant a "positive" trial that demonstrated a statistically significant benefit from experimental treatment. For example, there have now been several randomized trials in which oral anticoagulants produced very large, statistically significant reductions in the risk of stroke and death among patients with non-valvular atrial fibrillation. By "low false-negative (β) error (high power)" is meant a "negative" trial that demonstrated no effect of therapy, yet was large enough to exclude the possiblity of a clinically important benefit (i.e. had very narrow 95% confidence intervals, the upper end of which was less than the minimum clinically important benefit, thereby excluding any improvement due to the test treatment). For example, the ISIS-III randomized trial has ruled out any clinically significant difference in the efficacy of streptokinase, tPA, and APSAK in acute myocardial infarction. The elements of a valid and useful randomized trial are summarized in Table 1.

The advent of meta-analysis permits us to sharpen this classification further by generating a "pooled" estimate of the treatment's efficacy across all the high quality, relevant trials. Meta-analyses also reveal any inconsistencies in the estimates of efficacy between trials ("heterogeneity"), highlighting those that require further scrutiny before an overall treatment policy can be generated.

Level II: Randomized Trials with High False-Positive (α) and/or High False-Negative (β) Errors (Low Power)

By "high false-positive (α) error" is meant a trial with an interesting positive trend that is not statistically significant. For example, the HA-1A study by Ziegler and colleagues [9] generated a positive but not statistically significant trend favoring HA-1A in sepsis (placebo: 43% mortality; HA-1A: 39%, $p=0.24$). By "high false-negative (β) error (low power)" is meant a "negative" trial which concluded that therapy was not efficacious, yet was compatible with the real possibility of a clinically important benefit (i.e. had very wide 95% confidence intervals on the effect of experimental therapy). For example, several trials of anticoagulants in completed thrombotic stroke con-

Table 1. Elements of a valid and useful randomized trial

1. Are the results valid?
   a) Was the assignment of patients to treatments really randomized?
   b) Were all patients who entered the study accounted for at its conclusion?
   c) Were the clinical outcomes measured blindly?
2. Is the therapeutic effect important?
   a) Were both statistical and clinical significance considered?
   b) Were all clinically relevant outcomes reported?
3. Are the results relevant to my patient?
   a) Were the study patients recognizably similar to my own?
   b) Is the therapeutic maneuvre feasible in my practice?

cluded that such treatment was ineffective when, in fact, the confidence intervals on the treatment effect they observed ranged from virtually eliminating subsequent deterioration and death to doubling the risk of these outcomes. In this situation, the 95% confidence interval includes the minimal clinically important difference, and clearly the strength of inference is lower than would be the case for Level I studies.

The advent of meta-analysis has a major impact here, for it can show that two or more high-quality, homogeneous but small (and therefore Level II) trials really provide Level I evidence of treatment efficacy. Stated another way, when Level II studies are pooled, the lower limit of the confidence interval around the pooled estimate may then become greater than the minimal clinically important difference, rendering the aggregate of several Level II studies now Level I evidence.

Level III: Non-Randomized Concurrent Cohort Comparisons between Contemporaneous Patients who did and did not Receive Antisepsis Therapy

In this case, the outcomes of patients who receive (and complied with) antisepsis therapy would be compared with those of contemporaneous patients who did not (through contraindication, oversight, local practice, refusal, etc.) receive these same interventions. The biases described earlier are usually in play here. Although Level III–V data can be subjected to meta-analysis, such overviews are difficult to interpret, and we therefore do not recommend this approach.

Level IV: Non-Randomized Historical Cohort Comparisons between Current Patients who did Receive Antithrombotic Agents and Former Patients (from the Same Institution or form the Literature) who did not

In this case, the outcomes of patients who received antisepsis therapy (as a result of a local treatment policy) would be compared with those of patients treated in earlier era or at another institution (when and where different treatment policies prevailed). To the biases already presented, must be added those that result from inappropriate comparisons over time and space.

Level V: Case Series without Controls

In this situation, the reader is simply informed about the fate of a group of patients with sepsis. Such series may contain useful information about clinical course and prognosis but can only hint at efficacy.

Synthetic Research: Scientific Overviews

Primary studies are often limited by inadequate sample size, which leaves negative studies open to large false-negative (β) errors (in which important differences which actually exist may be missed). Moreover, even positive studies, when small, will generate such wide confidence intervals that clinicians are left uncertain as to whether the treatment effect is trivial or huge. The most compelling rationale for meta-analysis is its ability to generate more precise estimates (reflected in narrower confidence intervals) of the true treatment effect than can be provided by any individual trial.

A key element in interpreting this confidence interval is its relation to the "minimally important benefit" which, if met or exceeded, will lead clinicians to use the treatment [18]. A drug may be more effective than alternative management strategies, but if the difference is small enough, use of the agent may not be warranted. Deciding what constitutes a clinically important benefit is difficult, and is dependent on the baseline risk of an adverse event, side effects and cost, and what outcome is being averted (whether, for example, one is preventing death, or organ dysfunction). As a result, deciding on the minimal clinically important difference often generates controversy. Nevertheless, a decision about the likelihood that an intervention results in clinically important benefit is necessary for establishing a management recommendation.

If the entire confidence interval surpasses the minimal clinically important benefit (for example, a 10% reduction in mortality), then the inference that the treatment should be administered is very strong. If the lower limit of a 95% confidence interval of a relative risk reduction exceeds the minimal clinically important benefit, this means that there is at least a 95% chance that the true treatment effect is greater than the clinically important benefit. If, on the other hand, the confidence interval brackets the clinically important benefit, the strength of the inference that treatment should be administered in such patients is much weaker. Finally, when sample sizes are very small or events very rare, even though the point estimate of benefit may favor active treatment, the lower limit of the confidence interval may suggest not only the possibility that the treatment is harmful, but that the degree of harm is important. Under these circumstances, the strength of inference in a positive treatment recommendation is very weak.

Evaluating the Quality of Scientific Overviews

Just as there are explicit rules to rate primary studies with respect to their validity and usefulness, there are also explicit criteria for rating the quality of scientific overviews [19], which have been applied in a reproducible and valid fashion by epidemiologists, clinicians, and research assistants [18]. They are summarized in Table 2.

Table 2. Guidelines for assessing research overviews

1. Were the question(s) and methods clearly stated?
2. Were the search methods used to locate relevant studies comprehensive?
3. Were explicit methods used to determine which articles to include in the review?
4. Was the validity of the primary studies assessed?
5. Was the assessment of the primary studies reproducible and free from bias?
6. Was variation between the findings of the relevant studies analyzed?
7. Were findings of the primary studies combined appropriately?
8. Were the reviewers' conclusions supported by the data cited?

Useful overviews begin with a clear statement of the clinical question to be answered, followed by a description of the methods employed in carrying it out. The validity of an overview is compromised when it fails to begin with a successful, comprehensive, reproducible, and bias-free search for all potentially relevant articles. Variations in treatment effects among the studies must be sought and analyzed, and the statistical methods for aggregating their results must be appropriate. Finally, the reviewers' conclusions must be supported by the data!

Variations in treatment effects ("heterogeneity") among the studies being pooled in an overview is a special problem of scientific overviews that deserves comment. Heterogeneity exists when some individual studies document very favorable effects of treatment and other studies document no benefit or even harm. Even if the primary studies are both sound and large (with individually narrow confidence intervals), if their results are heterogeneous, then the strength of the inference about the overall effect of therapy may be substantially reduced.

When significant heterogeneity across studies is present, the inference that can be made is that the best estimate of the effect of treatment in the population is represented by the pooled relative risk reduction. This is the estimate of treatment efficacy that clinicians should assume when deciding whether or not to treat their patients. However, the credibility of the estimate is not as great when heterogeneity is present as when it is absent. It is likely that in a subset of patients, for example, or with the use of a higher or lower intensity of therapy, treatment effects are appreciably larger or smaller than the pooled relative risk reduction.

Nonetheless, the discovery of heterogeneity requires an exploration of why it has occurred. The causes include differences in patients enrolled in the trials, differences in the stage and severity of their primary and co-morbid disorders, differences in the treatments or the way that they are administered, differences in the nature or measurement of the outcomes used to determine efficacy, or differences in the methodologic rigor of the primary studies (by one or more of the criteria in Table 1). If this search convinces the overviewers that they have an explanation for the heterogeneity, they can then report separate pooled estimates for the treatment effects among subsets of studies separated according to the source of heterogeneity.

For example, suppose that an overview examines the frequency of superinfection among patients receiving multiples antibiotics, and discovers significant heterogeneity. One obvious possible explanation for this heterogeneity would be varying intensity of antibiotic therapy. If further analysis confirmed that the incidence of superinfection was systematically higher in the subset of studies in which patients received more intense antibiotic therapy, the heterogeneity would have a logical explanation and an appropriate action would be to conduct two meta-analyses: one restricted to studies using more intense antibiotic therapy, and one including only studies with less intense regimens.

However, if significant heterogeneity exists that cannot be explained by differences in patients, diseases, treatments, outcomes, or study methods, the resulting inference about the effectiveness of treatment is weakened, and clinical readers are less confident that the pooled result is applicable to their patient.

An overview which incorporates low-quality studies is worse than useless, for it may mislead. An overview that is not rigorously conducted (that is, does not meet the criteria presented in Table 2) adds little to the evaluation of evidence by traditional means and should not be considered. However, a rigorously conducted overview adds three important elements to the determination of Levels of Evidence. First, it generates narrower confidence intervals on estimates of the effectiveness of treatments (which can be related to the clinically significant differences that would trigger their clinical use). Second, it provides a more comprehensive assessment of the methodologic quality of the individual trials. Finally, it can detect and initiate the examination of heterogeneity in estimates of effectiveness among multiple trials of the same treatment.

Accordingly, if a rigorous overview is available, it becomes the basis for determining the level of evidence. Such a rigorous overview, in which the quality of the original studies also is high and there is no unexplained heterogeneity, can raise the designation of the level of evidence.

For example, if the lower limit of the confidence interval for a relative risk reduction (the estimate that was least favorable to active treatment, but still consistent with the trial results) exceeded the clinically significant benefit that would trigger its clinical use, the treatment effect was judged both large and important. Therefore, the treatment should be rated at Level I+ (regardless of whether the individual trials were Level I or Level II) if the result was homogeneous over a collection of high quality trials. This rating was lowered to I− if a rigorous overview documented heterogeneity in the trial results.

If the lower limit of the confidence interval for a relative risk reduction fell below the clinically significant benefit that would trigger its clinical use (but the point estimate of its effect was at or above the clinically significant benefit), the effect of treatment might be trivial. It would be rated at Level II+ (regardless of whether the individual trials were Level I or Level II) if the result was homogeneous over a collection of high quality trials. As before,

Table 3. Levels of evidence for therapy

If a high-quality overview is available	If no overview is available
When the lower limit of the confidence interval for the effect of treatment *exceeded* the clinically significant benefit, and: Individual study results are homogeneous: Level I+ Individual study results are heterogeneous: Level I−	Randomized trials with low false positive (α) and low false negative (β) errors (high power): Level I
When the lower limit of the confidence interval for the effect of treatment *fell below* the clinically significant benefit (but the point estimate of its effect was at or above the clinically significant benefit) and: Individual study results are homogeneous: Level II+ Individual study results are heterogeneous: Level II−	Randomized trials with high false positive (α) and high false negative (β) errors (low power): Level II
	Non-randomized concurrent cohort studies: Level III
	Non-randomized historical cohort studies: Level IV
	Case series: Level V

this rating would be lowered to II− if a rigorous overview documented heterogeneity (Table 3).

This system for establishing levels of evidence allows overviews to obtain a higher rating (1+) than can ever be achieved by individual trials. There are several reasons for this. First, relying on a single trial omits other evidence which will, inevitably, differ to some degree, leaving residual uncertainty. Second, in taking account multiple studies, the overview demands that results have been replicated. Consistent replication always strengthens inference. Third, since patients and clinical settings will inevitably differ somewhat between trials, replication with consistent results increases the generalizability and applicability of the findings.

We also recognize that these proposals place higher demands on overviews than on individual trials (one of the latter may be rated Level I even if its confidence interval brackets the clinically significant difference). It can be argued that this demand is justified, given the higher power of meta-analysis [20–25].

The Grading of Recommendations About Therapy

The relation between Levels of Evidence and Grades of Recommendations regarding therapy is presented here. Regardless of whether the levels of evidence were derived from overviews or individual trials, conference participants were encouraged to refer to this framework, and classify any recommendations of antisepsis therapy into 3 grades, shown in Table 4, depending on the level on evidence used to generate them:

- Grade A Recommendation: Supported by Level I Evidence.
- Grade B Recommendation: Supported by Level II Evidence.
- Grade C Recommendation: Support by Level III, IV or V Evidence.

Evaluating the Impact of Therapy: Number Needed to Treat

There is a very useful way of summarizing the efficacy of an intervention that you will see in some of the chapters in this book. The concept is the "Number Needed to Treat", or the number of patients that one would need to treat to prevent one event [20].

Suppose that the results of a trial or overview are generalizable to your patient, and the outcomes are important; the next question is what is the impact of the intervention? A relative risk reduction may be quite impressive, but if the baseline risk of an adverse outcome is low, the impact of treatment may be minimal. This notion of therapeutic impact can be captured in the concept called "the number needed to be treated" or NNT, which incorporates not only the relative risk reduction, but also the baseline risk. Let us take the example of beta blockers, which reduce the risk of death following myocardial infarction by approximately 25% (that is, the relative risk reduction that accompanics their use is 25%). Consider a 40 year old man with a small infarct, normal left ventricular function and exercise capacity, and no sign of ventricular arrhythmia who is willing to stop smoking and

Table 4. Grades of recommendations for therapy

Level of Evidence	Grade of Recommendation
Level I	Grade A
Level II	Grade B
Level III Level IV Level V	Grade C

take aspirin daily. This individual's risk of death in the first year after infarction may be as low as 1%. Beta blockers would reduce this risk by 25%, but the absolute risk reduction produced here is 25% of 1%, or only 0.0025. As it happens, the reciprocal of an absolute risk reduction (that is, the absolute risk reduction divided into 1) is the number of patients one needs to treat in order to prevent one event. In this case, one would have to treat 400 such low-risk patients for one year to save a single life (1/0.0025 = NNT 1 year of 40).

On the other hand, an older man with limited exercise capacity and frequent ventricular extrasystoles who continues to smoke following infarction may have a risk of dying in the next year of 10%. In this case, a relative risk reduction of 25% generates an absolute risk reduction of 0.025, and one would have to treat only 40 such individuals (1/0.025) for one year to save a life.

Closing Remarks

In this book, reference has been made to the level of evidence and the grade of recommendation supporting various treatments. Intensivists today must complement their knowledge of current literature with their clinical skills and knowledge of anatomy and pathophysiology. To that end, we hope that this book will serve as a useful reference for busy clinicians who want an up-to-date synthesis of clinical studies in sepsis.

References

1. Sackett DL (1981) How to read clinical journals: Why to read them and how to start reading them critically. Can Med Assoc J 124:555–558
2. Sackett DL, Haynes RB, Tugwell P (1985) Clinical epidemiology: A basic science for clinical medicine. Boston, Little Brown & Co Ltd
3. Cook DJ, Jaeschke R, Guyatt GH (1992) Critical appraisal of therapeutic interventions in the intensive care unit: Human monoclonal antibody treatment in sepsis. J Intens Care Med 7:275–282
4. Eddy DM (1990) Practice policies – what are they? Clinical decision making: From theory to practice. JAMA 263:877–880
5. Haynes RB, McKibbon KA, Fitzgerald D, et al (1986) How to keep up with the medical literature: V. Access by personal computer to the medical literature. Ann Intern Med 105:810–824
6. Bulpitt CJ (1987) Confidence Intervals. Lancet 1:494–497
7. Godfrey K (1985) Simple linear regression in medical research. N Engl J Med 313:1629–1636
8. Eddy DM (1990) Practice policies: Where do they come from? Clinical decision making: From theory to practice. JAMA 263:1265–1275
9. National Institutes of Health Consensus Development Conferences (1977–1978) 1:1–43
10. Sackett DL, Haynes RB, Guyatt GH, Tugwell P (1991) Clinical epidemiologyy: A basic science for clinical medicine. 2nd Edition. Boston: Little, Brown, pp 187–248

11. Cobb LA, Thomas GI, Dillard DH, Merendino KA, Bruce RA (1959) An evaluation of internal-mammary-artery ligation by a double-blind technique. N Engl J Med 260:1115–1118
12. Coronary Drug Project Research Group (1980) Influence of adherence treatment and response of cholesterol on mortality in the Coronary Drug Project. N Engl J Med 303:1038–1041
13. Asher WL, Harper HW (1973) Effect of human chorionic gonadotropin on weight loss, hunger, and felling of well-being. Am J Clin Nutr 26:211–218
14. Hogarty GE, Goldberg SC (1973) Drug and sociotherapy in the aftercare of schizophrenic patients. Arch Gen Psychiatry 28:54–64
15. Fuller R, Roth H, Long S (1983) Compliance with disulfiram treatment of alcoholism. J Chronic Dis 36:161–170
16. Pizzo PA, Robichaud KJ, Edwards BK, Schumaker C, Kramer BS, Johnson A (1983) Oral antibiotic prophylaxis in patients with cancer; a double-blind randomized placebo-controlled trial. J Pediatr 102:125–133
17. Horwitz RI, Viscoli CM, Berkman L, et al (1990) Treatment adherence and risk of death after myocardial infarction. The Lancet 336:542–545
18. Cook DJ, Guyatt GH, Laupacis A, Sackett DL (1992) Rules of evidence and clinical recommendations on the use of antithrombotic agents. Antithrombotic Therapy Consensus Conference III. Chest 102 (Suppl):305S–311S
19. Sackett DL (1989) Rules of evidence and clinical recommendations of the use of antithrombotic agents. Chest 95 (2 suppl):2S–4S
20. Fallen EL, Armstrong P, Cairns J, Dafoe W, et al (1991) Report of the Canadian Cardiovascular Society's Consensus Conference of the Management of the Postmyocardial Infarction Patient. Can Med Assoc J 144:1015–1025
21. L'Abbe KA, Detsky AS, O'Rourke K (1987) Meta-analysis in clinical research. Ann Intern Med 107:224–233
22. Guyatt GH, Berman LB, Townsend M, et al (1987) A measure of quality of life for clinical trials in lung disease. Thorax 42:773–778
23. Oxman AD, Guyatt GH (1988) Guidelines for reading literature reviews. Can Med Ass J 138:697–703
24. Oxman AD, Guyatt GH, Singer J, et al (1991) Agreement among reviewers of review articles. J Clin Epidemiol 44:91–98
25. Laupacis A, Sackett DL, Roberts RS (1988) An assessment of clinically useful measures of the consequences of treatment. N Engl J Med 318:1728–1733

Epidemiology of Sepsis

The Systemic Inflammatory Response Syndrome (SIRS)

R. C. Bone

Introduction

Sepsis and multiple organ failure remain as important causes of mortality and morbidity in hospitals around the world today, despite the innovative techniques that have been developed to deal with these illnesses and the vast body of knowledge accumulated regarding its causes and pathogenesis. Over the last decade, basic science researchers have determined that the systemic inflammatory response syndrome (SIRS) and a number of related clinical entities actually represent different phases and severities of a single pathologic dysfunction. This dysfunction affects the pathways of inflammation, a complex response that is normally beneficial in assisting the host to fight infecting pathogens. It is for this reason that the term sepsis – meaning a systemic infection – came into being: the adverse condition of sepsis was almost always associated with the presence of invading bacteria. The problem with this definition was that infection could not *always* be found when sepsis occurred; not only was infection simply not seen in some cases, but it could also be associated with certain other, non-infective states, such as fat embolism, burns, and trauma. With this and other discoveries about the pathogenesis of sepsis, it became apparent to researchers and clinicians that the old concepts and terminology regarding sepsis were not accurate. In order to develop a new terminology that complemented the new discoveries about the pathophysiology of sepsis, the American College of Chest Physicians/Society of Critical Care Medicine held a consensus conference on the terminology and medical treatment of sepsis [1]. The updated terminology for sepsis and its sequelae are presented in Table 1.

The new term for sepsis agreed upon at that conference, the "systemic inflammatory response syndrome" (SIRS), embodies their essential message. This new term underscores the discovery that "sepsis" is actually a condition associated with runaway inflammation that results in numerous adverse effects. While SIRS may often be associated with bacterial infection (in which case it may correctly be called "sepsis"), it is not the infecting pathogens that cause the life-threatening damage. Rather, it is the host response, through a profusion of molecular messengers and bacterial killing effects, that can cause the patient's death. Figure 1 schematically represents the relationship

Table 1. New definitions for sepsis and its sequelae. (Adapted from [1] and [17], with permission)

Infection
A microbial phenomenon characterized by an inflammatory response to the presence of microorganisms or the invasion of normally sterile host tissue by those organisms.

Bacteremia
This is the presence of viable bacteria in the blood. The presence of viruses, fungi, parasites and other pathogens in the blood should be described in a similar manner (i.e. viremia, fungemia, parasitemia, etc.).

Septicemia
In the past, this term has been defined as the presence of microorganisms or their toxins in the blood. However, this term has been used clinically and in the medical literature in a variety of ways which have added to confusion and difficulties in data interpretation. Septicemia also does not adequately describe the entire spectrum of pathogenic organisms which may infect the blood. We therefore suggest that this term be eliminated from current usage.

Systemic Inflammatory Response Syndrome (SIRS)
The systemic inflammatory response syndrome is a new term that broadly encompasses the essential disease process. The term emphasizes the fact that not all cases of runaway systemic inflammation can be tied to a specific infection.

Sepsis
This is the systemic inflammatory response to infection. In association with infection, manifestations of sepsis are the same as those previously defined for SIRS, and include, but are not limited to, more than one of the following:

1. a temperature $>38°C$ or $<36°C$,
2. an elevated heart rate >90 beats per minute,
3. tachypnea, manifested by a respiratory rate >20 breaths per minute or hyperventilation, as indicated by a $PaCO_2$ <32 mm Hg, and
4. an altered white blood cell count >12000 cells per ml^3, <4000 cells per ml^3, or the presence of $>10\%$ immature neutrophils ("bands").

To help identify these manifestations as sepsis, it should be determined whether they are a part of the direct systemic response to the presence of an infectious process. Also, the physiologic changes measured should represent an acute alteration from baseline in the absence of other known causes for such abnormalities.

Severe sepsis
This term is defined as sepsis associated with organ dysfunction, hypoperfusion abnormality, or sepsis-induced hypotension. Hypoperfusion abnormalities include lactic acidosis, or an acute alteration of mental status.

Sepsis-induced hypotension
Occurs in the presence of a systolic blood pressure <90 mm Hg or its reduction by $\geqslant 40$ mm Hg from the baseline, in the absence of other causes for hypotension (e.g. cardiogenic shock).

Septic shock
An exacerbation of sepsis and a subset of severe sepsis, this term is defined as sepsis-induced hypotension, persisting despite adequate fluid resuscitation, along with the presence of hypoperfusion abnormalities or organ dysfunction. Patients receiving inotropic or vasopressor agents may no longer be hypotensive by the time they manifest hypoperfusion abnormalities or organ dysfunction, yet they would still be considered to have septic shock.

Multiple Organ Dysfunction Syndrome (MODS)
Presence of altered organ function in an acutely ill patient such that homeostasis cannot be maintained without intervention.

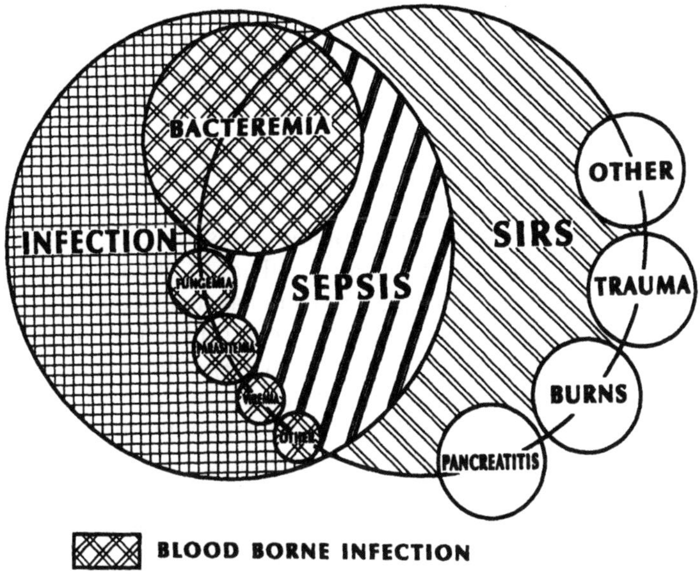

Fig. 1. The interrelationship between systemic inflammatory response syndrome (SIRS), sepsis, and infection. (From [1] and [17] with permission)

between sepsis, SIRS, infection, and their causes. As SIRS advances through several stages of severity that include hypotension, shock, and hypoxic and edema-related organ dysfunction termed "multiple organ dysfunction syndrome (MODS)", (terms defined in Table 1), the risk of mortality increases rapidly.

These new clinical definitions are relatively broad-based: they may include patients who might not have been considered septic under the definitions previously used by clinicians and researchers. This is of obvious importance in the treatment of critically ill patients; however, it may be of even greater importance in the performance of clinical trials of potential treatments for sepsis. Trials are frequently criticized on the grounds that the inclusion and exclusion of patients vary from trial to trial, making the results difficult to compare and restricting the conclusions. These broad-based, standardized definitions should make the rapid identification and treatment of septic patients practicable. Additionally, they should improve the quality of research into the pathophysiology and treatment of SIRS.

The development of severity-of-illness scoring systems, of which there are several, should be particularly important in the treatment of septic patients and should also be important in clinical trials of treatments for sepsis, allowing the subject's condition to be assessed in detail. In treating patients with sepsis, the use of these scoring systems should allow clinicians to allocate time and equipment to patients with a reasonable chance of reversibility, since they will predict, with reasonable reliability, which patients will not be able to survive their bout with SIRS. It will also allow clinicians to limit use of the more toxic agents to those patients less likely to improve without heroic therapy.

The Pathogenesis of SIRS

Inflammation is essentially an adaptive response that makes the individual better able to survive through an enhanced ability to fight infection. The response is extremely complicated and has many components; numerous endogenous, molecular mediators may control each of the steps within the individual components. These mediators may either enhance or inhibit a given reaction; in addition, they may affect another part of the inflammatory response or help to control the presence of another mediator that has a similar or a different action. With such complicated controls, it is not surprising that researchers have not fully revealed the mechanisms behind the deleterious effects of inflammation. However, a number of important findings have opened the door to our first, preliminary steps in finding a cure for SIRS, MODS, and other inflammation-related conditions.

A number of key mediators in the inflammatory process have been identified and are the subjects of current research studies. Tumor necrosis factor (TNF)-alpha, has been identified as one of the first endogenous mediators to be released in SIRS, along with IL-1, -6, and -8, a group of mediators that have been termed the cytokines. These molecules serve to activate leukocytes and stimulate their migration to sites of infection. These mediators are released from mononuclear phagocytes and other cells. The coagulation and complement systems are activated by these mediators. They also cause the breakdown of arachidonic acid to form leukotrienes, thromboxane A_2, and prostaglandins. IL-1 and IL-6 activate T-cells, causing them to produce interferon-γ, IL-2, IL-4, and granulocyte-monocyte colony stimulating factor. This cascade-like release of mediators is the essential underlying cause of SIRS and sepsis. Because some of these mediators can affect their own and other's release, the syndrome is capable of sustaining its own existence. This is why attempts to cure sepsis that relied simply on eliminating infective pathogens often failed to work: they could not affect the cascade of mediator releases.

While it sometimes cannot be determined how a particular inflammatory response was started, there are several conditions under which SIRS and sepsis are likely to be spawned. The presence of circulating titers of endotoxin is one such condition: this constituent of the cell walls of many gram-negative bacteria has been associated with sepsis in critically ill patients. Endotoxin, also known as lipopolysaccharide (LPS), has a number of potential antigenic sites, including a side chain known as the "O antigen". Figure 2 shows some of the events that may occur in the development of gram-negative sepsis. *In vitro* experiments have shown that endotoxin induces the release of pro-inflammatory mediators from monocytes, while *in vivo* injec-

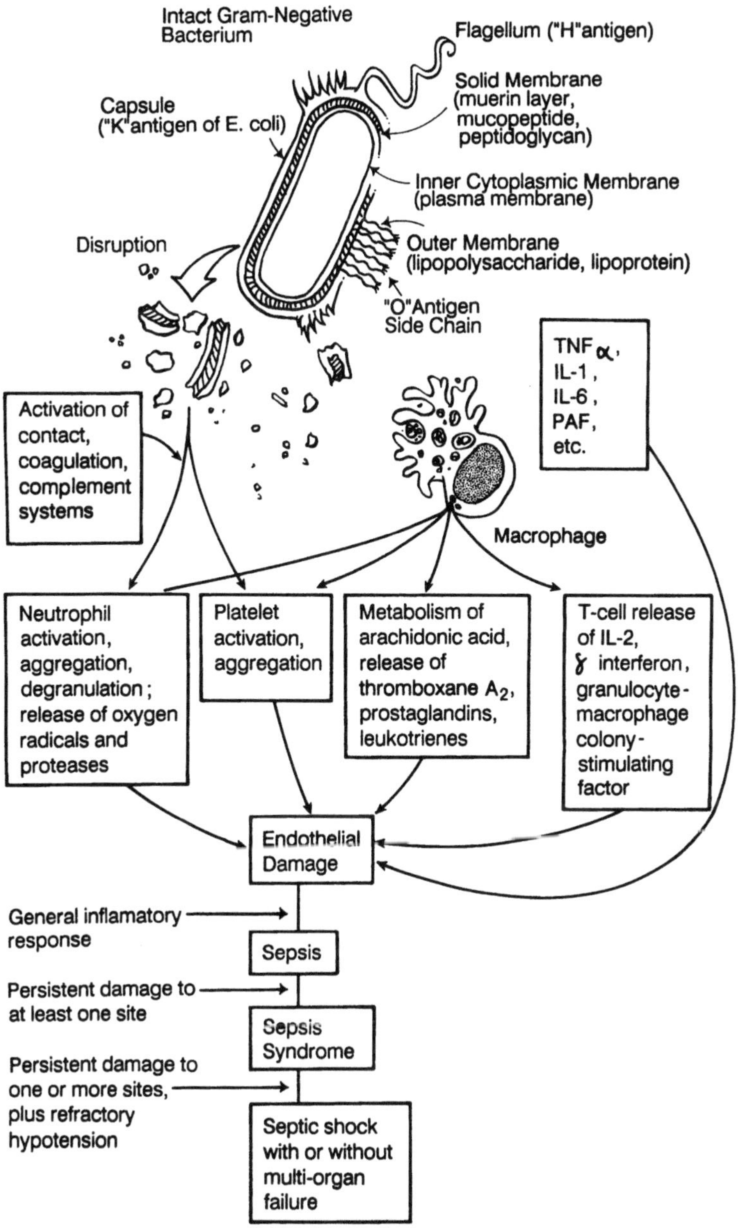

Fig. 2. Schematic of mechanisms underlying gram-negative sepsis. This figure provides a framework for understanding how sepsis and SIRS may occur. The pathways, however, are not distinct and effects may vary from individual to individual, depending on physiologic conditions. If general homeostasis is not restored, the systemic inflammatory response will produce clinical evidence of sepsis, and persistent endothelial damage at one site will ultimately result in organ dysfunction. (From [18]) with permission)

tions of endotoxin in volunteers produce symptoms of sepsis, including hypotension [2] and fever [3]. A system termed the "LPS-cytokine score" has been developed that can relate the presence of inflammatory mediators with a patient's chance of survival. In this system, endogenous TNF, IL-1, and IL-6 levels are rated as either non-detectable (0), low (2), or high (4). These scores are summed to obtain the LPS-cytokine score, a useful adjunct to the diagnostic process. There are a number of other products derived from pathogenic microorganisms that have the ability to foment inflammatory responses. These include enterotoxin, toxic shock syndrome toxin-1, teichoic acid residues from gram-positive bacteria, yeast cell wall products, and viral or fungal antigens.

These mediators can cause deleterious effects through a variety of effects. The most damaging effect, however, seems to be the destruction of the vascular endothelium at various sites throughout the host circulatory system. Although it is not known exactly what factors are involved in this event, many of the toxic effects are believed to come from neutrophils that have been activated by inflammatory mediators. This causes them to adhere to the vascular endothelium and release oxygen-derived free radicals. These highly-reactive particles are normally used to kill bacteria but, following release in the region of the endothelium, it is believed that they damage endothelial cells. This event could cause dire changes in the vascular system's permeability not only to water, but also to various ions and small proteins. It has also been shown that endotoxin is capable of affecting the clotting response, demonstrated by its effect in generating both the local and generalized Schwartzman reactions.

Further actions of endotoxin on the coagulation cascade include activation of factor XII (Hageman factor), which initiates the intrinsic clotting sequence. This causes the conversion of fibrinogen to fibrin. The continued activity of endotoxin can lead to thrombosis and reductions in the levels of platelets and coagulation factors II, V, and VII, a situation termed coagulopathy or disseminated intravascular coagulation (DIC). Hageman factor activation also causes complement activation via both the classic and alternative pathways. The complement system promotes the lysis and phagocytosis of pathogenic organisms; however, overstimulation of the system may result in the increased chemotaxis of polymorphonuclear leukocytes, an important step in leukocyte activation that can produce localized leukostasis, an event that may precede the development of organ system dysfunctions. Activated Hageman factor also stimulates the conversion of prekallikrein to kallikrein and bradykinin. This latter mediator has a number of adverse effects on the vascular system, including an increase in vascular permeability and a decrease in vascular resistance that can lead to hypotension [4].

It is believed that numerous other endogenous mediators are involved in SIRS, including such diverse species as catecholamines, endorphins, serotonin, and adrenal corticosteroids [5]. The mechanisms by which these mediators are released and the clinical significance of their release leave considerable work for further investigations.

Diagnosis

The early diagnosis of SIRS is of critical importance; in cases where bacterial etiology is present, prompt treatment with appropriate antibiotics has been shown to be effective, decreasing the mortality and morbidity resulting from sepsis by 50% [6]. The most common, early, overt signs of SIRS include hyperthermia, tachypnea, and tachycardia, as may be seen in Table 1. When these symptoms accompany a known or suspected site of infection, empiric treatment with antibiotics should be initiated immediately.

A dramatic decrease in systemic resistance and the resultant hypotension are classic characteristics of SIRS, despite an early increase in cardiac output. This hypotension can cause inadequate organ function and, occasionally, early signs of SIRS may include various organ dysfunctions that can result in altered mental state, elevated plasma lactate, and oliguria. Later in SIRS, cardiac function may be compromised resulting in a further drop in blood pressure and more profound evidence of organ dysfunction. Specific hematologic manifestations characteristic of SIRS include vacuolized neutrophils, eosinopenia, and DIC. Signs of liver dysfunction are likely to include increased serum bilirubin, while renal problems may present as azotemia and oliguria.

Management

As stated above, the early treatment of sepsis with appropriate antibiotics may be the most beneficial treatment we have today; when the inflammatory response is not allowed to start, the positive feedback mechanisms believed to be at work in SIRS are thwarted. The administration of empiric, broad-spectrum, parenteral antibacterial therapy is the generally accepted mode of therapy when sepsis is suspected [7]. However, drug selection can be improved by information about the site of the infection, the source of the infection (community- or hospital-acquired), the underlying disease status, and possible drug resistance of the microbes.

A combination of agents is usually recommended in the treatment of sepsis for a number of reasons: these regimes are active against a broader range of pathogens; often, sepsis-related infections are polymicrobial; and the possibility that a drug combination may work synergistically in its ability to kill pathogens. Such regimes reduce the likelihood of fostering drug-resistant forms of microbes. When a gram-negative infection is suspected, appropriate treatment may consist of an aminoglycoside in combination with a third-generation cephalosporin. The aminoglycosides most often used are gentamicin and tobramycin; however, if drug resistance is suspected, amikacin or netilmicin may be administered. Levels of these aminoglycosides should be kept high, although ototoxicity and nephrotoxicity are possible side effects and drug levels should be monitored. In nosocomial infection, *Pseudomonas* species are more likely to be found than are *Klebsiella* species and the cephalosporin-aminoglycoside drug combination is likely to be effective, while in community-acquired infection, the cephalosporin-antipseudomonal combination is likely to be the best treatment. The use of three-drug combinations, however, has not been shown to improve the outcome in sepsis and SIRS [8].

While the above antimicrobial treatment attempts to quell sepsis before it starts, the following discussion deals with treatments that are of a supportive nature and are to be applied when specific symptoms indicate their use. Hypotension is an early sign of SIRS that must be countered, if possible. Volume resuscitation should be the first strategy employed to this end. Crystalloid solutions are usually preferable, although solutions containing large colloids may be more appropriate when endothelial damage is suspected. Because of the circulatory dysfunctions in SIRS, even large infusions may fail to return a patient to normotension. Extreme care must be taken not to administer too much fluid, since this increases the tendencies toward edema and lung dysfunction. The administration of fluids is best monitored with the pulmonary artery catheter, which can alert the physician to the risk of pulmonary edema; a recommended target for the pulmonary capillary wedge pressure is 12 mm Hg [9].

If the circulatory pressure remains below 90 mm Hg despite optimized fluid resuscitation, vasoactive agents should be administered. The sympathomimetic amines can increase systemic blood pressure: dopamine (2–10 μg/kg/min), which activates both α- and β-adrenergic receptors, should cause peripheral vasoconstriction while maintaining blood flow to the kidney; higher doses increase the heart rate. Norepinephrine may be added to this regime to further increase peripheral vasoconstriction. If decreased myocardial contractility is suspected, an inotrope such as dobutamine may be infused. Isoproterenol should be reserved for use as an inotrope of last resort during severe bradycardia.

The enlistment of other supportive measures should occur as indicated. Often, the first organ to show signs of dysfunction is the lung, which is highly susceptible to the effects of endothelial damage and edema. Together whith hypotension, lung dysfunction can result in a decreased ability to carry oxygen to the tissues. Supplemental oxygen should be used as a first-line measure when arterial oxygen levels fall below 60 mm Hg. However, because of poor ventilation/perfusion matching, supplemental oxygen may not achieve this goal; in that case, mechanical ventilation must be instituted.

Other organs may be rendered dysfunctional in SIRS. Renal dysfunction may occur early in SIRS, usually resulting in oliguria, although polyuria may occasionally be observed in some cases. Oliguria is associated with renal hypoperfusion. When the complicated hemodynamic factors that dictate renal perfusion result in ischemic tubule damage, acute tubular necrosis may occur, further decreasing renal function. As stated above, low-dose dopamine helps to preserve renal circulation and should be used when oliguria is seen. Rarely, renal dysfunction may necessitate dialysis treatments. The central nervous system may be affected early in sepsis, probably as a result of altered perfusion or hypoxemia. Mental slowness, confusion, lethargy, and obtundation are signs of nervous system involvement. The liver also may show signs of dysfunction in sepsis: high bilirubin levels may be an early sign of sepsis. As each organ becomes involved in these specific effects of inflammation, the patient's outlook becomes incrementally worse.

Future Treatments

The nature of SIRS, as a disease mediated by the body's own defense system, makes its treatment difficult. The inflammatory mechanisms use complicated biological molecules that require biological counter measures. A number of such ideas have been developed and tested. For instance, the most simple idea – to blunt the entire inflammatory response with anti-inflammatory treatments – has been tested in animal and clinical trials. However, for reasons that are not clear, treatment with methylprednisolone does not positively affect the outcome of septic patients [10–13]. The use of other anti-inflammatory agents may hold some hope for the future.

A number of agents that work more specifically are now being developed and tested. For instance, a number of antibodies that bind to endotoxin have been developed. Unfortunately, the clinical trials of this monoclonal antibody have provided equivocable results, with only marginal benefits accruing [14–16]. Because the body's complicated system of endogenous messengers must be very finely tuned, many of the mediators involved in the inflammatory response have antagonistic counterparts – molecules that blunt or nullify the mediator's effects. Thus, the inflammatory system normally works as a whole, with the complex system of effects and countereffects leading to an ultimate result of enhanced ability to repel pathogenic invaders. Fortuitously, this has provided researchers with molecules that may be used to block the effects of many putative septic mediators. Such is the case for TNF and IL-1. It can easily be imagined that a large number of such effect and anti-effect molecules exists. In theory, at least, it should be possible to treat any case of SIRS, whatever the idiosyncracies of a particular case might be, with the appropriate combination of specific mediators and antibodies to block the numerous reactions that occur during SIRS. However, it should be remembered that inflammation is essentially a beneficial response that improves the body's ability to fight infection. There is a risk to blocking potentially beneficial responses, and careful research assessing the risk/benefit of each agent or combination of agents is needed.

Conclusion

Sepsis, SIRS, MODS, and the related conditions that have been discussed above can be characterized as a state of systemic inflammation that runs rampant, causing widespread hemodynamic deficiencies and damage to the delicate endothelial layer of the blood vessels. While mortality and treatment modes have changed little over the past 20 years, much has recently been learned about the pathogenesis of the condition. However, it seems likely that it will take researchers some time to completely understand and control the complicated molecular mechanisms that underlie SIRS.

References

1. Bone RC, Balk RA, Cerra FB, et al (1992) Definitions for sepsis and organ failure and guidelines for the use of innovative therapies in sepsis. Chest 101:1644–1655
2. Suffredini AF, Fromm RE, Parker MM, et al (1989) The cardiovascular response of normal humans to the administration of endotoxin. N Engl J Med 321:280–287
3. Wolff SM (1973) Biologic effects of bacterial endotoxins in man. J Infect Dis 128 (Suppl):251–264
4. Nies AS, Forsyth RP, Williams HE, Melmon KL (1968) Contribution of kinins to endotoxin shock in unanesthetized rhesus monkeys. Circ Res 22:155–164
5. Young LS (1990) Gram-negative sepsis. In: Mandell GL, Douglas RG Jr, Bennett JE (eds) Principles and Practice of Infectious Diseases, 3rd Edition. Churchill Livingstone, New York, pp 611–636
6. Kreger BE, Craven DE, McCabe WR (1980) Gram-negative bacteremia. IV. Re-evaluation of clinical features and treatment in 612 patients. Am J Med 68:344–355
7. Treadwell TL (1988) Gram-negative bacteremia: The current setting. Hosp Pract July:117–123
8. International Antimicrobial Therapy Project Group of the European Organization for Research and Treatment of Cancer (1983) Combination of amikacin and carbenicillin with or without cefazolin as empirical treatment of febrile neutropenic patients. J Clin Oncol 1:597–603
9. Packman MI, Rackow C (1983) Optimum left heart filling pressure during fluid resuscitation of patients with hypovolemic and septic shock. Crit Care Med 11:165–169
10. The Veterans Administration Systemic Sepsis Cooperative Study Group (1987) Effect of high-dose glucocorticoid therapy on mortality in patients with clinical signs of systemic sepsis. N Engl J Med 317:659–665
11. Sprung CL, Caralis PV, Marcial EH, et al (1984) The effects of high-dose corticosteroids in patients with septic shock: A prospective, controlled study. N Engl J Med 311:1137–1143
12. Schumer W (1976) Steroids in the treatment of clinical septic shock. Ann Surg 184:333–341
13. Rackow EC, Astiz ME (1991) Pathophysiology and treatment of septic shock. JAMA 266:548–554
14. Greenman RL, Schein RMH, Martin MA, et al and the XONA Sepsis Study Group (1991) A controlled clinical trial of E5 murine monoclonal IgM antibody to endotoxin in the treatment of gram-negative sepsis. JAMA 266:1097–1102
15. Ziegler EJ, Fisher CJ, Sprung CL, et al (1991) Treatment of gram-negative bacteremia and septic shock with a HA-1A human monoclonal antibody against endotoxin. N Engl J Med 324:429–436
16. Bone RC (1991) Monoclonal antibodies to endotoxin: New allies against sepsis? JAMA 266:1125–1126
17. Bone RC, Balk RA, Cerra FB, et al (1992) American College of Chest Physicians/Society of Critical Care Medicine Consensus Conference: Definitions for sepsis and organ failure and guidelines for the use of innovative therapies in sepsis. Crit Care Med 20:864–874
18. Bone RC (1991) The pathogenesis of sepsis. Ann Int Med 115:457–469

The "At Risk" Patient Population

J.L. Vincent

Introduction

Patients with severe sepsis represent a group of patients with a significant risk of morbidity and mortality. Although for many years, sepsis and infection have been used alternatively, recent investigations have more clearly separated the two entities [1] (Fig. 1). Infection is a microbiological event describing the invasion by pathogen bacteria, viruses, fungi or other organisms, and triggering a host reaction (In the absence of such reaction, one would refer only to colonization). Sepsis refers to the systemic response to infection and is recognized by a constellation of clinical, hemodynamic, hematologic, biochemical and inflammatory signs. Sepsis is triggered by the immunological response of the host, and it involves the release of a wide array of mediators. The same mediators may be released in association with a variety of diseases such as trauma, pancreatitis, ischemia and reperfusion, and even heart failure, in the absence of an identified infection [2, 3]. Hence,

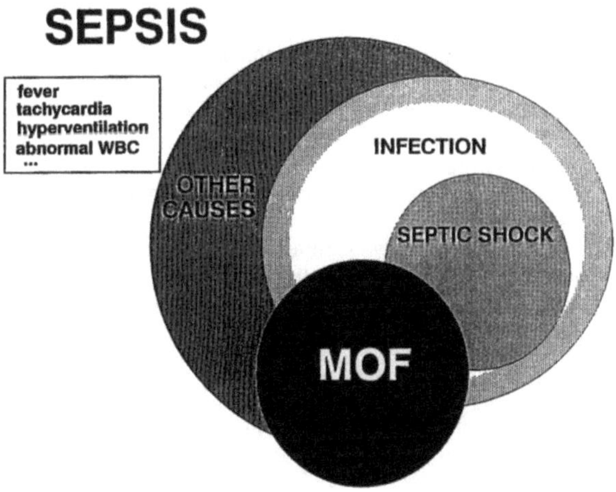

Fig. 1. Relation between sepsis, infection, septic shock and multiple organ failure. Infection is surrounded by a hatched zone corresponding to uncertainty about the presence of an infectious process (adapted with permission from [1])

although sepsis is the typical syndrome occurring in association with an infection, the presence of such an infection is not always demonstrated. Accordingly, the presence of positive blood cultures or an obvious source of infection is necessary to confirm the infectious nature of sepsis.

Undoubtedly, these recent developments have created a problem of definitions, and it is important for the members of the medical community to use the same language to describe patients. Nevertheless, the problems of definitions should not obscure the real problem, which is to recognize the patients "at risk" of development of major complications, who may benefit from new therapeutic interventions. To be successful, these new therapeutic approaches require a good understanding of the pathophysiologic process, and this is still lacking.

The purpose of this chapter is to review which groups of septic patients are "at risk" of severe complications and should therefore be included in clinical trials investigating the potentially beneficial effects of new therapeutic interventions.

The Importance of the Signs of Sepsis

The Table 1 presents the most important signs of sepsis. Clearly, no sign of sepsis is either sensitive or specific, especially in the critically ill patient [4].

Table 1. Signs of sepsis and septic shock

Sepsis
- Fever
- Tachycardia
- Tachypnea
- Elevated cardiac output, low systemic vascular resistance
- Hyperleukocytosis (with "left shift") or leukopenia
- Increased cellular metabolism, elevated oxygen consumption
- Increased insulin requirements
- Respiratory alkalosis
- Inflammatory signs: increased sedimentation rate, elevated C-reactive protein and fibrinogen levels
- Elevated cytokines levels: tumor necrosis factor, interleukin-6, interleukin-10...
- Cutaneous, ophthalmic manifestations
- Organ dysfunction: acute respiratory failure, acute renal failure, altered coagulation, mental obtundation...

Septic shock
- Arterial hypotension (systolic arterial pressure below 90 mm Hg or mean arterial pressure below 65 mm Hg) associated with signs of altered tissue perfusion:
  - altered organ function: oliguria, altered mentation, coagulation abnormalities, altered skin perfusion,...
  - increased blood lactate levels (>2 mEq/L)
  - abnormal VO_2/DO_2 dependency
  - decreased gastric intramucosal pH (tonometry)

Fever is an important sign of infection, but it can be absent in a number of cases. In recent clinical trials on sepsis, a common source of frustration for investigators was the absence of fever or hypothermia in patients who otherwise had obvious signs of severe infection. On the other hand, fever is often present in other conditions than infection, such as trauma or even myocardial infarction.

Failure to develop fever [5] or presence of hypothermia [6] have been related to increased fatality rates, as they probably reflect an impairment in the thermogenic mechanisms. Hypothermia occurs more often in the presence of circulatory failure. In a recent analysis including 519 patients, a temperature less than 35.5 °C was found in 5% of the survivors but 17% of the non-survivors ($p<0.01$) [7].

After fever, tachycardia is probably the most important systemic sign of infection [8, 9]. Tachycardia is related to the sympathetic response to sepsis and sometimes to hypovolemia. The degree of tachycardia has been related to mortality in septic shock [10, 11]. Nevertheless, tachycardia may be remarkably absent, especially in elderly patients, or those treated with anti-arrhythmic agents.

Hyperventilation associated with respiratory alkalosis has been identified for many years as a sign of infection [12–14]. However, this clinical sign is often lost in the critically ill patients, particularly since many patients with severe sepsis are mechanically ventilated. Interestingly, a cohort analysis of 519 septic patients included in the APACHE III database revealed that tachypnea was associated with a better outcome. Indeed, a spontaneous respiratory rate above 20/min was found in 63% of the survivors but only in 32% of the non-survivors ($p<0.01$) [7]. However, the prevalence of hyperventilation resulting in a $PaCO_2$ lower than 32 mm Hg was similar as it was found in 39% of the survivors and 44% on the non-survivors, respectively.

The white blood count is often increased in the presence of infection, but also in relation to a stress response to other stimuli. It is not well related to prognosis. A recent analysis of the septic patients included in the APACHE III system revealed that the white blood cell count exceeded 15000/mm^3 in 50% of the survivors and 49% of the non-survivors, respectively [7]. However, leukopenia, as defined by a white blood cell count below 4000/mm^3, had a stronger prognostic value, as it was found in 7% of the survivors, but in 15% of the non-survivors ($p<0.01$) [7].

In summary, the "at risk" patients can hardly be identified on the basis of their signs of sepsis. Only hypothermia and leukopenia are significantly related to a worse outcome, but these abnormalities are found in a minority of patients. Therefore, any categorical definition of sepsis is not likely to be useful in the stratification of patients according to their relative risk of mortality.

The Importance of Infection

In any patient who appears septic, an infectious process should be actively sought. The presence of an infection requires an appropriate antibiotic therapy, and the removal of the source by the appropriate procedure.

In some clinical conditions, an infectious source is presumed, but unproven. The severity of sepsis may be similar in patients dying with uncontrolled infection or without demonstrable infection [15]. In the absence of a demonstrable infection, some investigators believe that the translocation of bacteria and their products from the gut may plan an important role by stimulating the septic response [16]. This, however, remains a hypothesis. The prognosis may not be better in these patients without treatable infection. It may even be worse.

Since the same cascade of septic mediators can be activated in the absence of any demonstrable infection, one may thus wonder if the documentation of an infection is of any importance in the evaluation of therapeutic trials in septic patients. In other words, does the trial focus on severe sepsis or severe infection? We do not have a precise answer to this fundamental question. Before we have it, mixing together septic patients with and without documented infections should be avoided, as it may confound some important issues. A patient with polytrauma or a patient with pancreatitis who develop a "sepsis-like" syndrome in the absence of demonstrable infection should not be mixed with patients having undisputable infection. In addition, the type of acute event may have important qualitative and quantitative differences in the activation of the inflammatory cascade of mediators. For instance, the role of oxygen free radicals may be more important in the presence of trauma with ischemia-reperfusion and the role of proteases may be more important in the presence of severe pancreatitis.

Therefore, the effects of therapy of sepsis should be evaluated separately in infected and non-infected patients. For all patients included into clinical trials, it is essential to assure that whenever present, infection was recognized early, the source was actively sought and eradicated, and the appropriate antibiotic therapy was applied. Overlooking an infectious process can rapidly become fatal, regardless of the novel therapeutic option, which is introduced.

At time of inclusion in clinical trials, it is not sufficient to state that there is a clinical suspicion of infection (Table 2). This suspicion should be more supported by two elements. First, infection may be proven in a number of patients since admission into the trial. This is true for the patient with peritonitis found at laparotomy, or with drained abscess or purulent alveolar secretions. If the infection is severe, i.e. if it plays a significant role in the critical disease of the patient, there is no need to identify all signs of sepsis in these patients before starting a therapeutic trial. In other words, the therapeutic trial might be started even in the patient without fever or hypothermia. If no infectious process can be documented early, there should be documentation that this infection was sought not only by cultures but also by other procedures (e.g. abdominal CT-scan). The various procedures and tests that can

Table 2. Criteria used to define the presence of infection

Initial documentation of an infection
– Standard definition of the various types of infection (urinary tract infection, pneumonia, etc.)
– Gram stain of biological fluid
– Presence of pus
Final documentation of an infection
Idem +
– Bacteriological cultures.
Suspicion of infection
– Onset of (or change in) antibiotic therapy
– If infection cannot be readily documented: Documentation of an active search for infection (comprehensive microbiologic evaluation, CT-scan, etc.).
Final evaluation
– Infection documented, likely or absent.

be performed to evaluate the presence and the source of infection in patients "at risk" have been reviewed elsewhere [17].

Second, therapeutic implications should be also documented. These may involve the removal of a source of infection in some instances. In all patients, the institution of or a change in antibiotic therapy should take place. Failure to do so would indicate that the development of a new infection is not considered seriously.

Obviously, a major difficulty resides in the early identification of this infection, as the cultures results cannot be immediately obtained. Once this entire bacterial information is available, one may classify the patients in three groups [18]. A first group consists of patients in whom a source of infection is clearly documented. These patients may have a surgically confirmed peritonitis, a drained microbial abscess or positive blood cultures for a known pathogen. A second group of patients includes those for whom a source of infection is suspected, but not clearly demonstrated. These patients may have a suspected nosocomial pneumonia, a bacteriuria with less than 100000 col/field or blood cultures growing a *Staphylococcus epidermidis* of questionable significance. A third group of patients includes those for whom an infection is unlikely (we should not state *without infection*, because this is too strong a statement). This group may include patients with pancreatitis and/or those for whom all cultures remained negative. These distinctions may not be evident at entry of the clinical trial, but may be re-evaluated by the clinical evaluation committee.

In summary, although the septic response rather than the infection itself is thought to be deleterious to the host, therapies presently focus on "infected" patients. The likelihood of an infectious process should be clearly documented. Categorization of infection as documented, likely and unlikely is useful.

The Importance of the Source of Infection

The source of sepsis may have important influence on the exact nature and the severity of the septic response. In particular, patients with infections due to urosepsis may have a much lower mortality rate than those with other types of infection [19]. In a recent study including 519 septic patients out of 17440 patients included in the APACHE database, Knaus et al. [7] reported that the mortality rate was 55% when the source was gastrointestinal, 54% when it was pulmonary, but only 30% when it was urinary. Interestingly, the mortality rate was 50% when the source was unknown.

In summary, it is important to identify the source of infection. In particular, the urinary tract should be separated from the other sources of infection.

The Importance of Bacteremia

Septic patients with and without bacteremia have a similar presentation. The analysis of the data on 2568 septic patients included in the VA trial of corticosteroid therapy revealed that three factors were independently predictive of bacteremia: elevated temperature, low systemic blood pressure and low platelet count. Nevertheless, these criteria were not very accurate [20].

Clearly, the presence of demonstrable bacteria in the blood is not a requirement for the diagnosis of sepsis. Only about 50% of patients with severe sepsis have documented bacteremia [21]. Some studies reported a higher incidence of circulatory shock when bacteremia was present [21, 22], but others did not [23]. In a recent study from a major Dutch hospital [23], including 382 patients from whom blood was drawn for culture, signs of severe sepsis were found in 92 patients, including 31 patients with shock and 61 without shock. The mortality rate was markedly different in the two groups (55% and 28%, respectively), but the prevalence of positive blood cultures was similar (35% and 39%, respectively).

Recent studies found hardly any significant difference between patients with and without positive blood cultures [24–26]. The lack of significance of positive blood cultures is probably in part due to the fact that many patients develop severe infections while already treated with antibiotic therapy.

In summary, the presence or absence of positive blood cultures is not very important, beyond the clear documentation of an infection.

The Importance of the Type of Microorganisms

Severe infections due to gram-negative and gram-positive bacteria appear to have a similar pattern. Early studies on patients with septic shock suggested that the hemodynamic pattern may be different in patients with infections due to gram-negative and gram-positive infections [27], but more recent studies did not confirm these findings [28, 29]. A recent study reported a higher mortality rate in septicemia due to gram-positive than to gram-negative bacteria [8]. There may also be important interactions between gram-negative and gram-positive infections. A recent study by Walmrath et al. [30] indicated that endotoxin can prime rabbit lungs for enhanced prostanoid generation and pulmonary hypertension in response to *Staphylococcal aureus* toxin. Infections due to gram-positive microorganisms are also increasingly common [31, 32], and this evolution is at least in part a consequence of our antibiotic therapy.

Nevertheless, endotoxin is such a potent trigger of the septic response, that its importance cannot be neglected. Some studies indicated that the cytokines release may be greater in the presence of gram-negative septicemia [33]. The benefit from PAF antagonists may be more substantial in the presence of gram-negative infection [34].

The presence of bacteria versus other forms of microorganisms is also very important. On the one hand, bacteria may represent more potent triggers of the inflammatory cascade of mediators and thus more likely to induce septic shock. On the other hand, fungal infections are more likely to develop in more debilitated, immunocompromised patients, whose prognosis is very poor. There is also an increasing prevalence of fungal infections in critically ill patients, whose degree of debilitation and underlying immunosuppression is greater than before [35].

Thus, the type of microorganisms may play an important role in the nature and the severity of the septic process. These differences have been perhaps overlooked.

The Importance of the Acute Disease and the Underlying Health Status

The underlying disease and the functional health status of the patients are the most important determinant of outcome in severe sepsis. The debilitated patient with generalized arteriosclerosis admitted for the third time in the intensive care unit for another episode of septic shock has little chances to leave the hospital alive (Fig. 2). The prognosis in the patient with decompensated COPD due to lung infection and requiring another episode of mechanical ventilation is related to the chances of weaning from the respirator and these are essentially related to the underlying lung status of the patient [36]. In a recent report on 448 episodes of gram-negative bacteremia [37], the underlying disease was found to represent the most important prognostic factor. Thus one may expect any novel therapeutic intervention to have only a modest effect on outcome from severe sepsis.

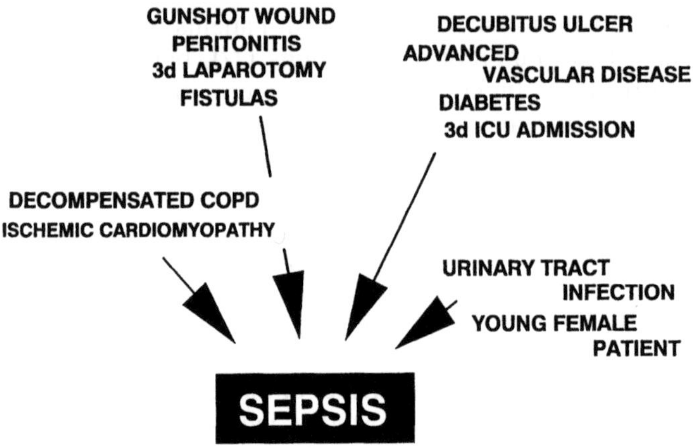

Fig. 2. Some examples stressing the heterogeneity of patients presenting with signs of sepsis

The type of acute disease may also influence the septic response. Infections may have a different pattern after trauma and in other forms of critical illnesses [38].

The Importance of Clinical Management

Obviously, treatment is a major determinant of survival. In the study by Kreger et al. [5], including 612 patients with gram-negative bacteremia, appropriate antibiotic therapy was associated with a 50% reduction in both circulatory shock and mortality rate. The management of underlying factors is also important. For instance, the early stabilization of the traumatized patient can have a significant influence on morbidity and mortality [39–41].

It remains difficult to define what "appropriate therapy" really means. There may be no consensus about the appropriate type of fluids to be administered, the type and the degree of adrenergic support and even the appropriate antibiotic therapy. There may be important differences in clinical management from one institution to another [42]. It is important to keep in mind that these factors are not included in severity indexes.

In randomized clinical trials, it must be assumed that the adequacy of therapy influenced similarly the treatment and the placebo arms of the study. Nevertheless, differences in management may represent a more significant variable if studies are so dispersed that they include only a few patients in each center. Accordingly, it is desirable for clinical trials to provide clear therapeutic protocols to standardize patient management.

How to Further Characterize the "At Risk" Population?

Is the "Sepsis Syndrome" a Valid Clinical Entity?

We all acknowledge the substantial contribution of Roger Bone, who attempted to define useful criteria to describe the "at risk" population. The term "sepsis syndrome" has been used to set a series of criteria applicable to multicenter studies [24–26]. It is supposed to represent a severe form of sepsis, refers to the association of sepsis with altered organ perfusion and/or altered organ function.

Several important problems have emerged with the use of the "sepsis syndrome" (Table 3). A first one is the inhomogeneity of the population studied. Patients with various sources of infection, various degrees of underlying impairment and medical, surgical and traumatic diseases are mixed together. The degree of severity is also quite variable. The experience revealed that a total of 36% of patients had the criteria of septic shock on admission, and another 23% developed septic shock after study admission. The mortality rate for the entire group was around 25%, but only 13% in the absence of shock, and 43% when shock developed after study admission [21]. More importantly, patients with minor degrees of severity can be included, because some of these criteria such as an alteration in mental status can be easily met, while others, such as a reduced systemic vascular resistance, may represent an appropriate response rather than a sign of cardiovascular failure (Table 1). A second major problem is that all criteria of sepsis may not be met in a patient with obviously severe infection. In particular, the core temperature may not be frankly abnormal in patients with very severe sepsis.

A North American consensus panel stated that "the term septic syndrome has been applied to a variety of inflammatory states and it now appears to be both confusing and ambiguous. We therefore recommend that the term septic syndrome no longer be used" [43].

Table 3. Problems with the use of common criteria used to define the sepsis syndrome

1. Heterogeneous populations: various sources of infection, mixing of medical, surgical and traumatized patients, various degrees of underlying impairment...
2. Patients with and without acute circulatory failure are different groups
3. Fever, tachycardia or tachypnea are not always present
4. Assessment of altered mental status is difficult, especially in patients who are sedated (or paralyzed)
5. Low systemic vascular resistance is not a reliable criteria, if shock is considered separately (It basically refers to an elevated cardiac output, which is not as such a sign of cardiovascular dysfunction)

Is "SIRS" a Valid Entity?

The same expert panel of North American colleagues then proposed to reserve the term "sepsis" for the host response to invading microorganisms and to introduce the new acronym SIRS ("systemic inflammatory response syndrome") to define a generalized inflammatory response in a broader sense. The introduction of this neologism may not be warranted for several reasons. First, the identification of the "at risk" population is not likely to improve with the introduction of another term. What is clearly needed is a better understanding of the pathophysiology of the disease, so as to base the identification process on mechanisms. Second, SIRS is conceptually a very sensitive entity mean to include a large number of critically ill patients with possible infection. Since most ICU patients do meet the SIRS criteria [9], there may be almost as many "SIRS" patients than there are "critically ill" patients. It is not warranted to "lump together" a large number of acutely ill patients with different disease states.

Third, clinical studies using these very broad criteria should then rely heavily on the use of a severity index to stratify the degree of severity of illness of the patients (Fig. 3). The clinical trial may want to include neither patients with low risk of death (who will probably do well with or without the tested therapy) nor those with end-stage organ failure (who will do poorly regardless of treatment). Therefore, the therapeutic intervention should be tested on patients with a relatively high range of severity scores but not those with the highest score. However, the use of scoring systems has several major limitations (Table 4).

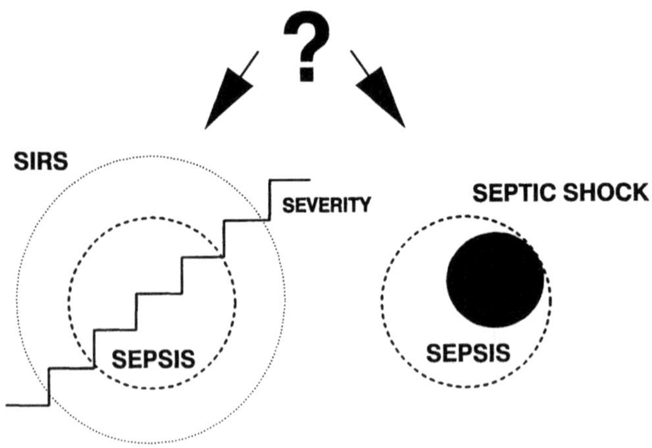

Fig. 3. Evolution of concepts related to severe sepsis. The use of broad criteria included in the "SIRS" concept results in a strong reliance on a scoring system to stratify patients. A second option is to focus more on a group of patients susceptible to benefit the most from the new therapeutic interventions, i.e. the patients with septic shock

Table 4. Ten problems associated with the use of scoring systems to evaluate "at risk" septic patients

1. Scoring systems are hardly applicable to all septic patients. The admission diagnosis and the underlying disease (e.g. cirrhosis) remain the major determinants of outcome.
2. Scoring systems primarily focus on the relative risk of death, whereas degree of organ dysfunction (or even quality of life) are also important.
3. Scoring systems are usually established within 24 h after ICU admission but severe sepsis may develop later.
4. Scoring systems can hardly combine accuracy and simplicity. More sophisticated systems may become cumbersome and yet the gain in accuracy may be limited.
5. Scoring systems are subject to selection bias and lead-time bias.
6. Scoring systems may not provide a better outcome evaluation than doctors and nurses.
7. Scoring systems are influenced by therapy (e.g. vasopressor agents, antipyretic agents...).
8. Scoring systems all remain somewhat subjective, especially in the selection of the primary diagnosis and the assessment of chronic health status.
9. Scoring systems are designed to compare patient population but cannot be applied in individual decision.
10. Scoring systems have no real pathophysiologic basis.

First, no scoring system is applicable to all groups of critically ill patients. Scoring systems are less reliable in patients with burns, trauma, coronary artery disease, hemodynamic pulmonary edema ... [44, 45]. The primary diagnosis remains the most important determinant of outcome. The presence of recent CPR, advanced cirrhosis or cancer with metastasis will influence prognosis more than any other parameter directly related to sepsis.

Second, severity indexes have been developed to evaluate the risk of death of a patient. New forms of therapy may not result in improvement in survival, but may reduce morbidity. A more complete and rapid reversal of organ failure or a lower complications rate may represent a major health achievement and may also reduce the ICU costs.

Third, these indexes have been used either on ICU admission or 24 h after ICU admission, but many patients do develop severe sepsis while they are treated in the ICU.

Fourth, to improve accuracy, some of these indexes have become quite complex, requiring sophisticated programs, and the access to these systems may even be protected. Furthermore, the degree of complexity may be out of proportion of the gain in accuracy, as any prognostic assessment will keep strong limitations.

Fifth, all scoring systems are subject to selection bias and lead-time bias. This is especially important in view of the changing pattern of sepsis in relation to the type of patients (e.g. patients with organ transplant) and the type of infection (e.g. resistance patterns of microorganisms).The lead time bias is also important, in view of the number of patients transferred from other institutions.

Sixth, the evaluation of the severity of the disease process may be as accurate when done by the doctors and even by the nurses rather than by the scoring system [46].

Seventh, the prognosis is very influenced by the therapeutic possibilities, which are not taken into account by the scoring system (e.g. the influence of vasopressor agents on the degree of hypotension).

Eighth, all scoring systems remain subjective, especially in the selection of the primary disease.

Ninth, the prognostic indexes are developed for the evaluation of groups of patients, but their use for individual therapeutic decisions is difficult.

Finally and most importantly, scoring systems do not have a pathophysiologic basis, since they take all possible factors into account. For instance, the origin of the patient may be strongly related to prognosis. In the APACHE III experience on septic patients, 47% of the survivors but 30% of the non-survivors were admitted from the emergency room ($p<0.01$). Conversely, 53% of the survivors but 70% of the non-survivors were transferred and 9% of the survivors but 16% of the non-survivors were readmitted (differences $p<0.01$) [7]. Can we consider that the origin of the patient will influence the decision to start a new therapy for sepsis?

In summary, even though great progress has been made (and will be further made) in the prognostic assessment of critically ill patients, the "at risk" patient is not likely a severity score. The use of new therapies of sepsis should remain based on relatively simple criteria obtained at the bedside. Our therapeutic approach should not fundamentally differ for severe sepsis and for other problems.

Is Septic Shock a Valid Entity?

The use of septic shock criteria may represent a valuable basis to identify the "at risk" patient, as it has a reasonable pathophysiologic basis and is identified relatively easily by the ICU physician (Fig. 3).

Pathophysiologic Basis: Like other forms of acute circulatory failure, septic shock can be defined by an imbalance between the oxygen demand and the oxygen supply to the tissues [47]. An increase in oxygen demand, an altered oxygen extraction and a reduced myocardial contractility have been implicated in this phenomenon, accounting for the presence of perfusion failure despite a normal or elevated cardiac output [42]. The release of the various mediators of sepsis have been implicated in all three alterations (Fig. 4). The stimulating effects of cytokines on the oxygen requirements have been well recognized. Similarly, the various mediators of sepsis are known to alter the oxygen extraction capabilities by altering the distribution of blood flow and

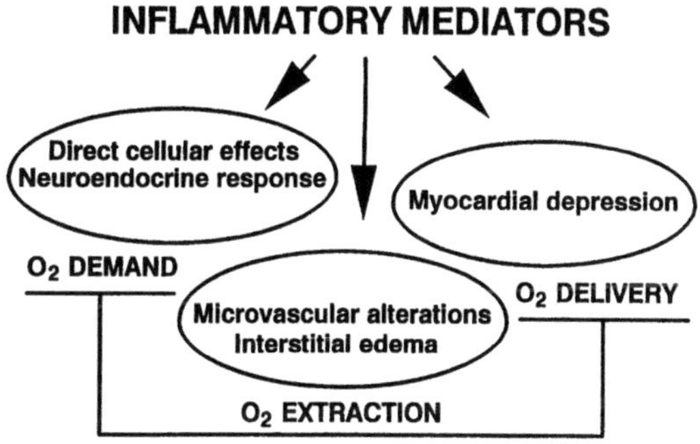

Fig. 4. The effects of the mediators of sepsis on oxygen demand, oxygen extraction and oxygen delivery

the endothelial cell function in the microcirculation. The role of nitric oxide in these peripheral alterations has been more recently recognized [48]. It has been recently shown that the cytokines can alter myocardial contractility. Tumor necrosis factor, interleukin-1 (IL-1), IL-2, platelet activating factor (PAF), arachidonic acid metabolites, nitric oxide and other oxygen free radicals have been all implicated [49–52]. Cytokines have been shown to alter myocardial contractility by interfering with the cellular response to adrenergic stimulation, resulting in a reduced intracellular calcium availability [53]. The degree of myocardial dysfunction has been directly related to the severity of sepsis in animal studies [54] as well as in clinical studies [55, 56].

Oxygen deprivation can also alter the immune response of the host. Hypoxia may alter the phagocytic cell function by a reduced generation of oxygen free radicals. Hypoxia may also enhance complement activation, alter neutrophil function [57]. Even brief episodes of hypoxia may also suppress the T-cell immune response for prolonged periods [58]. Human monocytes exposed to hypoxia spontaneously release TNF and TNF receptors [59]. Hypoxia also influences the immune response of the endothelial cell. Shreeniwas et al. [60] recently showed that hypoxia induces the synthesis and release of IL-1, resulting in an autocrine enhancement in the expression of adhesion molecules. Hence, one may hypothesize the development of a vicious cycle where tissue hypoxia may stimulate the immune system to release a higher amount of mediators, which may in turn alter the balance between oxygen demand and oxygen supply to the tissues and thereby further activate the immune response.

This hypothesis is supported by experimental studies showing the protection by antibodies to TNF in the presence of endotoxic shock but not in the presence of peritonitis [61]. It is also supported by the results of recent clinical trials with murine anti-TNF antibodies and IL-1ra [62].

It is difficult to predict the risk of development of shock in septic patients. In a recent study on 331 patients with bacteremia, Aube et al. [63] identified the following alterations to represent significant risk factors for septic shock: male gender or age older than 75 years, creatinine level greater than 2 mg/

dL, a prothrombin time less than 60% and the presence of an interstitial pattern on the chest roentgenogram. Nevertheless, none of these signs was very reliable.

Clinical Definition: Septic shock describes the clinical syndrome corresponding to acute circulatory failure. Even though the presence of bacteria may not always be demonstrated, septic shock is most commonly associated with a bacterial infection, which are equally attributed to gram-negative and gram-positive infections [63].

Arterial hypotension is an important clinical sign, which however is neither specific nor very sensitive. Hypotension can be associated with other forms of acute circulatory failure. In particular, the differential diagnosis between hypovolemic and septic shock is sometimes difficult, and it is generally the confirmation (or exclusion) of the infectious process that determines the eventual diagnosis. Transient hypotension can also occur in relation to a vagal reaction, or to some reduction in venous return associated with some degree of hypovolemia, in particular when the intrathoracic pressures are increased. These forms of transient hypotension are usually not associated with signs of organ failure. In some cases, signs of tissue hypoperfusion can be found in the absence of significant hypotension.

The recent onset of oliguria (urine output less than 20 mL/h in an adult patient) is an important sign of altered renal function. Respiratory failure is also usually present, and known to have a strong prognostic value [7]. Altered skin perfusion may also reflect the circulatory alterations, although the cutaneous examination may not reveal severe alterations. Hypothermia, when present is a strong clue in favor of the diagnosis of septic shock.

The presence of altered cellular function can be reflected by an increase in blood lactate levels. Hyperlactatemia in septic shock may represent the presence of other derangements than tissue hypoxia. For instance, endotoxin administration in animals results in an increase in blood lactate levels when the VO_2 is still well above the critical DO_2 value [64]. Also the administration of dichloroacetate, an activator of the pyruvate dehydrogenase, in animals [65] like in men [66] decreases the lactate levels, pointing to a metabolic disorder involving pyruvate metabolism [67]. Nevertheless, lactate levels are generally normal in stable, septic patients, and lactate levels can be correlated with the development of organ failure and mortality [68]. Therefore, regardless of the exact mechanism, an increase in blood lactate levels can reflect the presence of altered cellular function. Whenever possible, increased blood lactate levels should confirm the diagnosis.

It is important to note that cardiac output can be found elevated, normal or low in septic shock. Determinations of DO_2 or VO_2 are not very useful to predict survival [68].

Some investigators included some therapeutic aspects in the definition, such as "not responding to fluid therapy" or "requiring the use of vasopressor agents". Unfortunately, these therapeutic elements are non-specific and largely dependent on treatment protocols. How much fluids are required to state that there is no satisfactory response? To define an optimal level of cardiac filling pressures in septic shock is very difficult. Similarly, the use of vasopressors can differ substantially from one center to the other, as illustrated by some recent studies on the use of vasopressors in septic shock. In some studies, the administration of epinephrine was started in patients with a mean pulmonary artery occlusion pressure (PAOP) of 19 mm Hg [69] while in others the administration of either norepinephrine [70] or epinephrine [69] was started in patients with a mean PAOP of only 9 mm Hg.

The use of "refractory shock" to characterize a prolonged episode of circulatory shock is not helpful, because it is too imprecise, and too dependent on therapy [70]. It could even have a negative connotation, implying that the situation has become hopeless. We think important to consider that even the most severe shock state is potentially reversible. The degree of severity of shock can be assessed by the degree of concurrent organ dysfunction, the severity of lactic acidosis, and the amount of adrenergic therapy required to maintain an adequate blood pressure.

In summary, the definition of shock must include several elements. The best definition of septic shock remains the development of arterial hypotension associated with signs of altered tissue perfusion (Table 1). Although the degree of severity of septic shock should be assessed, the use of the term "refractory shock" is probably not useful, and even potentially misleading.

Is Organ Failure a Valid Entity?

Alterations in organ function can spread from some degree of organ dysfunction (e.g. moderate elevation in creatinine or bilirubin levels) to severe organ failure (e.g. severe acute respiratory failure or coma). The most severe form, multiple organ failure (MOF), often follows an episode of acute circulatory failure, but sometimes develops in the absence of frank circulatory shock.

Organ failure can be defined by three types of criteria:

1. Objective criteria, based on measurable parameters, such as the urea/BUN levels, the bilirubin levels. These are by far the preferred criteria.
2. Categorical diagnoses, such as cholecystitis or ARDS. These should be avoided, as these definitions may be somewhat arbitrary and subjective.
3. Criteria based on treatment, such as the level of PEEP to define the degree of respiratory failure or the requirements for hemodialysis or hemofiltration to define renal failure. These criteria should be avoided, as they may critically depend on the policy of the ICU. As a comparison, one would not like to define pneumonia by the requirements for penicillin. Nevertheless, they are sometimes unavoidable. As an example, the evalu-

ation of the PaO_2/FiO_2 ratio to assess the degree of respiratory failure must take the type of ventilatory support and especially the PEEP level into account.

The most reliable parameters to define the degree of failure of the organs are presented in the Table 5. Most of these criteria have their limitations. For instance, the BUN/urea and creatinine levels can be influenced by the use of extracorporeal renal replacement and hemofiltration may be started early in some centers, where clinicians believe that the removal of mediators may be beneficial. The use of the Glasgow coma scale is the best method to assess neurological function. However, many patients are treated with sedative agents, that can be responsible for the alteration in mental status. In addition, many patients are treated with mechanical ventilation so that the assessment of speach capabilities can become very subjective.

Many studies included the degree of cardiovascular dysfunction in the assessment of organ dysfunction [71, 72]. In most of these studies, cardiovascular failure referred to the presence of circulatory shock, which is so important that it should be considered separately. Shock can be considered as a consequence of sepsis, but its presence will rapidly induce the failure of the other organs so that it will represent by itself a cause of organ failure.

The other criteria used to describe cardiovascular failure, such as the presence of arrhythmias, a high or a low cardiac output, or the development of myocardial infarction or the presence of endocarditis are no specific complications of sepsis. The cardiac output is not a reliable prognostic factor in severe sepsis and the development of arrhythmias can be associated with underlying cardiac disease or to some electrolyte abnormalities rather than to the complications of the septic process.

Some investigators listed some diagnoses, such as cholecystitis or stress ulcer in the definition of multiple organ failure. This can be hazardous, as diagnoses are more subject to a subjective interpretation. This is also why the assessment of gastrointestinal failure is virtually impossible.

Table 5. Definition of organ dysfunction/failure for 5 organs

Respiratory: PaO_2/FiO_2 ratio, use of mechanical ventilation (including the level of positive end-expiratory pressure). In the assessment of the severity of the acute respiratory distress syndrome (ARDS), the degree of alteration of the chest roentgenogram and the thoracic compliance may be added.

Renal: Urea (or BUN) and creatinine concentrations, urine output.

Hematologic: Coagulation abnormalities: platelet count, prothrombin time (PT), activated partial thromboplastin time (APTT). A low hematocrit or a low white blood cell count may be also sometimes included.

Hepatic: Bilirubin level (probably the most reliable), elevated liver enzymes (SGOT, SGPT and alkaline phosphatase).

Neurologic: Glasgow coma score.

Another important consideration is whether or not some degree of organ failure was preexistant to the development of shock. Should the evaluation of renal failure be similar in a patient with chronic renal failure but stable renal function and in a patient whose a previously normal renal function deteriorated acutely? Should it be similar when hyperbilirubinemia is due to liver metastasis and when it is attributed to sepsis?

Finally, the degree of organ failure is an important determination of outcome, but hardly a useful basis to define the "at risk" population. Patients with hardly any sign of organ dysfunction should not be considered, since there is not much to gain from another therapeutic intervention. At the other extreme, patients with advanced multiple organ failure may not benefit either, since the novel intervention may be applied too late (Fig. 5). The presence of respiratory failure and oliguria may help to identify a group of patients at higher risk of death [7].

In summary, the assessment of the degree of organ failure should be based on objective, measurable parameters rather than on clinical signs or symptoms. This assessment is very important to quantify the severity of the disease process in the therapeutic trial. The frequence of sepsis-related organ failure can help to identify the "at risk" patient. In particular, the presence of respiratory failure (hypoxemia, need for endotracheal intubation and mechanical ventilation), disseminated intravascular coagulation or oliguria can help to recognize the "at risk" patient.

The Future of Clinical Trials in "At Risk" Patients

Despite the very encouraging experimental studies, the clinical trials in the field of sepsis have usually yielded only modest improvements, if any. A possible explanation is our lack of clear understanding of the pathophysiology of these disease states. The clinical, hematologic and biochemical signs that we

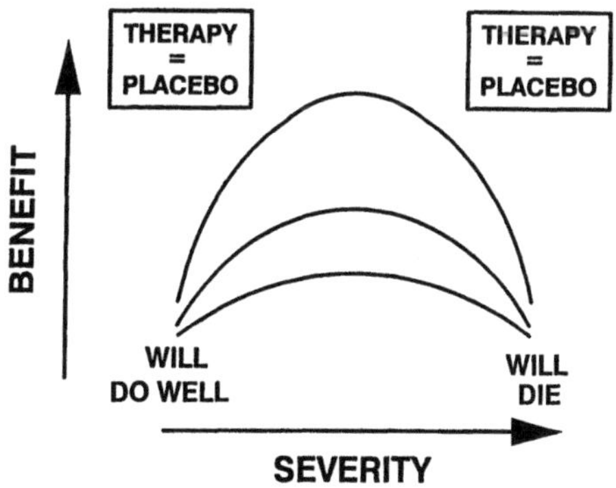

Fig. 5. The degree of benefit from new therapeutic interventions, in relation to the severity of the disease process. A novel intervention is not likely to benefit patients with the lowest severity (who are likely to do well with or without this intervention) and with the highest severity (who are likely to do poorly with or without this intervention)

can identify are only the "tip of the iceberg", the only visible portion of a complex but deep cellular-humoral reaction. Therefore, the criteria used to enter patients into the trials cannot be precise enough to permit to apply the right treatment at the right time in the right group of patients.

Nevertheless, we should be cautious and modest, but not overly pessimistic. Several trials showed an overall moderate beneficial effect, characterized by a moderate reduction in morbidity and mortality rates. We should realize that no substance will represent a miraculous agent, a "magic bullet" that will dramatically improve outcome.

Actually, we may be in the field of immunotherapy of sepsis where we stood a number of years ago, when thrombolysis of myocardial infarction was started. There were many discussions regarding the efficacy of this new form of therapy. Today, nobody doubts about the efficacy of thrombolytic therapy for myocardial infarction.

We may also find the situation analogous to that of chemotherapy of cancer, which also started with modest results. The combination of chemotherapeutic agents greatly improved the efficacy of these treatments. Similarly, the combination of immunomodulating agents may be the way in the future.

To maximize the chances of success of a novel therapeutic intervention, clinical trials may follow two different approaches. The first one is to include a very large number of patients into clinical trials so that confounding factors will be eventually eliminated. If a molecule is found effective, a subgroup analysis may then help to identify the patients who benefit the most. These large trials must have relatively broad criteria for entry, except that a severity index must be used to stratify the patients. These trials must be relatively simple to be practically feasible. This type of trials is sometimes preferred by the pharmaceutical industry, because it may result in wide indications of a therapeutic agent in large numbers of patients. A foreseeable problem is the availability of centers that will be ready to participate, in view of the multiplicity of the trials dealing with the same type of patients! The danger of this type of trials is to include too many small centers, possibly resulting in differences in management. This was the experience of the recent CHESS trial. A too large clinical trial may also mask the evidence of a beneficial effect in a subgroup of patients if this therapy has deleterious effects in another subgroup of patients.

The second approach is to focus any new therapeutic intervention on a specific group of patients with an identifiable disease process. Rather than mixing traumatized with non-traumatized patients, patients with early and advanced organ failure, these trials would include well defined groups of patients. Although the criteria need to be defined for each therapeutic intervention, it is likely that circulatory shock will represent a useful basis.

In any case, the clinical trials will need to stratify the patients according to the severity of the disease process and thus the chances of survival. Those patients with high chances of survival will be eliminated, because they are likely to do well in the absence of additional therapy. Furthermore, immunotherapy may even have deleterious effects by blocking the physiological septic response. At the other end of the spectrum, patients who are very debilitated, at the end of a long disease process should be also eliminated, because any form of investigational therapy is not likely to benefit those patients who are likely to die (Fig. 5).

Conclusions

The "at risk" patient presents a septic reaction that becomes excessive, resulting in significant damage to the host. The syndrome is typically found in association with severe infections, but in some instances, no infection can be demonstrated. In each patient, it is important to consider individually a number of factors, including the presence and the source of infection and the type of microorganisms, the severity of the underlying disease and the appropriate therapy. The search for an infection is essential of course not only for diagnostic purposes but also to eradicate the source whenever possible and to apply the appropriate antibiotic therapy. The identification of an infection due to gram-negative microorganisms may also enhance the chances of success of immunotherapy.

An identifiable "at risk" group is the group of patients with evidence of acute circulatory failure (septic shock). To define the "at risk" group by other clinical, hematologic or immunologic signs of sepsis has not been found very useful. The predominant use of scoring systems has major problems of complexity, and lack of pathophysiologic basis. To define the "at risk" group by the degree of organ failure may be misleading, as it may select a group of patients with end-stage disease for whom any new therapeutic trial may be ineffective. A definition based on acute circulatory failure has a sound pathophysiological basis, as indicated by many experimental and clinical studies. New forms of therapy of severe sepsis are most likely to find a therapeutic effect in the most severe forms of sepsis, i.e. those associated with circulatory failure.

References

1. Vincent JL, Bihari D (1992) Sepsis, severe sepsis or sepsis syndrome: Need for clarification. Intensive Care Med 18:255–257
2. Levine B, Kalman J, Mayer L, Fillit HM, Packer M (1990) Elevated circulating levels of tumor necrosis factor in severe chronic heart failure. N Engl J Med 323:236–241
3. McCurry KR, Campbell DA, Scales WE, Warren JS, Remick DG (1993) Tumor necrosis factor, interleukin 6, and the acute phase response following hepatic ischemia/reperfusion. J Surg Res 55:49–54
4. Harris RL, Musher DM, Bloom K, et al (1987) Manifestations of sepsis. Arch Intern Med 147:1895–1906
5. Kreger BE, Craven DE, McCabe WR (1980) Gram-negative bacteremia. Am J Med 68:344–355
6. Clemmer TP, Fisher CJ, Bone RC, Slotman GJ, Metz GA, Thomas FO (1992) Hyperthermia in the sepsis syndrome and clinical outcome. Crit Care Med 20:1395–1401

7. Knaus WA, Sun X, Nystrom PO, Wagner DP (1994) Evaluation of definitions for sepsis. Chest 101:1656–1662
8. Geerdes HF, Ziegler D, Lode H, et al (1992) Septicemia in 980 patients at a university hospital in Berlin: Prospective studies during 4 selected years between 1979 and 1989. Cl Infect Dis 15:991–1002
9. Metrangolo L, Fiorillo M, Friedman G, et al (1993) Hemodynamic profile in the first 24 hours of septic shock. Medicina Intensiva 17:S53 (Abstract)
10. Azimi G, Vincent JL (1986) Ultimate survival from septic shock. Resuscitation 14:245–253
11. Parker MM, Shelhamer JH, Natanson C (1987) Serial cardiovascular variables in survivors and nonsurvivors of human septic shock: Heart rate as an early predictor of prognosis. Crit Care Med 15:923–929
12. Simmons DH, Nicoloff J, Guze LB (1960) Hyperventilation and respiratory alkalosis as signs of gram-negative bacteremia. JAMA 174:196–199
13. Blair E (1969) Hypocapnia and gram-negative bacteremic shock. Am J Surg 117:433–439
14. MacLean LD, Mulligan GW, McLean AP, Duff JH (1967) Alkalosis in septic shock. Surgery 62:655–662
15. Marshall J, Sweeney D (1990) Microbial infection and the septic response in critical surgical illness. Arch Surg 125:17–23
16. Meakins JL (1990) Etiology of multiple organ failure. J Trauma 30:S165–S168
17. Norwood SH, Civetta JM (1987) Evaluating sepsis in critically ill patients. Chest 92:137–144
18. European Society of Intensive Care Medicine (1994) The problem of sepsis. An expert report. Intensive Care Med 20:300–304
19. Wong DT, Wagner DP, Knaus WA (1992) Lower ICU mortality in septic shock due to urosepsis compared to non-urosepsis. Anesthesiology 77:A318 (Abstract)
20. Peduzzi P, Shatney C, Sheagren J, Sprung C (1992) Predictors of bacteremia and gram-negative bacteremia in patients with sepsis. Arch Intern Med 152:529–535
21. Bone RC, Fisher CJ, Clemmer TP, Slotman GJ, Metz CA, Balk RA (1989) Sepsis syndrome: A valid clinical entity. Crit Care Med 17:389–393
22. McCabe WR, Treadwell TL, De Maria A (1983) Pathophysiology of bacteremia. Am J Med 75:7–18
23. Kieft H, Hoepelman AI, Zhou W, Rozenberg-Arska M, Struyvenberg A, Verhoef J (1993) The sepsis syndrome in a Dutch university hospital. Arch Intern Med 153:2241–2247
24. Bone RC, Fisher CJ, Clemmer TP, et al (1987) The methylprednisolone severe sepsis study group: A controlled clinical trial of high-dose methylprednisolone in the treatment of severe sepsis and septic shock. N Engl J Med 317:353
25. The Veterans Administration Systemic Sepsis Cooperative Study Group (1987) Effect of high-dose glucocorticoid therapy on mortality in patients with clinical signs of systemic sepsis. N Engl J Med 317:659–665
26. Ziegler EJ, Fisher CJ, Sprung CL, et al (1991) Treatment of gram-negative bacteremia and septic shock with HA-1A human monoclonal antibody against endotoxin. N Engl J Med 324:429–436
27. Blain CM, Anderson TO, Pietras RJ, Gunnar RM (1970) Immediate hemodynamic effects of gram-negative vs gram-positive bacteremia in man. Arch Intern Med 126:260–265
28. Wiles JB, Cerra FB, Siegel JH, Border JR (1980) The systemic septic response: Does the organism matter? Crit Care Med 8:55–60
29. Ahmed AJ, Kruse JA, Haupt MT, Chandrasekar PH, Carlson RW (1991) Hemodynamic responses to gram-positive versus gram-negative sepsis in critically ill patients with and without circulatory shock. Crit Care Med 19:1520–1525
30. Walmrath D, Griebner M, Kolb B, et al (1993) Endotoxin primes perfused rabbit lungs for enhanced vasoconstrictor response to staphylococcal α-toxin. Am Rev Respir Dis 148:1179–1186

31. Bone RC (1994) Gram-positive organisms and sepsis. Arch Intern Med 154:26–34
32. Barie PS (1993) Emerging problems in Gram-positive infections in the postoperative patient. Surg Gynecol Obstet 177:55–64
33. Fisher CJ, Opal SM, Dhainaut JF, et al (1993) Influence of an anti-tumor necrosis factor monoclonal antibody on cytokine levels in patients with sepsis. Crit Care Med 21:318–327
34. Tenaillon A, Dhainaut JF (1992) Administration of BN 52021 a PAF antagonist in patients with severe sepsis. 6th European Congress on Intensive Care Medicine (Barcelona) (Abstract)
35. Vincent JL, Bihari D, Suter PM, et al (1994) The prevalence of nosocomial infection in intensive care units in Europe – The results of the EPIC study. (UnPub)
36. Vincent JL (1994) Outcome from mechanical ventilation. Eur Respir J (In press)
37. Uzun O, Akalin HE, Hayran M, Unal S (1992) Factors influencing prognosis in bacteremia due to gram-negative organisms: Evaluation of 448 episodes in a Turkish university hospital. Cl Infect Dis 15:866–873
38. Polk HC (1993) Factors influencing the risk of infection after trauma. Am J Surg 165:2S–7S
39. Livingston DH (1993) Management of the surgical patient with multiple system organ failure. Am J Surg 165:8S–13S
40. Goris RJA, Gimbrere JSF, Van Niekerk JLM, Schoots FJ, Booy LHD (1982) Early osteosynthesis and prophylactic mechanical ventilation in the multitrauma patient. J Trauma 22:895–903
41. Roumen RM, Redl H, Schlag G, Sandtner W, Koller W, Goris JA (1993) Scoring systems and blood lactate concentrations in relation to the development of adult respiratory distress syndrome and multiple organ failure in severely traumatized patients. J Trauma 35:349–355
42. Vincent JL (1991) Diagnostic and medical management/supportive care of patients with gram-negative bacteremia and septic shock. Infect Dis Clin North Am 5:807–816
43. Bone RC, Balk RA, Cerra FB, et al (1992) Definition for sepsis and organ failure and guidelines for the use of innovative therapies in sepsis. Chest 101:1644–1655
44. McAnena OJ, Moore FA, Moore EE, Mattox KL, Marx JA, Pepe P (1992) Invalidation of the APACHE II scoring system for patients with acute trauma. J Trauma 33:504–507
45. Fedullo AJ, Swinburne AJ, Wah GW (1988) APACHE II score and mortality in respiratory failure due to cardiogenic pulmonary edema. Crit Care Med 16:1218–1223
46. Kruse JA, Thill-Baharozian MC, Carlson RW (1988) Comparison of clinical assessment with APACHE II for predicting mortality risk in patients admitted to a medical intensive care unit. JAMA 260:1739–1742
47. Vincent JL, Van der Linden P (1990) Septic shock: Particular type of acute circulatory failure. Crit Care Med 18:S70–S74
48. Moncada S, Palmer RM, Higgs EA (1991) Nitric oxide: Physiology, pathophysiology, and pharmacology. Pharmacol Rev 43:109–142
49. Horton JW, White J (1993) Free radical scavengers prevent intestinal ischemia-reperfusion-mediated cardiac dysfunction. J Surg Res 55:282–289
50. Heard SO, Perkins MW, Fink MP (1992) Tumor necrosis factor-alpha causes myocardial depression in guinea pigs. Crit Care Med 20:523–527
51. Vincent JL, Bakker J, Marécaux G, Schandene L, Kahn RJ, Dupont E (1992) Anti-TNF antibodies administration increases myocardial contractility in septic shock patients. Chest 101:810–815
52. Odeh M (1993) Tumor necrosis factor-α as a myocardial depressant substance. Int J Cardiol 42:231–238
53. Yokoyama T, Vaca L, Rossen RD, Durante W, Hazarika P, Mann DL (1993) Cellular basis for the negative inotropic effects of tumor necrosis factor-α in the adult mammalian heart. J Clin Invest 92:2303–2312

54. Goldfarb RD, Tambolini W, Wiener SM, Weber PB (1983) Canine left ventricular performance during LD50 endotoxemia. Am J Physiol 244:H370–H377
55. D'Orio V, Mendes P, Saad G, Marcelle R (1990) Accuracy in early prediction of prognosis of patients with septic shock by analysis of simple indices: Prospective study. Crit Care Med 18:1339–1345
56. Vincent JL, Gris P, Coffernils M, et al (1992) Myocardial depression characterizes the fatal course of septic shock. Surgery 111:660–667
57. Beachy J, Weisman LE (1993) Acute asphyxia affects neutrophil number and function in the rat. Crit Care Med 21:1929–1934
58. Zuckerberg AL, Goldberg LI, Lederman HM (1994) Effects of hypoxia on interleukin-2 mRNA expression by T lymphocytes. Crit Care Med 22:197–203
59. Scannell G, Waxman K, Kaml GJ, et al (1993) Hypoxia induces a human macrophage cell line to release tumor necrosis factor-α and its soluble receptors in vitro. J Surg Res 54:281–285
60. Shreeniwas R, Koga S, Karakurum M, et al (1992) Hypoxia-mediated induction of endothelial cell interleukin-1α. An autocrine mechanism promoting expression of leukocyte adhesion molecules on the vessel surface. J Clin Invest 90:2333–2339
61. Bagdy GJ, et al (1991) Anti-TNF antibodies. J Infect Dis 163:83
62. Fisher CJ, Dhainaut JF, Opal SM, et al (1994) Recombinant human interleukin 1 receptor antagonist in the treatment of patients with sepsis syndrome. JAMA 271:1836–1843
63. Aube H, Milan C, Blettery B (1992) Risk factors for septic shock in the early management of bacteremia. Am J Med 93:283–288
64. Zhang H, Vincent JL (1993) Oxygen extraction is altered by endotoxin during tamponade-induced stagnant hypoxia in the dog. Circ Shock 40:168–176
65. Preiser JC, Moulart D, Vincent JL (1990) Dichloroacetate administration in the treatment of endotoxin shock. Circ Shock 30:221–228
66. Stacpoole PW, Wright EC, Baumgartner TG, et al (1992) A controlled clinical trial of dichloroacetate for treatment of lactic acidosis in adults. N Engl J Med 327:1564–1569
67. Vary TC, Siegel JH, Nakatani T, Sato T, Aoyama H (1986) Effect of sepsis on activity of pyruvate dehydrogenase complex in skeletal muscle and liver. Am J Physiol 250:E634–E640
68. Bakker J, Coffernils M, Leon M, Gris P, Vincent JL (1991) Blood lactate levels are superior to oxygen derived variables in predicting outcome in human septic shock. Chest 99:956–962
69. Moran JL, O'Fathartaigh MS, Peisach AR, Chapman MJ, Leppart P (1993) Epinephrine as an inotropic agent in septic shock: A dose-profile analysis. Crit Care Med 21:70–77
70. Desjars Ph, Pinaud M, Bugnon D, Tasseau F (1989) Norepinephrine therapy has no deleterious renal effects in human septic shock. Crit Care Med 17:426–429
71. Knaus WA, Draper EA, Wagner DP, Zimmerman JE (1985) Prognosis in acute organ-system failure. Ann Surg 202:685–693
72. Marshall JC (1994) A scoring system for multiple organ dysfunction syndrome. In: Reinhart K, Eyrich K and Sprung C (eds) Update in Intensive Care and Emergency Medicine Vol 18 Sepsis. Current perspectives in pathophysiology and therapy, Springer Verlag, Berlin, Heidelberg, New York: pp 38–49

Outcome and Prognostic Factors in Bacteremic Sepsis

Y. Gasche, D. Pittet, and P. M. Suter

Introduction

Bacteremic sepsis accounts for about one-half of the 400000–600000 episodes of sepsis occurring each year in the United States; according to vital statistics, bacteremic sepsis – previously called "septicemia" – is the 13th leading cause of death nationwide [1–3]. The incidence of sepsis is increasing in hospitals, and is two to five times higher in intensive care than in other hospital wards [4–6]. At least 50% of all patients with bacteremic sepsis show evidence of organ dysfunction [7–9].

Mortality among patients with sepsis and associated positive blood culture remains high. It averages 35% in hospital-wide series (range 20–60%) and accounts for about 100000 deaths per year in the United States, i.e. half the 200000 deaths from all cases of sepsis [3, 7–15].

Appropriate antibiotic therapy influences the outcome of bacteremia [11, 12, 16]. However, despite the availability of potent antibiotics and modern intensive care, no change in the overall fatality rates has been noted for over a decade. The potential benefit of adjuvant immunotherapies using anti-endotoxin antibodies in the treatment of gram-negative sepsis has been investigated [8, 9, 17–19]. The real benefit of these newly developed compounds however has still to be defined. So far, a potential benefit has only been suggested in subsets of septic patients in clinical trials which were not designed for this specific patient subsets [20, 21]. Similar therapeutic approaches are currently under investigation with monoclonal antibodies against tumor necrosis factor or with an interleukin-1 receptor antagonist [22, 23]. It is of importance that the latter therapies might be of benefit not only to patients with gram-negative infections, but also to those with gram-positive, fungal, or parasitic diseases.

Organ dysfunction is frequent in sepsis and associated with a poor prognosis [7–9, 13, 14, 24–29]. Some of the high-technology immunotherapies may prevent the development of organ dysfunction [8, 9, 19, 22, 23] and thereby improve outcome. Reliable definitions of risk factors associated with poor outcome in sepsis are needed to help select candidates for these expensive agents.

In the present chapter, we review the evidence for relevant risk factors for mortality in patients presenting with clinical signs of sepsis with bacteremia.

We will use the term "bacteremic sepsis" to describe the association of sepsis and positive blood cultures. This definition is indispensable for an accurate understanding of the prognosis related to bacteremic sepsis and seems preferable to the older term "septicemia".

Terminology

The imprecise terminology used during the past 10 or 20 years led to considerable confusion and difficulties in the interpretation of comparative clinical investigations. Thus it has been necessary to establish a specific nomenclature with exact definitions of infection, bacteremia, sepsis and septic shock (see chapter by R. Bone in this book). Vital organ dysfunction syndrome (MODS) has also had to be redefined more precisely in this context (see chapter by G. Bernard in this book) and implies the presence of altered organ function in acutely ill patients to an extent that homeostasis cannot be maintained without medical intervention. Sepsis is a complex clinical entity and is a dynamic process associated with various complications. It affects a heterogeneous population of patients infected by a variety of causing pathogens. Complications from sepsis can be relatively non-specific, and making a distinction between alterations in direct relation to the causing pathogen or due only to the pathophysiologic sequence of the septic process may be very difficult. A number of factors have to be taken into consideration to analyse precisely the natural course and prognosis of bacteremic sepsis.

In our view, bacteremia, which refers to the presence of viable bacteria in the blood, does not represent the same clinical entity as sepsis accompanied by bloodstream infection, where patients present positive blood cultures in addition to the clinical manifestation of sepsis. Because bacteremia can occur in clinical settings without signs of sepsis, we propose using the term "bacteremic sepsis" to better discriminate between sepsis with or without positive blood culture. Our proposition follows the recommendation of the consensus conference of the American College of Chest Physicians/Society of Critical Care Medicine [3] which suggests that the term "septicemia" be eliminated from current usage (see chapter by R. Bone in this book) and should help clinicians to better define the populations of patients being studied.

Crude and Attributable Mortality

For an even better approach to the actual prognosis of bacteremic sepsis, it is vital to specify the concept of mortality. Patients may die as a direct result of the septic process but also as a result of the interaction between sepsis and other pre-existing conditions or even because of a pathologic event not related to sepsis. Thus the notion of crude and attributable mortality has to be defined.

Crude mortality ranges between 20 and 60% and represents the overall death rate of a cohort of patients who developed bacteremic sepsis in the course of their ICU or hospital stay. In other words, these patients might die because of sepsis, or with sepsis but because of unrelated medical conditions, or after sepsis resolution. Attributable mortality defines the mortality rate attributed to the infection, apart from the underlying disease or other confounding factors that contribute to death; these patients die directly *because of sepsis*. Attributable mortality from nosocomial bloodstream infection averages 26% in large hospital-wide series but varies according to the microorganisms causing the infection and patient population [30]. Fatality rate is higher in critically ill than in ward patients [30].

In a specifically designed pairwise matched (1/1) case control study, where cases were defined as patients with nosocomial bloodstream infection and controls were selected according to matching variables, crude mortality rates differed significantly between cases and controls, 50 and 15% respectively; thus, the estimated attributable mortality of nosocomial bloodstream infection was 35% (95% confidence intervals 25–45%) [31].

Prognostic Factors

Prognostic factors determining the outcome of bacteremic sepsis have been studied extensively. However, most studies identified variables possibly associated with poor outcome without appropriate adjustment for confounding variables. Two of the major concerns of epidemiologists when designing, analyzing and interpreting studies are correcting for confounding variables and identifying indirect and direct causes of disease, morbidity or mortality.

A confounder is a variable that is: a) causally related to the effect under study (i.e. mortality of sepsis); b) associated with the risk of disease (or the risk of death in the current discussion). A confounder is obviously not the cause of the disease (or of death), but affects its development. In the current discussion, a confounder will definitely affect the outcome of bacteremic sepsis.

Age and Sex

Age is a typical confounder for the association between bacteremic sepsis and mortality; it follows from a) that older age at the time of bacteremic sepsis is associated with increased odds of mortality. In this example, age is also associated b) with an increased risk of acquiring nosocomial bloodstream infection [30]. In epidemiological terms, age is a strong confounder of prediction of mortality from bacteremic sepsis and must be considered in any outcome analysis.

The different studies which have analyzed the risk of death in bacteremic sepsis according to age have shown that the elderly die more frequently. The cut-off value for increased risk ranges generally between 60 and 70 years

[7, 30, 32], but Weinstein et al. [12] have noted that the risk increased according to decade categories (<20 years, 21–40, 41–50, >50) and became significantly higher in the 5th decade and thereafter. The same authors observed a significant difference in mortality (48 versus 33%) between male and female patients, but these results could not be confirmed in later studies [33].

Associated Morbidities

Co-morbid conditions predict the length of stay and the number of infectious and non-infectious complications, independent of primary diagnosis, both in general hospital as well as in medical ICU populations. Reviewing the hospital stay of 2647 surgical patients, Munoz et al. [34] clearly demonstrated a relationship between the number of co-morbidities and increased morbidities, hospital cost and mortality. Gross et al. [35] quantified the number of co-morbidities in 148 patients admitted to a combined medical intensive care-coronary care unit who stayed in the unit at least three days, and found that this index was directly correlated with increased length of stay and the development of infectious and non-infectious complications. Obviously, the presence of co-morbidities at the time of diagnosis of sepsis appears to be a determinant risk factor for death.

The initial stratification of patients according to underlying disease was created by McCabe in 1962 in order to estimate the prognosis of gram-negative bacteremia [36]. Subsequent studies by Freid et al. [37] confirmed that the associated underlying disease was a major determinant of fatality in patients with gram-negative bacteremia. The APACHE [32, 38, 39] scoring system, developed by Knaus et al. for patients admitted to ICU in general, has allowed in its 3rd development (APACHE III) to confirm and quantify the influence of severe co-morbidities such as AIDS, hepatic failure, cirrhosis, hematologic malignancies, metastatic cancer or immune suppression on the mortality due to sepsis.

More recently, we demonstrated, using a specific scoring system which takes into account active pre-existing co-morbidities in addition to the diagnosis at admission, the importance of underlying medical conditions in the prognosis of mortality in ICU patients with bacteremic sepsis [40]. Among co-morbidities recorded at ICU admission, 9 conditions (active smoking, alcoholism, non-cured malignancy, previous antibiotic therapy, splenectomy or major surgery prior to admission, diabetes mellitus, previous cardiogenic shock and cardiopulmonary resuscitation before admission) were associated with a higher risk of death, but only 4 of them reached statistical significance by univariate analysis: non-cured malignancy, previous antibiotic therapy, previous cardiopulmonary resuscitation, and cardiogenic shock. A specific scoring system for co-morbidities named *"active pre-existing co-morbidities" (APC)* was created by summing the total number of these conditions present in one patient. The mean number of APC were significantly higher in non-survivors than in survivors, and the APC score was identified by multivariate analysis with logistic regression procedures as an independent predictor of mortality at ICU admission in addition to the APACHE II score. Importantly, taking into account the above-cited co-morbidities assessed at admission to the ICU significantly improved the prediction of mortality from bacteremic sepsis as assessed with the APACHE II score alone (Fig. 1). By linear regression analysis, the number of co-morbidities demonstrated a highly significant correlation with hospital mortality (Fig. 2). However, this new score has still to be validated and perhaps refined, but its merit is that it opens the way for a specific, standardized quantification of co-morbidities.

Patient's Location

Patients who develop nosocomial bacteremia have been shown to be at greater risk of death than patients with community-acquired bacteremia [12, 30, 33]. Prognosis is also related to the type of hospital (review [30]). Bryan et al. [16] found a lower mortality of gram-negative bacteremia in non-teaching community hospitals compared to teaching community hospitals which is probably due to the presence of fewer patients with serious underlying disease in the former type of institution.

Rates of nosocomial infections in selected ICU are 3 to 4-fold higher than in the general hospital [30, 41]. On the other hand, the rate of infection may differ according to the type of ICU considered, with a tendency to be higher

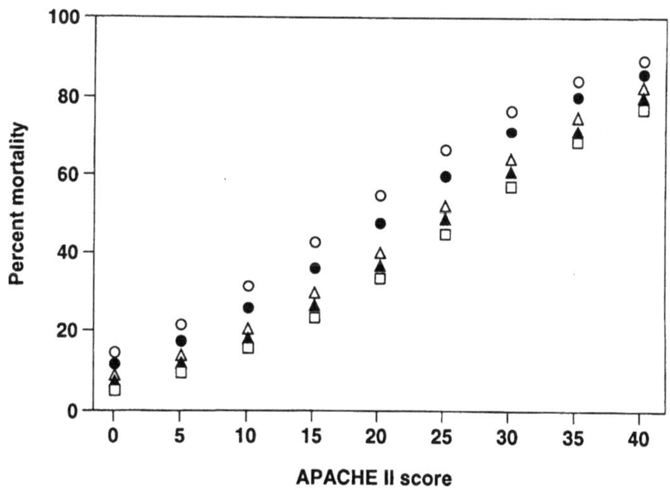

Fig. 1. Impact of preexisting co-morbidities on the mortality predicted by APACHE II score. Predicted mortality (vertical axis) have been calculated taking into account APACHE II scores on admission to the ICU (horizontal axis) in patients without (□) or with one (▲), two (△), four (•), or six (○) preexisting co-morbidities. The figure illustrates the influence of preexisting co-morbidities on mortality rates predicted by APACHE II scores. (From [40] with permission)

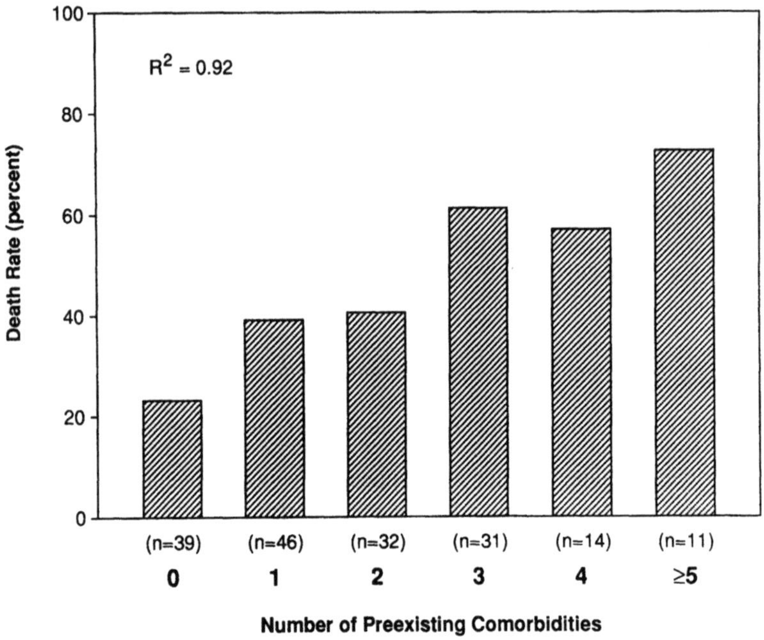

Fig. 2. Death rates from bacteremic sepsis according to the number of co-morbidities in 173 ICU patients. Patient stratification is presented according to the number of pre-existing co-morbidities recorded on admission to the ICU. A good correlation between number of co-morbidities and fatality rates was observed ($R^2=0.92$). For details, see text. (From [40] with permission)

in the surgical ICU than in the medical and pediatric ICU [41]. This high but variable prevalence of nosocomial infections is partly related to the recent development of monitoring and therapeutic technology requiring the use of invasive devices [41].

Patient's location immediately prior to ICU admission is of great importance in the evaluation of outcome from sepsis. Knaus et al. [32] noted that patients directly admitted from the emergency departments have a better prognosis. This phenomenon is in agreement with previous reports concerning the scoring systems used in ICU [42], where this difference in mortality was attributed to *"lead-time bias"*.

Origin of Sepsis and Type of Microorganisms

The origin of bacteremic sepsis greatly influences outcome; bacteremia associated with bone and joint infections generally results in no death [15], and urinary sepsis has a much better prognosis [15, 43, 44] than respiratory, gastrointestinal or other sources of bacteremic sepsis, whatever the degree of the initial physiologic disturbance [32].

Overall rates of nosocomial bloodstream infections increased markedly over the past decade in all types of hospitals in the United States [30, 45]; the rates of bacteremia increased significantly for each type of pathogen except for gram-negative bacteria. The most important progression in rates of bloodstream infections occurred for the following groups of pathogens: coagulase-negative *Staphylococci* (CNS), *Candida* species, *Staphylococcus aureus* and *Enterococci.* Upon stratification, no variation in this increase according to type of institution was found [30, 45]. The analysis of data from the National Nosocomial Infections Surveillance System [46] for the period of October 1986 to December 1990 showed that CNS were the most frequently reported bloodstream pathogens accounting for 27.9% of infections, followed by *Staphylococcus aureus* (16.5%), *Enterococci* (8.3%), *Candida* species (7.8%) and *E. coli* (5.6%). In ICU patients, the same distribution was found except that *Enterobacter* species rather than *E. coli* were the 5th leading cause of bloodstream infection. Nosocomial bloodstream infections have a worse prognosis than community-acquired infections [30].

Mortality attributable to nosocomial bloodstream infection varies according to the type of microorganism responsible for the infection, reaching 14% for CNS, 31% for *Enterococci,* and 38% for *Candida* species (review [30] and [47]). The particularly high fatality rate associated with *Candida* species and *Pseudomonas aeruginosa* bloodstream infections has been widely recognized [48, 49]. Miller et al. [50] found that infection with either *Candida* species or *Pseudomonas aeruginosa* is an independent predictor of death. They also showed that etiologic organism(s) contribute to morbidity and that consequently infections with *Pseudomonas aeruginosa, Candida* species, *Enterococcus, Enterobacter, Klebsiella pneumoniae* and *Serratia marcescens* are predictors of the clinical parameters associated with shock.

Bacteremic or Non-Bacteremic Sepsis; Polymicrobial or Unimicrobial Bacteremia

Sepsis is currently defined as a systemic response to infection, either in presence or absence of bacteremia. Patients with sepsis and positive blood cultures, bacteremic sepsis in the present chapter, in particular polymicrobial bacteremia, have been traditionally considered to have a higher risk of death due to sepsis [12, 30, 49, 51, 52]. The proportion of polymicrobial bacteremias ranges from 6 to 21% [12, 15, 30, 51]; higher rates have been reported in the geriatric population as well as in newborns [30]. In a population of critically ill patients [53], polymicrobial bacteremia was found to represent 8.4% of all bacteremic episodes. Over three-quarters of these polymicrobial episodes were nosocomial.

Weinstein and colleagues [54], comparing polymicrobial episodes to unimicrobial episodes of bloodstream infections, confirmed that the former were significantly more likely to be hospital-acquired than unimicrobial bacteremias. Mortality associated with polymicrobial bacteremia was 63%, while mortality related to unimicrobial bacteremia was 38%. Mortality attributable to bacteremic sepsis in polymicrobial episodes was two times higher than in unimicrobial episodes.

Roberts et al. [15] reported an analysis of bacteremia spanning a period of 3 years. In this study, organisms associated with lower mortality (*E. coli, CNS*) in unimicrobial bacteremia were found to be associated with higher mortality in polymicrobial episodes reaching the fatality rates of bacteremic sepsis caused by *Pseudomonas aeruginosa* or *Candida spp.* Furthermore, polymicrobial bacteremic sepsis was always associated with higher mortality even after stratification for the type of microorganism.

In a cohort study of 364 patients with nosocomial bloodstream infections, we confirmed that polymicrobial infections had a worse prognosis than unimicrobial infections, even when corrected for confounding factors using multiple logistic regression procedure [55]. This analysis indicated that the best predictor of bloodstream infection mortality in the population studied was a model composed of 4 variables including polymicrobial bloodstream infection.

In bacteremic sepsis, secondary episodes have also been shown to have a worse prognosis than primary infections [12, 30, 33, 55], but again the source of infection and the class of microorganism were found to be of great importance. In the study by Roberts and colleagues [15], striking differences in mortality rates were apparent when the source of secondary bloodstream infection was considered.

Blood culture positivity appears to be an important risk factor for mortality in sepsis, but recent studies [7, 8, 13, 14, 56, 57], conducted to evaluate the efficacy of new therapies, question this theory. In these large clinical trials, bacteremia was identified in less than 50% (Table 1) of patients with sepsis, and the admission demographic data (including physiologic variables modified by sepsis) did not allow a reliable discrimination between bacteremic and non-bacteremic patients [7]. Furthermore, the overall mortality rates among septic patients with and without positive blood culture did not differ [13, 14] (Table 2). Such findings should, however, be evaluated in large cohort studies including patients with bacteremic and non-bacteremic sepsis; the analysis of patients included in clinical trials only is somewhat biased by the exclusion criteria used to select the patient population, and may sometimes not reflect the real clinical setting. The incidence of shock development after admission was nevertheless significantly higher in bacteremic patients included in such trials as a whole. With regard to shock development, no significant difference could be found between bacteremic sepsis due to gram-negative and that due to gram-positive organisms [7].

Physiologic Alterations and Shock

Several pathophysiologic modifications can be associated with sepsis and those known to be related with poor outcome are: hypoxemia, metabolic

Table 1. Incidence of positive blood cultures, gram-negative, gram-positive and fungal infections in 5 major recent clinical trials in sepsis [8, 9, 13, 14, 56]

	Methylprednisolone (Bone [13])		Glucocorticoid (Veterans Adm [14])		HA-1A (Ziegler [8])	E5* (Greenman [9])		Anti-TNF (Fischer [56])
	placebo n=191	steroïd n=191	placebo n=106	steroïd n=110	all patients n=543	placebo n=226	E5 n=242	all patients n=80
Positive blood culture (%)	45	50	37	46	—	—	—	36
Gram-negative (%)	30		21	26	37	34	39	21
Gram-positive (%)	15		16	17	—	—	—	15
Fungal (%)	1		0	3	—	—	—	—

* In the E5 study, the overall number of patients randomized to active treatment and placebo is not presented. Those numbers are used here to allow comparison with other studies (source: K Goerlick, PJ Scannon, J Hanningen, et al. (1990). Randomized placebo controlled study of E5 monoclonal antiendotoxin antibody. In: Larrick J, Borreback C (eds.). Therapeutic monoclonal antibodies. Stockton Press, New York, NY)

Table 2. Mortality in 4 recent clinical trials in sepsis. Comparison between bacteremic and non-bacteremic populations [8, 9, 13, 14]

	Methylprednisolone (Bone [13])	Glucocorticoid (Veterans Adm [14])	E5 (Greenman [9])		HA-1A (Ziegler [8])
Mortality at →	14 days	14 days	14 days	30 days	28 days
All patients					
No of patients	191	111	226	226	276
mortality (%)	26	22	28	41	43
Gram-positive sepsis					
No of patients		41			
mortality (%)		15			
Gram-negative sepsis					
No of patients		67	152	152	
mortality (%)		25	28	41	
With bacteremia					
No of patients	84	40			
mortality (%)	28	23			
Without bacteremia					
No of patients	104	66			
mortality (%)	23	21			
Gram-positive bacteremia					
No of patients	29	17			
mortality (%)	24	18			
Gram-negative bacteremia					
No of patients	55	22			95
mortality (%)	29	27			

acidosis, alteration of mental status, leukopenia (<4000/mm^3), severe leukocytosis (>20000/mm^3), hypothermia and acute renal failure [32]. Hypotension is another important prognostic factor; shock complicates about 40% of sepsis and obviously worsens the prognosis of septic patients [7, 11, 13].

These physiologic alterations have been collected together in different scoring systems such as the APACHE [38, 39, 58] or SAPS [59] for critically ill patients. The accuracy of these scoring systems in predicting mortality in septic populations has been shown in different studies [60–62]. A system for the specific quantification of physiologic alterations due to sepsis and grouping 7 organ functions (lung, kidney, cardiovascular system, coagulation, liver, gastrointestinal tract and neurologic system) has been developed by Stevens [63] and validated [62, 63], attesting once more the close relation between physiologic alterations and prognosis of sepsis.

Severe complications of sepsis are acute respiratory distress syndrome (ARDS) [7] and multiple organ dysfunction syndrome (MODS) [64] which significantly worsen the prognosis. The association of organ failure with infection has long been evident, but this relationship was clearly demonstrated by Fry et al. [64] in a study of 553 consecutive patients who had undergone major surgery or who had sustained severe trauma. Thirty-eight patients developed MODS; 63% (24 patients) had uncontrolled infections. The most common primary sites of infection were pulmonary and intra-abdominal.

Marshall et al. [65] recently pointed out the importance of the gastrointestinal tract as a reservoir of pathogens. In 35 of 54 surgical patients developing MODS, infection originated in the peritoneal cavity or biliary tract. Whereas intestinal flora was responsible for most of the initial infections, *Candida spp, CNS* and *Pseudomonas aeruginosa* were the most common ICU-acquired pathogens. In this study, mortality of patients with MODS was more strongly correlated with infections caused by *Candida spp* and *CNS* than with infections caused by other organisms.

The close relation between MODS and mortality during the evolution of sepsis has been confirmed by Hebert et al. [66]. A strong linear association between the number of organ failures on day 1 of sepsis and 30-day mortality has been found. Furthermore, patients who had MODS (defined as 3 or more organ failures) at the onset of sepsis were significantly more likely to die than the other patients. The overall mortality in this study was 34%; 70% of patients with MODS died, compared to 20% of patients without MODS. Another study suggests that the incidence of MODS during septic shock may be lowered by the administration of steroids without, however, increasing the overall survival rate [67]. ARDS is frequently associated with sepsis as part of a MODS or in isolation. It occurs in almost 20% of sepsis episodes [68, 69]. According to the study of Fein et al. [68], ARDS was more likely to follow gram-negative bacteremic sepsis than gram-positive bacteremic or fungal sepsis. The development of ARDS clearly worsened the prognosis of sepsis, reducing survival from 65 to 19%. Sustained shock identified patients at very high risk for developing subsequent ARDS (64% of shocked patients, none of non-shocked patients). The type of infecting organism had little influence on the apparition of ARDS. These statements need however to be confirmed in large studies involving a sufficient number of bacteremic episodes to ensure adequate statistical significance.

More recently, Bone et al. [70] studied the effect of high-dose corticoids on the mortality of sepsis syndrome in a prospective, randomized, double-blind, placebo-controlled study; they also analyzed the influence of corticotherapy on the incidence and reversibility of ARDS developing in relation to the septic process. The results of the study showed that the overall incidence of ARDS was 29%, and no significant difference was found between the placebo-treated and steroid groups (32 and 25%, $p=0.1$). The corticotherapy did not increase the reversibility of ARDS, and mortality was greater in patients treated with corticoids (14-day mortality: 52 and 21%).

Antimicrobial Therapy

The influence of antimicrobial therapy on the prognosis of bacteremic and non-bacteremic sepsis has still to be defined. In 1980, Kreger et al. [11] reviewed 612 bacteremic patients and found that early institution of appropriate antibiotic treatment was associated with a 50% reduction in fatality rate compared to that observed in patients treated with antibiotics to which the infecting organisms were resistant. The authors also noted that, with appropriate antibiotic treatment, there was a 2-fold reduction at least in the frequency of shock. On the other hand, in this series, antibiotic combination therapy did not correlate with a better prognosis than single antibiotherapy.

Other authors have identified the benefit of appropriate antibiotherapy on bacteremic sepsis prognosis [12, 30, 33]. Bryan et al. [16] confirmed the overall lower mortality in patients treated with appropriate antimicrobials; however these authors found that mortality attributed to infection was not lowered by either initial adequate antibiotherapy or subsequent adequate therapy for episodes of bacteremia complicated by clinically diagnosed shock. Similar unfavorable results have been seen during infections in patients suffering from ARDS [71], in experimental gram-negative sepsis [72], and recently during nosocomial bacteremia in a medical-surgical ICU [49].

Furthermore, antimicrobial treatment prior to the apparition of sepsis has been recently identified as a risk factor for death [40]. One explanation of this fact could be that sepsis in these patients represents secondary bacteremia complicating incompletely-treated primary sites of infections; secondary bacteremia has been associated with higher mortality in several large series [11, 12, 14, 27, 51].

The prognosis of sepsis remains poor in spite of well conducted antibiotherapy and sophisticated management of hemodynamic instability.

Conclusions

Outcome in bacteremic sepsis is determined by a number of factors: age and preexisting chronic morbidities; physiologic disorders at ICU admission and acute organ dysfunction at this time; organ dysfunctions developing after onset of sepsis; microbiological factors such as class of microbial pathogens causing the infection (i.e. *Candida spp* and *Pseudomonas*), origin of sepsis, multiple-organism bacteremia, and finally the adequacy of antimicrobial therapy.

The respective importance of preexisting co-morbidities is not well known, but the number of co-morbid conditions affecting the patients (i.e. COPD, cancer, diabetes, liver cirrhosis, etc. ...) seems crucial. Other factors not yet studied, such as nutrition or genetic predisposition, are probably of great importance in the evaluation of the prognosis of sepsis.

Recommendations

To design, conduct and analyze clinical studies on mortality prediction for either bacteremic or non-bacteremic sepsis, the following points should be considered. Recommendations have been graded as A+ (highest priority grade), A, B+ and B.

- Severity scoring systems such as APACHE, SAPS, MPM must be used when evaluating new therapies for bacteremic or non-bacteremic sepsis (Grade A+].
- A number of variables have been demonstrated as significant predictors of outcome from bacteremic or non-bacteremic sepsis. Most of them are already included in the above listed severity scoring systems. Some variables however are not sufficiently weighed by these scoring systems in the context of sepsis; recently, Knaus and colleagues [57] modified the currently used APACHE III score into a sepsis severity scoring system to correct for this discrepancy. For example, in the case of a white blood cell count $<1.5\times10^9$/L, 36 points had to be added to the calculation of APACHE III in order to allow a more accurate outcome prediction in the presence of sepsis. All currently used severity scoring systems have to be adapted for adequate prediction of outcome [Grade B+].
- The presence of positive blood cultures during sepsis ("bacteremic sepsis") has to be considered when comparing morbidity and mortality [Grade A+].
- Outcome of sepsis must be corrected for confounding factors [Grade A+].
- Bacteremic sepsis caused by multiple organisms (polymicrobial bacteremia) must also be identified [Grade B+].
- The types of microbial pathogens (*Candida spp* and *Pseudomonas aeruginosa*) [Grade B] and the origin of the septic process are crucial [Grade B+].
- Surgical or non-surgical drainage of an abscess certainly constitutes one of the major therapeutic procedures to consider, particularly in case of bacteremic or non-bacteremic sepsis of abdominal origin [Grade B+].
- Location of the patient, as well as the duration of hospital or ICU stay at the time of the onset of sepsis are crucial [Grade A].
- The adequacy of patient management should be assessed based on the advice of an expert clinical review committee; adequate hemodynamic resuscitation and correct antimicrobial and nutrition therapy are among the most important factors when comparing mortality [Grade A].
- Antibiotic treatment at the time of bacteremic sepsis is important [Grade A].
- Preexisting co-morbidities must be taken into account for the evaluation of prognosis [Grade A+].
- The number of organ dysfunctions at onset of sepsis as well as those evolving after the onset of sepsis must be recorded [Grade A].

References

1. Centers for Disease Control (1990) Increase in national hospital discharge survey rates for septicemia – United States, 1979–1987. MMWR 39:31–34
2. National Center for Health Statistics (1989) Annual summary of births, marriages, divorces and deaths: United States 1988. Hyattsville, Md: US dept of Health and Human Services 37:7
3. American College of Chest Physicians/Society of Critical Care Medicine Consensus Conference (1992) Definitions for sepsis and organ failure and guidelines for the use of innovative therapies in sepsis. Crit Care Med 20:864–874
4. Daschner FD, Frey P, Wolff G, Baumann PC, Suter PM (1982) Nosocomial infections in intensive care wards: A multicenter prospective study. Intensive Care Med 8:5–9
5. Donowitz LG, Wenzel RP, Hoyt JW (1982) High risk of hospital-acquired infection in the ICU patient. Crit Care Med 10:355–357
6. Duggan JM, Oldfield GS, Ghosh HK (1985) Septicemia as a hospital hazard. J Hosp Infect 6:406–412
7. Bone RC, Fisher CJ Jr, Clemmer TP, et al (1989) Sepsis syndrome: A clinical valid entity. Crit Care Med 17:389–693
8. Ziegler EJ, Fisher CJ Jr, Sprung CL, et al and the HA-1A Sepsis Study Group (1991) Treatment of gram-negative bacteremia and septic shock with HA-1A human monoclonal antibody against endotoxin. N Engl J Med 324:429–436
9. Greenman RL, Schein RMH, Martin MA, et al and the XOMA Sepsis Study Group (1991) A controlled clinical trial of E5 murine monoclonal IgM antibody to endotoxin in the treatment of gram-negative sepsis. JAMA 266:1097–1102
10. McGowan JR Jr, Barnes MW, Filand MJ (1975) Bacteremia at Boston City Hospital: Occurrence and mortality during 12 selected years (1935–1972) with special reference to hospital-acquired cases. J Infect Dis 132:316–335
11. Kreger BE, Craven DE, McCabe WR (1980) Gram-negative bacteremia. IV: Re-evaluation of clinical features and treatment in 612 patients. Am J Med 68:344–355
12. Weinstein MP, Murphy JR, Reller LB, Lichtenstein KA (1983) The clinical significance of positive blood cultures: A comprehensive analysis of 500 episodes of bacteremia and fungemia in adults. II. Clinical observations with special reference to factors influencing prognosis. Rev Infect Dis 5:54–70
13. Bone RC, Fisher CJ Jr, Clemmer TP (1987) A controlled clinical trial of high-dose methylprednisolone in the treatment of severe sepsis and septic shock. N Engl J Med 317:653–658
14. The Veterans Administration Systemic Sepsis Cooperative Study Group (1987) Effect of high-dose glucocorticoid therapy on mortality in patients with clinical signs of systemic sepsis. N Engl J Med 317:659–665
15. Roberts FJ, Geere IW, Coldman A (1991) A three-year study of positive blood cultures, with emphasis on prognosis. Rev Infect Dis 13:34–46
16. Bryan CS, Reynolds KL, Brenner ER (1983) Analysis of 1186 episodes of gram-negative bacteremia in non-university hospitals: The effects of antimicrobial therapy. Rev Infect Dis 5:629–638
17. Ziegler EJ, McCutchan JA, Fierer J, et al (1982) Treatment of gram-negative bacteremia and shock with human antiserum to a mutant Escherichia coli. N Engl J Med 307:1225–1230
18. Calandra Th, Glauser MP, Schellekens J, Verhoef J, and the Swiss-Dutch J_5 Immunoglobulin Study Group (1988) Treatment of gram-negative septic shock with human IgG antibody to Escherichia coli J5: A prospective, double-blind, randomized trial. J Infect Dis 158:312–319
19. Wenzel R, Bone R, Fein A, et al (1991) Results of a second double-blind, randomized, controlled trial of antiendotoxin antibody E5 in gram-negative sepsis. 31st Interscience Conference on Antimicrobial Agents and Chemotherapy, American Society for Microbiology, Washington DC., p. 194

20. Warren HS, Danner RL, Munford RS (1992) Anti-endotoxin monoclonal antibodies. N Engl J Med 326:1153–1157
21. Wenzel RP (1992) Anti-endotoxin monoclonal antibodies – A second look. N Engl J Med 326:1153–1157 (editorial)
22. Tracey KJ, Fong Y, Hesse DG, et al (1987) Anti-cachectin/TNF monoclonal antibodies prevent septic shock during lethal bacteremia. Nature 330:662–664
23. Ohlsson K, Björk P, Bergenfeldt M, Hageman R, Thompson RC (1990) Interleukin-1 receptor antagonist reduces mortality from endotoxin shock. Nature 348:550–552
24. Baue AE (1975) Multiple, progressive, or sequential systems failure. Arch Surg 110:779–781
25. Eiseman B, Beart R, Norton L (1977) Multiple organ failure. Surg Gynecol Obstet 144:323–326
26. Polk HC Jr, Shields CL (1977) Remote organ failure: A valid sign of occult intra-abdominal infection. Surgery 81:310–313
27. Bell RC, Coalson JJ, Smith JD, Johanson WG (1983) Multiple organ system failure and infection in adult respiratory distress syndrome. Ann Intern Med 99:293–298
28. Montgomery AB, Stager MA, Carrico J, Hudson LD (1985) Causes of mortality in patients with the adult respiratory distress syndrome. Am Rev Respir Dis 132:485–489
29. Knaus WA, Draper EA, Wagner DP, Zimmerman JE (1985) Prognosis in acute organ-system failure. Ann Surg 202:685–693
30. Pittet D (1993) Nosocomial bloodstream infections. In: Wenzel RP (ed) Prevention and Control of Nosocomial Infections. Williams and Wilkins, pp 512–555
31. Pittet D, Tarara D, Wenzel RP (1994) Nosocomial bloodstream infection in critically ill patients: Excess length of stay, extra costs, and attributable mortality. JAMA (in press)
32. Knaus WA, Sun X, Nystrom PO, Wagner DP (1992) Evaluation of definitions for sepsis. Chest 101:1656–1662
33. Gatell JM, Trilla A, Latorre X, et al (1988) Nosocomial bacteremia in a large Spanish teaching hospital: Analysis of factors influencing prognosis. Rev Infect Dis 10:203–210
34. Munoz E, Sterman H, Cohen J, et al (1988) Financial risk, hospital cost, complications and comorbidities in surgical non complication- and non-comorbidity-stratified diagnostic related groups. Ann Surg 207:305–309
35. Gross PA, De Mauro PJ, Van Antwerpen C, et al (1988) Number of comorbidities as a predictor of nosocomial infection acquisition. Infect Control Hosp Epidemiol 9:497–500
36. McCabe WR, Jackson GG (1962) Gram-negative bacteremia. II. Clinical, laboratory and therapeutic observations. Arch Intern Med 110:856–864
37. Freid MA, Vosti KL (1968) The importance of underlying disease in patients with gram-negative bacteremia. Arch Intern Med 121:418–423
38. Knaus WA, Zimmerman JE, Wagner DP, Draper EA, Lawrence DE (1981) APACHE – acute physiology and chronic health evaluation: A physiologically based classification system. Crit Care Med 9:591–597
39. Knaus WA, Draper EA, Wagner DP, Zimmerman JE (1985) APACHE II: A severity of disease classification system. Crit Care Med 13:818–829
40. Pittet D, Thiévent B, Wenzel RP, Li N, Gurman G, Suter PM (1993) Importance of pre-existing co-morbidities for prognosis of septicemia in critically ill patients. Intensive Care Med 19:265–272
41. Pittet D, Herwaldt L, Massanari RM (1992) The intensive care unit. In: Benett JV and Brachman JR (eds) Hospital Infections. Little Brown Co, pp 405–439
42. Dragsted L, Jorgenson J, Jensen NH, et al (1989) Interhospital comparisons of patients outcome from intensive care: Importance of lead-time bias. Crit Care Med 17:418–422
43. Krieger JN, Kaiser DL, Wenzel RP (1983) Urinary tract etiology of bloodstream infection in hospitalized patients. J Infect Dis 148:57–62
44. Bahnson RR (1986) Urosepsis. Urol Clin North Am 13:627–635

45. Banerjee SN, Emori TG, Culver DH, et al (1991) Secular trend in nosocomial primary bloodstream infections in the United States, 1980–1989. National Nosocomial Infection Surveillance System. Am J Med 91:86S–89S
46. Jarvis WR, Martone WJ (1992) Predominant pathogens in hospital infections. J Antimicrob Chemother 29 (Suppl A):19–24
47. Wenzel RP (1988) The mortality of hospital-acquired bloodstream infection: Need for a new vital statistic? Int J Epidemiol 17:225–227
48. Spengler RF, Greenough WB, Stolley RP (1978) A descriptive study of nosocomial bacteremias at Johns Hopkins Hospital, 1968–1974. Johns Hopkins Med J 142:77–84
49. Rello J, Ricart M, Mirelis B, et al (1994) Nosocomial bacteremia in a medical-surgical intensive care unit: Epidemiologic characteristics and factors influencing mortality in 111 episodes. Intensive Care Med 20:94–98
50. Miller PJ, Wenzel RP (1987) Etiologic organisms as independent predictors of death and morbidity associated with bloodstream infections. J Infect Dis 156:471–477
51. Hermans PE, Washington JA II (1970) Polymicrobial bacteremia. Ann Intern Med 73:387–392
52. Cooper GS, Havlir DS, Shlaes DM, Salata RA (1990) Polymicrobial bacteremia in the late 1980s: Predictors of outcome and review of the literature. Medicine (Baltimore) 69:114–123
53. Rello J, Quintana E, Mirelis B, et al (1993) Polymicrobial bacteremia in critically ill patients. Intensive Care Med 19:22–25
54. Weinstein MP, Reller LB, Murphy JR (1986) Clinical importance of polymicrobial bacteremia. Diagn Microbiol Infect Dis 5:185–196
55. Pittet D, Li N, Wenzel RP (1993) Association of secondary and polymicrobial nosocomial bloodstream infections with higher mortality. Eur J Clin Microbiol Infect Dis 12:813–819
56. Fisher CJ, Opal SM, Dhainaut JF, et al (1993) Influence of an anti-tumor necrosis factor monoclonal antibody on cytokine levels in patients with sepsis. Crit Care Med 21:318–327
57. Knaus WA, Harrell FE, Fisher CJ, et al (1993) The clinical evaluation of new drugs for sepsis. A prospective study design based on survival analysis. JAMA 270:1233–1241
58. Knaus WA, Wagner DP, Draper EA, et al (1991) The APACHE III prognostic system. Risk prediction of hospital mortality for critically ill hospitalized adults. Chest 100:1619–1636
59. Le Gall JR, Lemeshow S, Saulnier F, and the study participants (1993) Development of a new scoring system, the SAPS II, from a European/North American multicenter study. JAMA 270:2957–2963
60. Bohnen JMA, Mustard RA, Oxholm SE, Schouten BD (1988) APACHE II score and abdominal sepsis. Arch Surg 133:225–229
61. Meakins JL, Solomkin JS, Allo MD, Dellinger EP, Howard RJ, Simmons RL (1984) A proposed classification of intra-abdominal infections. Arch Surg 119:1372–1376
62. Skau T, Nyström PO, Carlsson C (1985) Severity of illness in intra-abdominal infection. A comparison of two indexes. Arch Surg 120:152–158
63. Stevens LE (1983) Gauging the severity of surgical sepsis. Arch Surg 118:1190–1192
64. Fry DE, Pearlstein L, Fulton RL, et al (1980) Multiple organ systems failure. The role of uncontrolled infection. Arch Surg 115:136–140
65. Marshall JC, Christou NV (1988) The microbiology of multiple organ failure. The proximal gastrointestinal tract as an occult reservoir of pathogens. Arch Surg 123:309–315
66. Hebert PC, Drummond AJ, Singer J, Bernard GR, Russell JA (1993) A simple multiple system organ failure scoring system predict mortality of patients who have sepsis syndrome. Chest 104:230–235
67. Sprung C, Caralis P, Marcial E, et al (1984) The effect of high dose corticosteroids in patients with septic shock: A prospective controlled study. N Engl J Med 311:1137–1143

68. Fein AM, Lippmann M, Holtzmann H, et al (1983) The risk factors, incidence and prognosis of ARDS following septicemia. Chest 83:40–42
69. Kaplan RL, Sahn SA, Petty TL (1979) Incidence and outcome of the respiratory distress syndrome in gram-negative sepsis. Arch Intern Med 139:867–869
70. Bone C, Fisher CJ, Clemmer TP, et al (1987) Early methylprednisolone treatment for septic syndrome and the adult respiratory distress syndrome. Chest 92:1032–1036
71. Seidenfeld JJ, Pohl DF, Bell RC, Harrys GD (1986) Incidence, site and outcome of infections in patients with the adult respiratory distress syndrome. Am Rev Respir Dis 134:12–16
72. Greisman SE, Dubuy JB, Woodward CL (1979) Experimental gram-negative bacterial sepsis: Prevention of mortality is not preventable by antibiotics alone. Infect Immun 25:538–557

ARDS and Sepsis: Resemblances and Differences

M. Lamy, G. Deby-Dupont, and P. Damas

Introduction

While sepsis is an old problem, particularly in ICU, acute respiratory distress syndrome (ARDS) is a younger entity, first described in 1967 [1]. However, old or young, the two topics, sepsis and ARDS, are still the subject of numerous studies [2–4]. Among the infectious problems faced today by hospital physicians, gram-negative sepsis is perhaps the most serious one, with a frustrating high mortality rate, particularly when sepsis is complicated by shock. This is true despite intensive care, surgery, potent antibiotics and the new treatment modalities [5].

In their original article, Ashbaugh et al. described a series of 12 patients who developed a syndrome of acute respiratory failure [1]. Most of these patients were young, without history of pulmonary disease, and were victims of severe trauma. Acute respiratory distress appeared rapidly between 1 and 96 h after the initial aggression. A particularly important observation of Ashbaugh et al. was that a similar syndrome appeared after various etiologies. It was also rapidly recognized that, in addition to playing a major role in the development of ARDS, infections commonly complicated the clinical course of established ARDS.

Thus ARDS and sepsis are frequently associated, often in such a strong manner that the differences between the two syndromes are not clear. However, despite a host of resemblances, differences exist, and these have important consequences in the therapeutic approach. The first difference between the two syndromes can be found in their definition. Other differences appear in the mortality rate (particularly when ARDS remains uncomplicated by infection), in the pathophysiological mechanisms at the origin of these syndromes (especially the sequence of appearance of inflammatory mediators), and in the possible therapies related to these pathophysiological mechanisms. Despite these differences, the similarities in their evolution and mechanisms are so important that, in biochemical studies or clinical trials of new therapies, an overlapping of patients is always present, with an important proportion of ARDS patients in sepsis studies and *vice versa.*

Definitions

The terms "sepsis"" and "ARDS" have frequently been the subject of discussions and are often used with relative imprecision. Recent consensus conferences have proposed broad definitions that could make early detection and treatment of sepsis and ARDS possible and which should facilitate a better organization of clinical trials by defining categories of patients, and allowing standardization of research protocols. This, in turn, should permit comparisons of patient populations, leading to easier interpretation of clinical trials designed to study pathophysiological mechanisms and evaluate conventional or innovative therapies for these syndromes.

Sepsis is the term used to describe the progressive systemic inflammatory response to infection. It is often associated with organ damage; it has, however, often been misused, what explains the recent attempts to provide a clear definition, taking into account the relation of sepsis with infection and the systemic inflammatory response [6, 7]. Systemic inflammatory response syndrome (SIRS) was defined recently in a 1991 consensus conference [8] with the purpose of reaching an agreement about the diagnostic criteria for sepsis. Many patients with sepsis who never develop shock yet die some time later of organ dysfunction. Bacteremia occurs in less than half of all patients with sepsis, and in a minority (still at least 15%), no source of infection can ever be found. A similar, even identical, disorder is known to result from non-infectious causes such as severe burns, trauma, hemorrhagic shock, pancreatitis ... A common pathway is believed to underlie sepsis and other related disorders such as ARDS which corresponds to the clinical manifestation of an endothelial cell disorder [5, 9]. The American College of Chest Physicians/Society of Critical Care Medicine (ACCP/SCCM) Consensus Conference [8] and the Expert Report of the European Society of Intensive Care Medicine [10] both presented recommendations for the organization of clinical trials and for the quantification of the severity of the disease process (severity index), the degree of organ dysfunction, and the presence or absence of underlying diseases (cancer, cirrhosis, diabetes mellitus, HIV ...).

ARDS also lacks a uniform definition. This leads to difficulties in comparing studies, owing to the variability of patient selection; the comparison is particularly biased for clinical trials using conventional or innovative therapies. The European-American Consensus Conference on ARDS recently tried to present a useful definition of ARDS to allow comparisons of studies on mediators, risk factors, incidences of mortality and of multiple organ failure [11]. Such a definition could help to compare studies on new therapies [2]. The first description of acute respiratory failure, which was named ARDS a few years later, was based on a clinical description: obvious respiratory distress with tachypnea, severe hypoxemia, decreased compliance, diffuse infiltrates on chest X-ray [12]. Numerous other names have been proposed (shock lung, pump lung, "DaNang lung" ...). It was recently decided to return to the original term "acute" rather than "adult" since ARDS is not limited to adults, as was already noted in the original description by Ashbaugh et al. [1]. ARDS is now considered as a spectrum of lung injury with a continuum of arterial blood gases and radiographic abnormalities. The term "acute lung injury" (ALI) should be applied to the entire spectrum of lung injury and the term ARDS should be reserved for the most severe manifestation, so that all patients with ARDS have ALI, but not all patients with ALI have ARDS [13]. ALI is defined as a syndrome of inflammation and increased permeability associated with clinical, radiologic and physiologic abnormalities: arterial hypoxemia resistant to oxygen therapy (PaO_2/FiO_2 < 300 mm Hg) and diffuse bilateral radiologic infiltrates without signs of cardiac failure or pulmonary capillary hypertension. The term ARDS is reserved for the most severe forms of ALI with a cut-off value of PaO_2/FiO_2 < 200 mm Hg. This definition of ARDS as the most severe form of ALI implies that this syndrome is part of a generalized inflammatory reaction. As is the case for sepsis, ARDS patients present a SIRS, but SIRS is not a synonym of ARDS, since it includes a large number of patients who will not develop ARDS.

When inflammation progresses, organ dysfunction will ensue, leading to the multiple organ dysfunction syndrome (MODS). This term thus describes the continuum from early dysfunction through severe organ failure [14], including ALI and ARDS. In these conditions, ARDS may be a complication of sepsis, and in a similar manner, when MODS developing after the onset of ARDS is characterized by sepsis, sepsis may be a complication of ARDS (Fig. 1) [3, 4]. These complex interactions and resemblances between sepsis and ARDS in the course of their evolution explain why, despite consider-

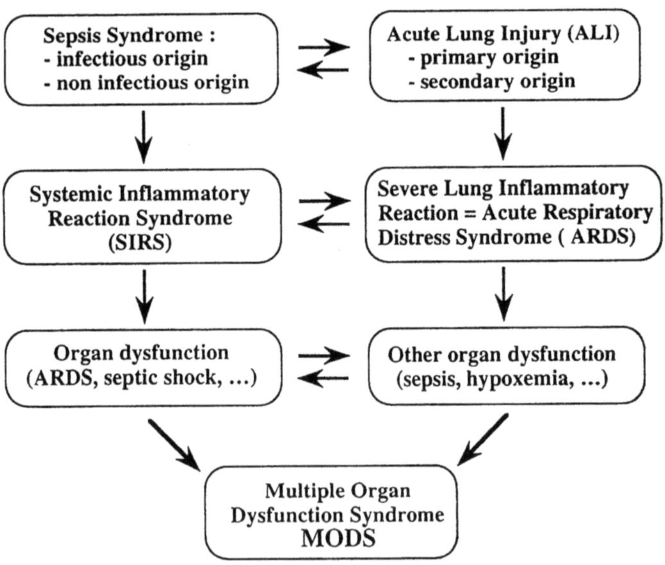

Fig. 1. Meeting points of ARDS and sepsis

able differences in their respective definitions, many of the patients selected for specific sepsis or ARDS studies actually belong to the two syndromes.

Incidence, Risk Factors, Prognosis and Mortality

The estimated incidence of sepsis in the US covers a large range from 70000 to 300000 cases each year with an increase of gram-negative sepsis from 0.75 episodes in 1951 to 13 per 1000 admissions in 1974 [4]. From recent data obtained from a stratified sample of acute-care hospitals, the annual number of discharge diagnoses of septicemia increased from 164000 in 1979 to 425000 in 1987 with the greatest increase among persons older than 65 years and about 40% of cases due to gram-negative bacteria, representing 170000 cases in 1987 [4]. Its occurrence is still increasing, in relation with increased use of invasive techniques, immunosuppression and cytotoxic chemotherapy, and by an increased occurrence of nosocomial infections [15–16]. A wide array of underlying medical conditions predispose patients to develop sepsis, including older age, chronic diseases (obstructive lung disease, congestive heart failure), immunosuppression (malignancy, AIDS, diabetes or auto-immunity), surgery or trauma, and invasive procedures (central venous catheters, endotracheal intubation). The organisms and site of infections are also diverse.

This syndrome carries an average mortality of 40–45% (80000 deaths each year in the US), with 60% of deaths in association with gram-negative bacteria. Table 1 shows that the mortality related to sepsis was increased in 1991 compared to 1987, remaining stable thereafter [17–21]. This difference in mortality observed between 1987 and 1991 can perhaps be attributed to better criteria for the selection of patients, enrolling more gram-negative bacteria patients. Among septic patients, the incidence of ARDS ranges from 15 to 38% (with a mortality as high as 90%) [4] and is increased in septic patients with sustained hypotension (septic shock) (Table 2); this incidence is doubled when endotoxemia is present [20–30]. Septic shock is a frequent complication of sepsis, present in 47% of bacteremic patients and in 30% of

Table 1. Mortality in septic patients from recent studies (last 7 years)

Authors	Reference	No of patients Total	Deaths	%
Bone RC et al. (1987)	[17]	382	113	30
Veterans Study Group (1987)	[18]	223	47	21
Greenman et al. (1991)	[19]	468	189	40
Ziegler et al. (1991)	[20]	531	218	41
Fisher CJ et al. (1993)	[21]	25	11	44

Table 2. Incidence of ARDS in sepsis and sepsis syndrome studies: A selection out of 15 years literature data [20–30]

Authors	References	Diagnosis	No of patients ARDS/total (%)
Kaplan et al. (1979)	[22]	Gram-bacteremia	20/86 (23%)
Pepe et al. (1982)	[23]	Sepsis syndrome	5/13 (38%)
Fein et al. (1983)	[24]	Bacteremia	21/116 (18%)
Weinberg et al. (1984)	[25]	Sepsis syndrome	10/40 (25%)
Langlois et al. (1988)	[26]	Sepsis syndrome	22/87 (25%)
Luce et al. (1988)	[27]	Septic shock	27/75 (36%)
Bone et al. (1989)	[28]	Sepsis syndrome	38/152 (25%)
Martin et al. (1989)	[29]	Gram-negative sepsis	65/316 (21%)
Danner et al. (1991)	[30]	Septic shock	37/100 (37%)
Ziegler et al. (1991)	[20]	Sepsis and septic shock	1/9 (22%)
Fisher et al. (1993)	[21]	Sepsis syndrome and septic shock	15/99 (15%) at entry

non-bacteremic patients, and is associated with a 40 to 75% mortality [7, 16]. Organ failure is also a frequent complication of sepsis, occurring in at least 40% of patients; the mortality rate from sepsis is directly related to the number of organs failing, with 100% mortality if 3 or more organ failures are present. Moreover, clinically important morbidity is common among survivors of sepsis, such as cardiac and renal failure and permanent brain injury [16].

The incidence of **ARDS** is still controversial. The reported annual incidence for the United States is 150000 cases (75 cases for 100000 inhabitants) [31], but these data have been challenged, and the real incidence may be lower, about 5 cases per year for 100000 inhabitants [32]. A more realistic estimation comes from a study in Gran Canaria (700000 inhabitants): the incidence of ARDS is estimated to be around 1.5 to 4.5 annual cases for 100000 inhabitants [33]. These fluctuations in the estimation of the incidence of ARDS reflect the lack of definition and consistent criteria for diagnosis in most studies performed in the last decade. In 1988, the score published by Murray et al. [34] was a first attempt to reach a uniform definition of ARDS. In this scoring system, all patients with a value above 2.5 were considered as suffering severe ARDS. This scoring system presented two major difficulties: use of chest X-ray evaluation in quadrants, and PEEP applied, owing to the numerous ventilatory modes used in the treatment of ARDS. The proposed definition of the syndrome by the European-American Consensus Conference [11] should allow better estimation of the exact incidence of the syndrome.

ARDS is associated with one or more risk factors, categorized as direct or indirect [30]. These risk factors are often sepsis, aspiration of gastric content, severe pneumonia, multiple trauma, and more rarely cardiopulmonary bypass, multiple transfusions, fat embolism, pancreatitis, severe burns … Sepsis and multiple trauma are associated with a high risk of ARDS, accounting for 30 to 50% of cases, and the 3 risk groups of aspiration of gastric content, trauma and sepsis account for nearly 75% cases [35–36]. Infection with gram-negative organisms is a more common cause of ARDS than infection with gram-positive organisms [37–38]. Taken together, gram-negative and gram-positive sepsis result in ARDS and multiple organ failure (MOF) in as many as 30–50% of cases. In the European Collaborative Study including 583 patients, sepsis and trauma were also the most common causes of ARDS (Table 3) [39]. Infectious etiologies (from pulmonary and abdominal sources) were the causes of ARDS in 57% of patients. Sepsis syndrome, in the absence of documented bacteremia, results in an incidence of ARDS and MOF similar to that of documented sepsis. Aspiration of gastric content is another important cause of ARDS. Following aspiration, ARDS occurs in 1 of 3 patients after a short median delay of 3 h [35]. Trauma, without hypotension or blood transfusions, is an uncommon cause of ARDS, unless trauma is thoracic. However, trauma, associated with hypotension and massive transfusions in the first 24 h, is frequently complicated by ARDS.

The prognosis for ARDS is based on the underlying diagnosis (cancer, head trauma ...), the etiology, the age, the presence of other diseases (AIDS, leukemia ...) and the severity of the illness as measured by a scoring system: Injury Severity Score (ISS) for trauma patients, APACHE and Simplified Acute Physiologic Score (SAPS) for all patients [40]. The onset of ARDS is acute; ARDS persists for days to weeks, and is frequently the first manifestation (the "easiest" to observe) of MODS [41]. ARDS has a high morbidity ranging from 41 to 74%, with a mortality rate of 15 to 20% when ARDS develops alone, increasing to more than 80–90% when complications, particularly MOF and sepsis, occur [38]. Table 4 indicates that since the syndrome was first described, the mortality has been high [1, 23, 37, 38, 42–45]. A small decrease in this mortality seems to appear in the last 5 years, but it can be essentially attributed to the patient selection: ARDS resulting from trauma has a lower mortality, as shown in the European Collaborative Study where total mortality was 59%, with the lowest mortality (38%, 41/109 patients) in trauma patients without complications during their clinical management (Table 3) [39]. Most deaths occurring in the first days of the syndrome can be attributed to the presence of an underlying illness or injury, later death cor-

Table 3. Incidence of ARDS and mortality related to the initial risk factor in the 583 patients of the European Collaborative Study [38]

Risk factor	Incidence (%)	Deaths (%)
Pneumonia	179 (31)	110 (62)
Extra- or intra-abdominal infection	142 (24)	103 (73)
Trauma	109 (19)	41 (38)
Miscellaneous	88 (15)	51 (59)
Aspiration pneumonia	65 (11)	39 (60)

Table 4. Mortality in ARDS patients: A selection out of 27 years literature data

Authors	References	No of patients	
		ARDS	Deaths (%)
Ashbaugh et al. (1967)	[1]	12	7 (58%)
Lamy et al. (1976)	[42]	45	30 (67%)
Pepe et al. (1982)	[23]	109	67 (61%)
Bell et al. (1983)	[37]	141	104 (74%)
Fowler et al. (1983)	[43]	88	57 (65%)
Montgomery et al. (1985)	[38]	47	32 (68%)
Pontoppidan et al. (1985)	[44]	46	41 (89%)
European study (1991)	[39]	583	344 (59%)
Suchyta et al. (1992)	[45]	215	114 (53%)

relating more with patient age and the extent of MOF; mortality increases to more than 80% when 3 or more complications are present. Infection has been shown to be a particularly important complication in ARDS and the highest mortality (about 90%) is associated with sepsis from nosocomial pneumonia [15]. Approximately 90% of deaths in ARDS patients occur within 2 to 3 weeks after onset of the syndrome and result from sepsis and MOF [30, 45].

Thus, less than 15% of ARDS patients die from refractory hypoxemia, most of patients dying from complications. When ARDS and sepsis are compared, it appears that as far as risk factors are concerned, the major difference is the mandatory presence of infection in sepsis, while the presence of infection is only one (albeit the most important) of the numerous risk factors for ARDS. The 2 syndromes are quite comparable in terms of their morbidity and mortality, but the mortality in ARDS appears higher than in sepsis. The general incidence, however, seems greater for sepsis than for ARDS (Table 5).

Pathophysiological Mechanisms

Sepsis and SIRS are characterized by metabolic derangements (acidosis, hyperglycemia, hypertriglyceridemia ...), and often by disseminated intravascular coagulation, hypotension, peripheral and pulmonary edema, and death of cells in various tissues [4, 46]. Gram-negative and gram-positive organisms, fungi, parasites and viruses can all induce sepsis implying a final common pathway which is only partially understood, but in which toxins seem to play a major role. For gram-negative organisms, endotoxins are a major trigger of the sepsis response. For gram-positive organisms, toxins coming from the wall constituents are also released. However, in many patients with a diagnosis of sepsis, no site of infection can be documented. In all these cases of

Table 5. Sepsis and ARDS: Comparison in their etiology, incidence, evolution and mortality

	Sepsis	ARDS
Etiology	infection	variable: aspiration of gastric content, trauma and sepsis = 75% of cases
Incidence	70000 to 425000 cases/year (US, 1987)	– 150000 cases/year (US): debated – 5 cases/100000 inhabitants (US, 1992) – 1.5 to 4.5 cases /100000 inhabitants (Europe, 1992)
Evolution	ARDS: 18 to 38% Shock: 30 to 47% MODS: ±40%	sepsis: 20 to 70% MODS: 20 to 70%
Mortality	40–45% = 80000 deaths/year (US, 1989) +ARDS: 90% +shock: 40 to 75% +MODS (≥3 organs): 100%	41 to 74% with sepsis and/or MODS: 80–90%

sepsis or SIRS, TNF plays a central role in their pathogenesis regardless of whether it is of infectious or non-infectious origin; the severity of sepsis is related to the magnitude of TNF expression [47]. TNF is able to orchestrate different events necessary for the successful initiation, maintenance and resolution of inflammation, via the release of several other cytokines. TNF can cause expression of IL-1, 6 and 8, and monocyte chemotactic protein in a number of immune and non-immune cells (fibroblasts, endothelial cells, pulmonary type II-like epithelial cells) [48]. TNF receptors are present on all somatic cells allowing their participation in inflammation. TNF is thus the essential factor, the central cause of endotoxic shock and thus of the sepsis syndrome, acting by the way of specific receptors [49]. It is produced in response to many infectious organisms, by endotoxins in gram-negative sepsis and by cell wall constituents (lipoteichoic acids) in gram-positive sepsis [50]; it may exert a beneficial or a deleterious effect depending on the quantity produced and the time period over which its production is sustained. TNF exerts its effects on endothelial cells by inducing their procoagulant activity (production of tissue factor, PAF, von Willebrand factor, downregulation of thrombomodulin expression), by inducing their expression of cell adhesion molecules (particularly ICAM-1), and/or by triggering a change in conformation or affinity state of cell surface molecules [51]. TNF also acts on chemotaxis of leukocytes, causing their attraction and margination, but not their transmigration (since it upregulates adhesion molecules). However, TNF-activated endothelial cells produce IL-8, a promoter of leukocyte transmigration, which counterbalances the effects of TNF on neutrophil function. TNF also triggers the release of PGE_2, PGI_2, TXA_2, nitric oxide (NO), and endothelin by endothelial cells, exerting conflicting effects on vascular tone and on platelet aggregation [52].

The pathophysiological mechanisms of **ARDS** are similar regardless of the etiology of the syndrome, with modifications of the permeability of alveolo-capillary walls and edema as pivotal points [53–55]. ARDS is characterized by injury to both lung endothelium and epithelium, but it may start with specific injury to either one of these two lung barriers [56, 57]. When the etiology is direct lung injury, the pathophysiological mechanisms are essentially a direct activation of alveolar macrophages or their activation by damaged lung epithelial cells. This cellular activation progresses to the release of inflammatory and chemotactic factors for polymorphonuclear granulocytes. This extends the inflammatory reaction to endothelial cells, with the release of mediators into the blood flow, and their transport to other organs, further extending inflammation and often leading to MOF. ARDS can also be an indirect result of an acute systemic inflammatory response to extra-thoracic injury, involving cellular and humoral factors [41]. The mediators, released at distant body sites, are transported by the blood flow to the lungs and micro-aggregates are trapped in capillary vessels. Blood cells (monocytes, PMN, lymphocytes, platelets and even erythrocytes) are the active elements, but the cellular response also involves the endothelial cells. The endothelium normally plays a role as an active barrier favoring or inhibiting the transport of substances from blood to adjacent tissues. It synthetizes and metabolizes compounds with effects on blood pressure, homeostasis, immune response and angiogenesis. In inflammatory conditions, under the action of endotoxins or cytokines, the normal functions of endothelium are altered, with the development of a procoagulant activity, the release of inflammatory mediators (cytokines, oxidant species, lipid compounds, proteases ...), some of which are specific, such as endothelin or NO. Endothelial cell activation plays a particular role in the release of chemotactic factors and the expression of receptors of adhesion, and thus in the chemotaxis and chemokinesis of neutrophils [51, 58]. These cells also play an essential role in ARDS. They are quickly trapped in the lung capillaries where they are activated. They then release potent mediators and active enzymes damaging the endothelium and leading to alterations of permeability and cellular diapedesis [59]. They represent up to 80% of cells found in broncho-alveolar lavage fluid of ARDS patients and products of their degranulation (elastase, myeloperoxidase ...) have been measured in the same fluids.

The humoral response includes complement, coagulation-fibrinolysis and kinin activation, together with the release of inflammatory factors. All these compounds are transported by the blood flow to the lung where they are responsible for cellular damage and functional alterations. However, no priority can be attributed in the development of ARDS to one of these inflammatory events, and it is likely that the pathogenesis of ARDS is different in relation with the different etiologies of the syndrome.

For **ARDS** as well as for **sepsis**, the pathophysiological mechanisms are complex, but the pivotal points have been more precisely elucidated for sepsis than for ARDS. In sepsis, toxins released by microorganisms (gram-negative or gram-positive) constitute the triggering mechanism. They directly activate endothelial cells and polymorphonuclear granulocytes, but essentially act on macrophages and on the release of cytokines, which, by activating other cellular elements, lead to a generalized inflammatory reaction. In ARDS, the triggering mechanisms vary with the cause of the syndrome; generalized inflammatory reactions are very often at the origin of ARDS. In these situations, the pathophysiological mechanisms are similar to those observed in sepsis (Table 6).

Mediators of Sepsis or ARDS

Sepsis presents a group of specific and early markers: endotoxin and cytokines. Endotoxin is an early specific marker of gram-negative sepsis, but its presence in blood is not easy to detect and it has often disappeared when the sepsis syndrome is clinically well defined. It activates a multitude of endogenous cascades that lead to the development of increased microvascular permeability. Directly or indirectly, it causes the release of TNF, IL and PAF. However, it is absent in gram-positive sepsis; in this case, other toxins appear to play a similar role to that of endotoxins, with the same early activation of macrophages and cytokine release as the triggering events. Cytokines are early markers of sepsis, and their sequential release has been largely studied [47]. Their role is undoubtedly essential, leading to intense activation of pha-

Table 6. Sepsis and ARDS: Comparison of mechanisms, mediators and clinical trials

	Sepsis	ARDS
Mechanisms	release of toxins: → phagocyte activation → release of cytokines: TNF as a pivotal point ⇒ inflammatory reaction	*lung etiology*: epithelium and endothelial alterations → excessive permeability, edema → cellular activation ⇒ inflammatory reaction *non lung etiology*: acute systemic inflammatory reaction → cellular and humoral mediators → transport to lungs → PMN trapping, endothelium damage ⇒ lung injury
Mediators	numerous: – (endo)toxins and cytokines as triggering mediators – (endo)toxins and cytokines: early release	numerous: – no specific marker – no hierarchy
Clinical trials	often common to the two syndromes (overlapping of patients)	
	more specific: monoclonal antibodies against endotoxins, TNF	more specific: surfactant

gocytes, and triggering an intense inflammatory reaction with the release of a host of mediators. TNF is one of the body's primary mediators of inflammation, probably acting early in the sequence of events that produce inflammation and related conditions, such as sepsis and MOF. The exaggerated production of TNF is associated with high morbidity and mortality rates. Inappropriate production of TNF has emerged as a key factor in the deterioration of patients with septic shock, and high levels of TNF have been associated with mortality during this state [47, 60]. These mediators are not, however specific markers of sepsis, since their presence has been described in non-septic situations and in ARDS [61]: in this latter condition, cytokines are not necessarily released early in the evolution of the syndrome.

Since the 1970's, a host of humoral and cellular mediators have been identified in plasma or broncho-alveolar lavage fluids from **ARDS** patients [53, 61–63]. A role as predictive factor has been attributed to many of them, such as complement fragments, prostanoids and coagulation factors. Abnormal levels of complement fragments (C3a and C5a) have been measured in plasma of patients with ARDS, sometimes early in the onset of the syndrome, and a role as a marker for ARDS was even attributed to the terminal complex of complement [26]. This role was rapidly challenged. It is now evident that no correlation exists between the presence of complement fragments in plasma and ARDS. Disseminated intravascular coagulation, proof of activation of the coagulation cascade, is also a frequent phenomenon in ARDS, but is not specific for this syndrome. In the 1980's, early release of prostanoids (particularly thromboxane) was described in animal models of ARDS, and as a consequence, a major role was attributed to these lipid mediators in the onset of human ARDS. Ten years later, it clearly appears that the role of these compounds is not pivotal to the development of human ARDS, even if highly abnormal concentrations of prostanoids have been measured in plasma from ARDS patients. TNF detected in plasma has been associated with a greater incidence of ARDS, a greater severity, and a higher mortality [64], but without specificity for early detection of the syndrome. Many other mediators are released during the inflammatory reaction associated with ARDS, but they are not specific markers of this process. Despite this array of biochemical mediators measured during ARDS, none of them can be considered to be specific, none have been proven to be early markers characteristic of this syndrome, and none have been well enough characterized so that they can be considered to play a pivotal role and to be a main target for therapy. Many inflammatory mediators have been measured in abnormal concentrations during the development of ARDS, in blood as well as in other fluids such as broncho-alveolar lavage fluids, but a general scheme of their appearance and time course does not exist. It appears that the nature of the early mediators varies with the origin of ARDS. Rather than one mediator, the cooperation and interactions of a variety of mediators and mediator systems, persisting over a long period of time, seem to be responsible for causing the permeability and vascular tone disturbances and the morphological alterations that finally may result in MOF. Circulating or resident inflammatory cells are now increasingly considered to be responsible for this persistant, excessive inflammatory state leading to MODS.

Sepsis and **ARDS** are thus characterized by the release and mutual interactions of a host of humoral and cellular mediators present from the beginning of the syndrome until its terminal evolution in MODS. The same mediators are present in the 2 syndromes, since sepsis patients are often also ARDS patients and *vice versa*; in sepsis, an appearance of hierarchy and a sequence in the release of mediators seem to exist, at least in gram-negative sepsis, where endotoxins and cytokines (especially TNF) appear as the first actors in the development of the excessive inflammatory reaction, despite the fact that their early presence in blood is not always detectable (Table 6).

Clinical Trials

For both sepsis and ARDS, as our understanding of the pathophysiological mechanisms has progressed, many interventions have been proposed with the purpose of altering morbidity and mortality rates. Many treatment modalities have been applied to these two syndromes after successful studies using *in vitro* or animal models. Among these treatments are the use of corticosteroids, PGE_1, non steroidal anti-inflammatory drugs, anti-PAF, antioxidants, and antibodies against endotoxin, cytokines, TNF or IL-1 receptors [64–71]. New drugs will soon be ready to be evaluated, such as antibodies against adhesion molecules or compounds active on polymorphonuclear leukocytes activation.

For clinical trials in **sepsis**, only critically ill patients with documented infections should be selected, excluding patients with low severity illness and those with terminal disease. For these 2 groups of patients, no convenient data will be obtained, since the first will recover and the last have a hopeless prognosis whatever the therapy applied. It is now possible to select a convenient population to enroll on the basis of the recent definitions proposed for sepsis and SIRS. However, these studies will generally also enroll ARDS patients owing to the frequency of this complication in sepsis. Therapeutic strategies for ARDS are highly variable from one patient to another, due to the wide variability in the causes of the syndrome and in the chronology of cascade activation and complications. On the other hand, a general treatment of sepsis seems possible, since the triggering cascades are similar, involving toxin release and macrophage/monocyte activation with release of cytokines. Early therapies applied in sepsis would thus be essentially directed against endotoxins and cytokines [72, 73]. Treatment with antibodies against endotoxins have been attempted recently with frustrating results [19, 20]; this could perhaps be explained by the transient lifespan of endotoxins in plasma. It is entirely possible, that in most patients, the antibody treatment, even if administered early, comes too late, when endotoxins have already triggered the inflammatory cascades. The variability of endotoxin biochemical structure can also explain the weak effect of monoclonal antibodies directed against a particular type of bacterial endotoxin [73]. The use of natural human antibodies would perhaps lead to better results.

Treatment with antibodies against TNF has also started [21, 74]. However, if the acute release of large quantities of TNF together with other cytokines (enhancing its toxic effects) may lead to shock, in more modest quantities the protective effect of TNF is undeniable: it thus has both helpful and harmful immunologic functions, and is useful in low concentrations for defense against granulomatous infections and several intracellular pathogens. This fact must be kept in mind when considering suppression and containment therapeutic strategies for TNF in sepsis as well as in ARDS.

Many other possibilities for future therapy directed against excessive TNF or IL-1 production exist, such as the use of anti-TNF receptors. These have the advantage of being non-antigenic. However all these therapies, if particularly convenient for septic patients, could also be useful for ARDS patients.

For studies of the treatment of **ARDS**, the heterogeneity of population is the most important problem, leading to maldistribution of risk for morbidity and mortality independently of the tested treatment. This heterogeneity is due to the variability in the severity of ARDS, some studies having enrolled mild ARDS patients with a better prognosis, and others severe terminal ARDS with a poor prognosis regardless of treatment used. However, the recent proposed definition of ARDS should reduce this problem. The heterogeneity of ARDS patients is also due to the variability in etiology and to the presence of an underlying disease, two aspects which will be difficult to avoid despite careful selection of patients. A thorough clinical description of the patients, allowing categorization into convenient subgroups, would permit an improvement of clinical trials; but this requires that each study enrolls a large number of patients. These difficulties can explain the frustrating results consistently obtained in recent clinical trials and the general overlapping of ARDS studies with sepsis studies.

Conclusions

Sepsis and ARDS are two syndromes with strong association and numerous resemblances. Some differences do exist at the level of their definitions as recently proposed by consensus conferences. These more precise definitions of ARDS, sepsis, SIRS and MODS, if generally accepted, will place clinicians in a better position to initiate appropriate therapy; researchers will be better able to compare studies covering treatment modalities.

Sepsis and ARDS carry significant morbidity and mortality, which is on the increase and comparable for the two syndromes. Their evolution often leads to MOF, with sepsis complicating ARDS and ARDS complicating sepsis. Many risk factors are common to the two syndromes, but sepsis requires the underlying presence of infection. The pathophysiological mechanisms of ARDS and sepsis are complex and similar, involving cellular activation and the release of humoral and cellular inflammatory mediators, of which none is characteristic of one of the two syndromes. However, for gram-negative sepsis, an early and precise pivotal point exists: the release of endotoxin, which triggers the activation of leukocytes and endothelial cells.

From the failure of previous clinical trials, it appears that the complexity of sepsis and ARDS requires the use of more than one therapeutic agent; future therapies may thus include a "cocktail" approach using various mediator antagonists, anti-oxidants, antiproteases and specific neutralizing antibodies. The overlapping of patients in sepsis and ARDS studies means that similar therapeutic interventions will be tested for the two syndromes, with perhaps differences in the timing of application of specific anti-endotoxin or anticytokine antibodies, which should be used as early as possible in sepsis in order to avoid further leukocyte activation.

Recommendations

- The definitions of ARDS and sepsis, as recently precised by consensus conferences, must be respected in order to obtain a good selection of patients, leading to comparable studies from one hospital to another, from where precise data about incidence, mortality and effectiveness of particular treatments will be collected.
- The incidence of sepsis in ARDS studies must be indicated and *vice versa*, since the presence of sepsis in ARDS patients largely influences their outcome (and *vice versa*), the mortality rate in ARDS alone being higher than in sepsis alone (near that of septic shock), but reaching a maximal value when sepsis (and/or MODS) complicates ARDS.
- In studies on ARDS, the rate of mortality must be described taking into account the etiology; indeed mortality rate of ARDS after trauma is lower than that observed in ARDS occurring with sepsis and/or MODS.
- In sepsis studies, a particular care must be taken to avoid confusion between true infection and SIRS.

References

1. Ashbaugh DG, Bigelow DB, Petty TL, Levine BE (1967) Acute respiratory distress in adults. Lancet 2:319–323
2. Demling RH (1993) Adult respiratory distress syndrome: Current concepts. New Horizons 1(3):388–401
3. Goldsberry DT, Hurst JM (1993) Adult respiratory distress syndrome and sepsis. New Horizons 1(2):342–347
4. Martin MA, Silverman HJ (1992) Gram-negative sepsis and the adult respiratory distress syndrome. Clin Infect Dis 14:213–218
5. Bone RC (1993) Gram-negative sepsis: A dilemma of modern medicine. Clin Microbiol Rev 6:57–68
6. Bone RC (1992) Toward an epidemiology and natural history of SIRS (systemic inflammatory response syndrome). JAMA 268:3452–3455

7. Bone RC (1992) Sepsis and multiple organ failure: Consensus and controversy. In: Lamy M, Thijs LG (eds) Mediators of Sepsis. Update in Intensive Care and Emergency Medicine, vol 16, Springer-Verlag, Berlin, pp 3–12
8. American College of Chest Physicians/Society of Critical Care Medicine Consensus Conference (1992) Definitions for sepsis and organ failure and guidelines for the use of innovative therapies in sepsis. Crit Care Med 20:864–874
9. Bone RC (1991) The pathogenesis of sepsis. Ann Intern Med 115:457–469
10. The European Society of Intensive Care Medicine (1994) The problem of sepsis. An Expert Report. Intensive Care Med 20:300–304
11. Bernard GR, Artigas A, Brigham KL, et al (1994) The American-European Consensus Conference on ARDS. Definitions, mechanisms, relevant outcomes, and clinical trial coordination. Crit Care Med 149:818–824
12. Petty TL, Ashbaugh DG (1971) The adult respiratory distress syndrome: Clinical features, factors influencing prognosis and principles of management. Chest 70:233–239
13. Beale R, Grover ER, Smithies M, Bihari D (1993) Acute respiratory distress syndrome ("ARDS"): No more than a severe acute lung injury? Br Med J 307:1335–1339
14. Hudson LD (1989) Multiple systems organ failure (MSOF): Lessons learned from the adult respiratory distress syndrome (ARDS). Crit Care Clin 5:697–705
15. Martin AM (1993) Nosocomial infections in intensive care units: An overview of their epidemiology, outcome, and prevention. New Horizons 1:162–171
16. Wherry JC, Pennington JE, Wenzel RP (1993) Tumor necrosis factor and the therapeutic potential of anti-tumor necrosis factor antibodies. Crit Care Med 21:S436–S440
17. Bone RC, Fisher CJ, Clemmer TP, Slotman CJ, Metz CA (1987) A controlled clinical trial of high-dose methylprednisolone in the treatment of severe sepsis and septic shock. N Engl J Med 317:653–658
18. Veterans Administration Systemic Sepsis Cooperative Study Group (1987) Effect of high-dose glucocorticoid therapy on mortality in patients with clinical signs of systemic sepsis. N Engl J Med 317:659–665
19. Greenman RL, Schein RMH, Martin MA, et al (1991) A controlled clinical trial of E5 murine monoclonal IgM antibody to endotoxin in the treatment of gram-negative sepsis. JAMA 266:1097–1102
20. Ziegler EJ, Fisher CJ, Sprung CL, et al (1991) Treatment of gram-negative bacteremia and septic shock with HA-1A human monoclonal antibody against endotoxin. N Engl J Med 324:429–436
21. Fisher CJ, Opal SM, Dhainaut JF, et al (1993) Influence of an anti-tumor necrosis monoclonal antibody on cytokine levels in patients with sepsis. Crit Care Med 21:318–327
22. Kaplan RL, Sahn SA, Petty TL (1979) Incidence and outcome of the respiratory distress syndrome in gram-negative sepsis. Arch Intern Med 139:867–869
23. Pepe PE, Potkin RT, Reus DH, Hudson LD, Carrico CJ (1982) Clinical indications of the adult respiratory distress syndrome. Am J Surg 144:124–130
24. Fein AM, Lippmann M, Holtzman H, Eliraz A, Goldberg SR (1983) The risk factors, incidence, and prognosis of ARDS following septicemia. Chest 83:40–42
25. Weinberg PF, Matthay MA, Webster RO, et al (1984) Biologically active products of complement and acute lung injury in patients with the sepsis syndrome. Am Rev Respir Dis 130:791–796
26. Langlois PF, Grawryl MS (1988) Accentuated formation of the terminal C5b-9 complement complex in patient plasma precedes development of the adult respiratory distress syndrome. Am Rev Respir Dis 138:368–375
27. Luce JM, Montgomery AB, Marks JD, Turner J, Metz CA, Murray JF (1988) Ineffectiveness of high-dose methylprednisolone in preventing parenchymal lung injury and improving mortality in patients with septic shock. Am Rev Respir Dis 138:62–63
28. Bone RC, Slotman G, Maunder R, et al (1989) Randomized double-blind multicenter study of prostaglandin E1 in patients with the adult respiratory distress syndrome. Chest 96:114–119
29. Martin MA, Wenzel RP, Gorelick KJ, et al and the Xoma Sepsis Study Group (1990).

Prospective US study of gram-negative bacterial sepsis-natural history in the 1980s. Circ Shock 31:245 (Abst)
30. Danner RL, Elin RJ, Hosseini JM, Wesley RA, Reilly JM, Parillo JE (1991) Endotoxemia in human septic shock. Chest 99:169–175
31. Hyers TM (1991) Adult respiratory distress syndrome: Definition, risk factors and outcome. In: Zapol WM, Lemaire F (eds) Adult respiratory distress syndrome, Marcel Dekker Inc, New York, pp 23–36
32. Thomsen GE, Morris AH, Danino D, Ellsworth J, Wallace CJ (1993) Incidence of the adult respiratory distress syndrome in Utah. Am Rev Respir Dis 147:A347 (Abst)
33. Villar J, Slutsky AS (1989) The incidence of adult respiratory distress syndrome. Am Rev Respir Dis 140:814–816
34. Murray JF, Matthay MA, Luce JM, Flick MR (1988) An expanded definition of the adult respiratory distress syndrome. Am Rev Respir Dis 138:720–723
35. Hyers TM (1993) Prediction of survival and mortality in patients with adult respiratory distress syndrome. New Horizons 1:466–470
36. Moore FA, Moore EE, Read RA (1993) Postinjury multiple organ failure: Role of extrathoracic injury and sepsis in adult respiratory distress syndrome. New Horizons 1:538–549
37. Bell RC, Coalson JJ, Smith JD, Johansonn WG (1983) Multiple organ system failure and infection in the adult respiratory distress syndrome. Ann Intern Med 99:293–298
38. Montgomery AB, Stager MA, Carrico CJ, Hudson LD (1985) Causes of mortality in patients with adult respiratory distress syndrome. Am Rev Respir Dis 132:485–489
39. Artigas A, Carlet J, Le Gall JR, Chastang CL, Blanch L, Fernandez R (1991) Clinical presentation, prognostic factors and outcome of ARDS in the European Collaborative Study (1985–1987): A preliminary report. In: Zapol WM, Lemaire F (eds) Adult respiratory distress syndrome, Marcel Dekker, New York, pp 23–36
40. Thomas MH (1993) Prediction of survival and mortality in patients with adult respiratory distress syndrome. New Horizons 1:466–470
41. Rinaldo JE, Heyman SJ (1990) ARDS, a multisystem disease with pulmonary manifestations. Crit Care Rep 1:174–183
42. Lamy M, Fallat RJ, Koeninger EL, et al (1976) Pathologic feature and mechanisms of hypoxia in adult respiratory distress syndrome. Am Rev Respir Dis 114:267–284
43. Fowler AA, Hamman RF, Good JP, et al (1983) Adult respiratory distress syndrome: Risk with common predispositions. Ann Intern Med 98:593–597
44. Pontoppidan H, Hüttemeier PC, Quinn DA (1985) Etiology, demography and outcome. In: Zapol WM, Falke KJ (eds) Adult respiratory distress syndrome, Marcel Dekker, New York, pp 1–21
45. Suchyta MR, Clemmer TP, Elliott CG, Orme JF, Weaver LK (1992) The adult respiratory distress syndrome. A report of survival and modifying factors. Chest 101:1074–1079
46. Parrilo JE (1993) Pathogenetic mechanisms of septic shock. N Engl J Med 328:1471–1477
47. Damas P, Reuter A, Gysen P, Demonty J, Lamy M, Franchimont P (1989) Tumor necrosis factor and interleukin-1 serum levels during severe sepsis in humans. Crit Care Med 17:975–978
48. Standiford TI, Kunkel SL, Phan SH, et al (1991) Alveolar macrophage-derived cytokines induce monocyte chemoattractant protein-1 expression from human pulmonary type II-like epithelial cells. J Biol Chem 266:9912–9918
49. Tracey KJ, Cerami A (1993) Tumor necrosis factor: An update review of its biology. Crit Care Med 21:S415–S422
50. Wakabayashi G, Gelfand JA, Burke JF, Thompson RC, Dinarello CA (1991) A specific receptor antagonist for interleukin 1 prevents *Escherichia coli* – induced shock in rabbits. FASEB J 15:338–343
51. Zimmerman GA, Prescott SM, McIntyre TM (1992) Endothelial cell interactions with granulocytes: Tethering and signaling molecules. Immun Today 13:93–99
52. Beutler B, Grau GE (1993) Tumor necrosis factor in the pathogenesis of infectious disease. Crit Care Med 21:S423–S435

53. Rinaldo JE, Christman JW (1990) Mechanisms and mediators of the adult respiratory distress syndrome. Clin Chest Med 11:621–632
54. Neuhof H (1991) Actions and interactions of mediator systems and mediators in the pathogenesis of ARDS and multiorgan failure. Acta Anaesthesiol Scand 35 (Suppl 95):7–14
55. Lamy M, Deby-Dupont G, Deby C, et al (1992) Measurements of mediator cascades during adult respiratory distress syndrome. In: Artigas A, Lemaire F, Suter PM, Zapol WM (eds). Adult respiratory distress syndrome, Churchill Livingstone, London, pp 71–88
56. Tomasheski JF (1990) Pulmonary pathology of the adult respiratory distress syndrome. Clin Chest Med 11:593–619
57. Matthay MA, Folkesson HG, Campagna A, Kheradmand F (1993) Alveolar epithelial barrier and acute lung injury. New Horizons 1:613–623
58. Wortel CH, Doerschuk CM (1993) Neutrophils and neutrophil-endothelial cell adhesion in adult respiratory distress syndrome. New Horizons 1:631–637
59. Tagan M, Markert M, Schaller M, Feihl F, Chiolero R, Perret C (1991) Oxidative metabolism of circulating granulocytes in adult respiratory distress syndrome. Am J Med 91:72S–78S
60. Strieter RM, Kunkel SL, Bone RC (1993) Role of tumor necrosis factor-a in disease states and inflammation. Crit Care Med 21:S447–S463
61. Suter PM, Suter S, Girardin E, et al (1992) High bronchoalveolar levels of tumor necrosis factor and its inhibitors, interleukin-1, interferon, and elastase, in patients with adult respiratory distress syndrome after trauma, shock, or sepsis. Am Rev Respir Dis 145:1016–1022
62. Chollet-Martin S, Montravers P, Giebert C, et al (1993) High levels of interleukin-8 in the blood and alveolar spaces of patients with pneumonia and adult respiratory distress syndrome. Infect Immunol 61:4553–4559
63. Donnelly SC, Strieter RM, Kunker SL, et al (1993) Interleukin-8 and development of adult respiratory distress syndrome in at-risk patient groups. Lancet 341:643–647
64. Marks JD, Marks CB, Luce JM, et al (1990) Plasma tumor necrosis factor in patients with septic shock. Am Rev Respir Dis 141:94–97
65. Said SI, Foda HD (1989) Pharmacologic modulation of lung injury. Am Rev Respir Dis 139:1553–1564
66. Goldstein G, Luce JM (1990) Pharmacologic treatment of the adult respiratory distress syndrome. Clin Chest Med 11:773–787
67. Lamy M, Deby-Dupont G, Deby C, Faymonville ME, Damas P (1990) Why is our present therapy for adult respiratory distress syndrome so ineffective? In: Aochi O, Amaha K, Takeshita H (eds) Intensive and critical care medicine, Elsevier, Amsterdam, pp 11–26
68. Jepsen S, Herlevsen P, Knudsen P, Bud MI, Klausen NO (1992) Antioxidant treatment with N-acetylcysteine during adult respiratory distress syndrome: A prospective, randomized, placebo-controlled study. Crit Care Med 20:918–923
69. Christman BW, Bernard GR (1993) Antilipid mediator and antioxidant therapy in adult respiratory distress syndrome. New Horizons 1:623–630
70. Slotman GJ, Fisher CJ, Bone RC, et al (1993) Detrimental effects of high-dose methylprednisolone sodium succinate on serum concentrations of hepatic and renal function indicators in severe sepsis and septic shock. Crit Care Med 21:191–195
71. Zapol WM, Hurford WE (1993) Inhaled nitric oxide in the adult respiratory distress syndrome and other lung diseases. New Horizons 1:638–650
72. Dinarello CA, Gelfand JA, Wolff SM (1993) Anticytokine strategies in the treatment of the systemic inflammatory response syndrome. JAMA 269:1829–1835
73. Fink MP (1993) Adoptive immunotherapy of gram-negative sepsis: Use of monoclonal antibodies to lipopolysaccharide. Crit Care Med 2:S32–S39
74. Exley AR, Cohen J, Buurman W, et al (1990) Monoclonal antibody to TNF in severe septic shock. Lancet 335:1275–1277

Monitoring the Treatment of Sepsis

Microbiological Requirements for Studies of Sepsis

W. A. Lynn and J. Cohen

Introduction

The development of novel treatment strategies for septic shock requires critical and accurate evaluation of new therapeutic agents. Much attention has focused on the nomenclature and clinical definitions of sepsis used to select patients for therapeutic trials [1–5]. This is particularly important as large multicenter trials are needed to detect a significant effect of therapy. Less attention, however, has been directed towards the bacteriological evaluation of patients with sepsis. Precise microbiological investigation of patients with sepsis is important because the techniques used both in the detection and definition of infection will influence the selection of patients, presentation of data and interpretation of results in these trials.

The microbiologic evaluation of patients has direct relevance to the design and interpretation of studies of sepsis for several different reasons. Firstly, some trials may target certain infections, for example meningococcal septicemia or gram-negative bacteremia [6, 7]. In these conditions the detection of pathogenic bacteria plays a critical role in the entry criteria for the study. Secondly, although many studies of sepsis have used clinical entry criteria irrespective of the infecting organism, microbiological factors may become important in analysis of data. For example, in the first study evaluating the anti-endotoxin monoclonal antibody HA-1A, bacteremia was not required for entry to the trial [8]. However, in the data analysis results from the subgroup of patients with gram-negative bacteremia were presented to demonstrate an apparently beneficial effect of HA-1A. Clearly, variations in the rate of detection of bacteremia in this study would have had an important impact on the final interpretation of results. Similarly, the first two studies with the anti-endotoxin monoclonal antibody E5 enrolled patients with a variety of different infectious causes of the sepsis syndrome [9, 10] but the third multicenter trial, which has just started, will concentrate on patients with proven gram-negative infection. Thirdly, the definition and recording of different infections is important and may affect the assessment of trial outcome. In studies of gram-negative sepsis, pneumonia is often the most commonly cited underlying infection and the application of different diagnostic criteria may result in variations in the rate of diagnosis [11]. In addition some therapies, for example corticosteroids [12, 13], can lead to infectious complications, and accurate documentation of secondary infections is of great importance. Finally, when applying the results of clinical trials to routine patient management, an accurate description of the methods used and infections found within the trial is essential in targeting the patients that are most likely to benefit from such treatment.

In view of the importance of the microbiological evaluation of patients for trials of sepsis, it is surprising that many of the published trials give very few details of the methods involved in documenting infection [7–9, 14–16]. Other studies have provided more detailed definitions of infection but few have detailed the methods used in sample collection and bacterial culture and isolation [12, 13, 17]. Indeed when the study protocols of some trials are examined, there is often only a brief passage dedicated to the assessment of infection with many of the variables left to the discretion of the individual investigators.

General Considerations

The clinical microbiology laboratories at participating trial centers should be licensed and certified by appropriate supervisory national organizations in accordance with the guidelines laid down by the Infectious Diseases Society of America [18]. It will be assumed that all laboratories involved in trials of sepsis will use standard, approved methods for the routine culturing of bacteriological specimens and the identification of organisms as detailed by their regulatory bodies. In any one study, all culture collection and laboratory techniques should be standardized as far as possible. However, in large multicenter trials, it is not reasonable to expect that the techniques will be identical at all centers, particularly where large capital expenditure would be required, for example in the processing of blood cultures. Variation in the detection rate or in the definition of different infections could seriously skew the presentation and interpretation of trial data, therefore, it is essential that the techniques used are clearly documented in the study methods. The following recommendations apply predominantly to immunocompetent patients with sepsis or to the critically ill patient. Patients with specific immune defects, such as neutropenia or immunodeficiency syndromes, may have particular culture requirements and should be the subject of specific clinical trials. A detailed discussion of the investigation of those patients is beyond the scope of this chapter.

The clinical definition and microbiological evaluation of many common infections, such as urinary tract infection, are not controversial and guidelines have been issued by the Centers for Disease Control (Atlanta, Ga, USA) and by the British Society for the Study of Infection (Table 1) [19, 20]. The three main areas that deserve more detailed discussion are the detection and significance of bacteremia, the diagnosis of intravascular line-related infections, and the diagnosis of pneumonia particularly in the ventilated patient.

Table 1. Definition and evaluation of common infectious causes of sepsis

Infection	Signs of infection	Evaluation
Upper respiratory tract	Inflammation plus exudate, ±Swelling ±Lymphadenopathy	Throat swab for aerobic culture
Lower respiratory tract	See Table 2	
Urinary tract	Fever, urgency, dysuria, loin pain	Microscopy >50 WBC/hpf: *Plus* – Midstream urine specimen: $>10^5$ organisms/ml – Suprapubic aspirate: $>10^3$ organisms/ml – Catheter specimen: Pure culture of $>10^5$ organisms/ml
Wound infection including burns	Breach in the epithelium Signs of inflammation, edema, erythema, discharge of pus	Gram-stain and culture of draining pus Wound swabs are not reliable
Skin/soft tissue	Signs of inflammation, spreading erythema, edema, lymphangitis	Culture any blister fluid or draining pus Role of tissue aspirates not proven
Central nervous system	Signs of meningeal irritation	CSF microscopy, protein and glucose CSF culture Bacterial antigen detection if available
Gastrointestinal	Abdominal pain, distension, diarrhea and vomiting	Stool culture on selective media for isolation of Salmonella, Shigella and Campylobacter
Intraabdominal infection	Specific abdominal symptoms/signs	Culture of peritoneal fluid, percutaneous aspiration of pus and intra-operative specimens must be cultured aerobically and anaerobically
Peritoneal dialysis infection	Cloudy PD fluid, abdominal pain, fever	Definite: >100 WBC/ml plus a positive culture Probable: >100 WBC/ml but no growth
Genital tract	Signs of infection plus low abdominal pain and vaginal discharge	Endocervical and high vaginal swabs onto selective media

Blood cultures should be performed in all cases. Specific radiological investigations may aid the localization and diagnosis for certain infections

Bacteremia

For the reasons outlined above, the detection of microorganisms in the blood stream is of major significance in trials of sepsis. Thus, blood cultures are the most important single microbiological investigation in these patients and it is somewhat surprising that more details regarding blood cultures are not given in most reports of clinical studies. Important variables that can affect the detection rate for bacteremia include the site of venupuncture, preparation of the skin, number and volume of blood cultures and the culture media, and the techniques of bacterial isolation used within individual laboratories. The isolation of any highly pathogenic organism from the blood, for example *Escherichia coli* is clearly significant, however, for less pathogenic organisms such as *Staphylococcus epidermidis* deciding whether it is pathogenic or merely a contaminant depends on the methods used and the definitions employed.

Site and Technique of Venupuncture

The frequency of contaminated blood cultures is increased when blood is taken from a femoral site, through abnormal skin or when drawn from an indwelling arterial or venous catheter [21–23]. Thus, if possible, these sites should be avoided for patients entering clinical trials. There is no advantage of taking cultures from arterial over venous sites [24]. Assiduous skin preparation and disinfection of the top of the blood culture bottles is very important in reducing the level of contamination. The skin should be swabbed twice with either 70% isopropyl or ethyl alcohol or with an iodine containing solution. Blood should then be drawn by a 'no touch' technique but there is no need for full sterile precautions such as gowns or masks. The culture bottles should be inoculated before any other sample tubes with the anaerobic bottle first. It has been demonstrated that changing the venupuncture needle prior to inoculating the culture bottles does not reduce the contamination rate [25]. With correct technique from a peripheral vein, a contamination rate of no more than 3% can be achieved [23]. In most studies of sepsis only 'clinically significant' bacteremias are reported making it impossible to comment on contamination rates within clinical trials.

Volume and Number of Blood Cultures

In adults with bacteremia, the volume of blood taken is crucial because most patients have less than 10 colony forming units (CFU) of bacteria per ml of blood and the figure may be as low as 0.1 CFU/ml [23, 26]. Therefore, inadequate sampling may fail to detect significant bacteremia. In a recent study of bacteremic adults, Mermel and Maki demonstrated a significantly higher yield when 8.7 ml of blood was taken vs 2.7 ml per culture (92 vs 69%) [27].

Data from this and other studies indicate that there is approximately a 3% increase in the detection of bacteremia per ml of blood using a variety of standard isolation techniques [27–32]. The total volume of blood required from adults is between 20 and 30 ml with no significant increase in yield seen with volumes above 30 ml [23, 32]. Children tend to have higher numbers of circulating bacteria (up to 100 CFU/ml) and, therefore, much smaller volumes of blood, 2–5 ml are acceptable [33].

Regardless of the volume of blood taken, one venupuncture is considered to be one blood culture. The volume of blood per culture will be determined by the laboratory system in use but is generally between 5 and 15 ml. A single culture should not be performed because it will make the assessment of possible contamination very difficult. However, there is no need for more than three separate cultures in patients entering into the trial; in cases with proven bacteremia 80% are positive with the first culture, 90% with the second and 99% by the third [34]. The timing of cultures has not been studied in great detail. In the context of bacterial sepsis, it is inappropriate to delay therapy whilst taking cultures over a protracted period of time.

Therefore, in clinical trials of sepsis, 20–30 ml of blood should be taken from at least two, and preferably three, distinct venupuncture sites on entry into the trial, whether or not the patient is on antibiotics and regardless of previous cultures. After entry into the trial, there is no consensus of opinion as to how often blood cultures should be repeated. After entry into the trial, further blood cultures should be taken as indicated by the clinical situation.

Techniques of Bacterial Culture from Blood

There is no consensus as to the best culture media and detection system for the isolation of bacteria from blood. There are a number of commercially available manual or automated blood culture systems in widespread use. These have broadly comparable bacterial isolation rates but there have not been large comparative trials of all these systems. Therefore, it is not possible to give specific recommendations as to the correct system to use in clinical trials. Furthermore, most trials in sepsis will involve several different centers and it is very unlikely that all of these will use the same system, and it is not reasonable to expect a uniform blood culture technique within any one study. However, it is important that the isolation techniques used are documented in the methods to allow accurate evaluation and comparison of studies.

Culture Media: There is no one isolation medium which is ideal for the isolation of all microorganisms and a detailed discussion of media composition is beyond the scope of this chapter. Broadly speaking, all of the media in widespread use have similar performance in the isolation of common bacterial pathogens [23, 35–37]. As a minimum requirement, the culture broth should dilute the blood at least 1/5 and contain an additive such as sodium polyanetholesulfonate which acts as an anticoagulant and also inhibits the antibacterial properties of human serum [22]. The use of more specific additives to inhibit antibiotics is discussed below.

Culture Conditions: Blood culture bottles should be incubated at 37°C as soon as possible after venupuncture. Therefore, it is important to ensure that appropriate incubation facilities are available outside of normal working hours. If possible, the bottles should be agitated during incubation as this increases the bacterial yield [38, 39], and most modern automated systems will agitate the bottles. Cultures should be incubated both aerobically and anaerobically. There have been recent suggestions that routine anaerobic cultures are not indicated [40]. In trials of sepsis, where a relatively high proportion of patients are likely to have intra-abdominal infection, it is essential that anaerobic cultures are performed. Routine subculturing onto selective media and terminal subcultures do not appear to be necessary in the more recently developed automated systems such as the BACTEC (Becton Dickinson Diagnostic Instrument Systems, MD, USA) or the BacT altert (Organon Teknika, Durham, NC, USA) [36–38]. However, in manual systems routine subcultures and terminal subculture at seven days will increase the diagnostic yield. The Roche Septi-Chek system allows daily subcultures to be performed without opening the bottles [38]. The optimal duration of culture has not been studied in patients with sepsis but the overwhelming majority of positive cultures will be obtained within seven days and some of the newer systems may only require a five day-incubation [36, 41].

Special Processing: A number of modifications to standard culture techniques have been described which will increase the yield of bacterial isolation. Of these lysis-centrifugation techniques and inhibition of antibiotics have been the most widely applied.

Lysis of blood cells followed by centrifugation and plating of the microbial pellet onto selective media will increase the yield of bacterial isolation particularly for fastidious organisms and in the presence of antibiotics [42, 43]. This technique is also more effective for the isolation of fungi, mycobacteria and unusual bacteria such as *Rochalimaea* spp. Currently there is only one commercial product that is widely available (Isolator, Wampole Laboratories, NJ, USA) and some laboratories have devised their own methods. Unfortunately this system is labor-intensive and relatively expensive and as such is not in widespread use. Therefore, in multicenter trials, it will not be possible to insist that all institutions use a lysis-centrifugation system.

The isolation of fungi may be enhanced by the lysis-centrifugation system or through the use of selective fungal media such as those available for the BACTEC systems [43, 44]. Of the available methods, the highest yields for fungemia have been consistently reported using lysis-centrifugation [23, 44]. In most clinical trials of sepsis, there would be a relatively small proportion of patients with fungal infections and the routine use of these systems is probably not indicated.

Antibiotic removal systems such as the Antibiotic Removal Device (ARD, Becton Dickinson) or BACTEC resin-containing medium may improve isolation rates [45] but not all researchers have found an improvement [46] and currently there is no agreement regarding their use [23].

In conclusion we would recommend that two or three separate blood cultures, with a total of 20–30 ml of blood, should be inoculated into one of the standard commercial blood culture media. The bottles should be incubated aerobically and anaerobically at 37 °C, and preferably agitated, for a period of seven days. If the system is not automated, the bottles should be inspected twice daily and routine subcultures and terminal subculture performed. The use of lysis-centrifugation or antibiotic removal systems have not been fully evaluated in comparison to the automated blood culture systems. As their use is not uniform and trials of sepsis are by necessity, multicenter routine use of such systems cannot be advocated at the current time. If some trial centers are using these methods then the results obtained should be included in the trial but this information must be stated clearly in the methods to allow adequate evaluation of the results and comparison with other trials.

Once isolated, bacteria should be identified in accordance with standard procedures such as described in the "Manual of Clinical Microbiology" [47] or with appropriately verified commercial identification systems. Antimicrobial sensitivity testing should also be performed using techniques standardized and recognized within the country where the trial is being conducted [18].

Interpretation of Positive Blood Cultures: If a high-grade pathogen is isolated from a single blood culture, for example *S. aureus, Streptococcus pneumoniae, Neisseria meningitidis, Haemophilus influenzae,* enteric gram-negative bacilli or *Candida* spp., then it is reasonable to conclude that this is a significant isolate. If a commensal organism such as *S. epidermidis, Bacillus* spp. or alpha-hemolytic streptococci are isolated, then two or more positive blood cultures, from separate sites, are required to conclude that the organism is a pathogen.

Intravascular Catheter-related Infection

Septic shock frequently occurs in hospitalized patients with indwelling vascular catheters. The recognition of the catheter as the source of infection is important in clinical trials as these patients may form a distinct subgroup and these data will be needed for correct trial interpretation. In addition, blood drawn through catheters and catheter tips are prone to contamination with skin organisms and misinterpretation of these positive cultures as pathogens may confound the trial results. Thus, a uniform definition of catheter-related infection is essential.

Despite the description of various techniques for quantitative culture, semiquantitative culture and direct staining of catheters to identify infecting organisms, there is no agreement as to the correct way to culture a catheter tip [48–51]. Clinical practice varies, including not culturing any catheters, qualitative culture of central venous catheters only, and quantitative culture of arterial and venous lines. This varied practice means that guidelines cannot be based on catheter tip culture alone but rather on a combination of clinical and microbiological factors.

We recommend that all central venous lines, pacing wires and pulmonary artery catheter tips are subject to culture on standard selective media as for blood isolates. If catheter infection is suspected clinically and pus is present, then the line site should be swabbed, the line should be removed and the tip cultured and at least two peripheral venous blood cultures drawn as described earlier. Arterial lines should be cultured only when infection at the line site is suspected. Culture of peripheral venous lines is seldom indicated unless gross infection is present at the site.

The isolation of a high-grade pathogen from the line tip indicates significant infection. If there are no other sources for this organism then the line can be presumed to be the focus of infection. However, if the patient is bacteremic from an alternative site, then the line should only be incriminated if there is gross infection at the line site. If a low-grade pathogen is isolated from a line tip, then it should only be considered significant if the same organism is recovered from a peripheral blood culture or from pus at the catheter site.

As discussed earlier, intravascular lines should be avoided for blood culture unless absolutely necessary. Although if carefully taken blood cultures through central lines only have an 8–10% contamination rate [52, 53], in large clinical trials this rate is likely to be much higher. The role of "through the line" blood cultures in diagnosing catheter-associated infection is unclear but the results of such blood cultures should be treated in the same way as a positive catheter tip culture.

Pneumonia

The diagnosis of pneumonia is predominantly clinical with supportive data from microbiological investigation. As such the diagnosis is open to variations in interpretation that may then alter the assessment and emphasis of trial data. For example, underdiagnosis of secondary bacterial pneumonia could obscure a potentially deleterious effect of a novel therapy.

In the non-ventilated patient, pneumonia is relatively straightforward to diagnose clinically and suitable criteria (Table 2) [54, 55]. However, in many cases a bacteriological diagnosis is not made despite adequate investigation. The microbiological evaluation of non-ventilated patients with pneumonia involves examination and culture of sputum, blood cultures, culture of pleural fluid if present and, if indicated serological investigations. The examina-

Table 2. Guidelines for the diagnosis of pneumonia

Clinical features

Major
- Fever/hypothermia: Temp >38 °C or <35.6 °C
- Inflammatory response:
- WBC $>15\times10^9$/L
- C-reactive protein > twice normal
- New infiltrate on chest radiograph

Minor
- Expectoration of purulent sputum
- Physical signs of consolidation
- Change in oxygen requirement[a]

Microbiological features
- Positive blood culture with a respiratory pathogen
- Good quality sputum[b] with a predominant growth of a presumptive pathogen (non-ventilated patients only)
- Positive culture of a deep lung specimen from a protected bronchial lavage[c], trans-tracheal aspiration[d] or a percutaneous lung aspirate (ventilated patients)
- Pneumococcal antigen detected in blood, sputum or urine
- Serological diagnosis[e]

Definite pneumonia
All major clinical criteria or
2 major plus 2 minor clinical criteria
plus
At least one microbiological criterion

Probable pneumonia
2 major plus 1 or more minor clinical criteria

[a] Not explicable by other means
[b] Murray and Washington criteria [57]
[c] Quantitative culture with at least 10^3 CFU/ml [64, 65]
[d] Quantitative culture with at least 10^6 CFU/ml [67]
[e] Only acceptable for the diagnosis of Legionella, Mycoplasma and Chlamydia pneumonia

tion of sputum is controversial and some authors feel that sputum gram-stain and culture is of little use [55, 56]. However, there is no doubt that these procedures can provide a diagnosis in a proportion of patients and we would support their use in the evaluation of the septic patient with pneumonia. Sputum should be examined by gram-stain according to the guidelines of Murray and Washington [57] and if of suitable quality, i.e. greater than 25 granulocytes and less than 10 epithelial cells per low power field, cultured aerobically on standard selective media. There is no point in anaerobic cultures of sputum. The isolation of a pathogenic bacteria from sputum, or blood culture in the context of a clinical diagnosis of pneumonia is presumptive evidence of causality. Samples from the lower airways obtained by trans-tracheal aspirate, bronchoalveolar lavage or lung aspiration are likely to be more reliable but these techniques are more invasive and not routinely available in all centers [58–61]. Therefore, the latter tests tend to be reserved for patients without sputum production or who are failing to respond to therapy or who are immunocompromised. The detection of bacterial antigens, particularly pneumococcal antigen, in sputum, blood and urine may increase the presumptive diagnosis rate for community-acquired pneumonia but is not available at all centers and its clinical significance is open to debate [54, 62].

The ventilated patient provides a difficult diagnostic challenge particularly if lung injury due to ARDS is also present [11, 63, 64]. There are a number of confounding issues that complicate both the clinical and microbiological examination of these patients. Firstly, the clinical criteria of alteration in oxygenation and chest X-ray changes may be very difficult to interpret, and secondly, the presence of an endotracheal tube or tracheostomy bypasses the physical barrier of the vocal cords [64]. This allows the trachea and other airways to become colonized with bacteria which are often hospital-acquired potentially pathogenic organisms [11]. Furthermore, the sputum is frequently purulent due to a low-grade tracheiitis making sputum gram-stain unreliable. Thus, a positive sputum culture alone cannot be taken as evidence of pneumonia. Invasive techniques including protected brush bronchoscopy and lung aspiration or biopsy have been found by some investigators to aid in the diagnosis of certain patients, particularly those with anaerobic infections [58, 65–67]. In many but not all centers, samples are routinely obtained from the lower airways by bronchial lavage to aid in the diagnosis of pneumonia in the intubated patient. It is essential to ensure that the same diagnostic evaluation is applied at all centers involved in the clinical trial, and we would propose that the ideal evaluation of the ventilated patient with suspected pneumonia should include culture of specimens obtained directly from the lower airways.

In many studies of patients with sepsis, the diagnosis of pneumonia has been left to the "clinical judgement of the assessing doctor". There is a need to provide clear definitions for pneumonia, along with other infections, in the setting of clinical trials. Not only will this allow comparison of different trial data but it will also help to minimize variation between participating centers within the trial. We suggest that the diagnostic scheme laid out in Table 2 provides such a framework encompassing both clinical and microbiological data to provide a reasonable clinical definition of pneumonia.

Non-bacterial Infections as Causes of Sepsis

The sepsis syndrome is most commonly associated with pyogenic bacterial pathogens but can occur with a variety of infecting organisms including atypical bacteria, ricketsia and viruses. In the majority of multicenter trials of novel therapeutic modalities in sepsis, these organisms are likely to represent a very small number of cases and should not adversely influence the trial outcome. Therefore, for the routine evaluation of patients, specific culture or serologic techniques for unusual pathogens do not need to be applied. However, in specific circumstances where particular organisms are prevalent locally, or for certain patient groups such as those with AIDS, additional microbiological investigations may be required.

Conclusion

We have attempted to provide a framework of basic microbiological evaluation for the septic patient to aid in the design and execution of clinical trials. Such a framework needs to be adaptable as diagnostic tests are refined and also has to acknowledge the limitations inherent in performing large multicenter trials. Our recommendations for the minimum evaluation of patients entering into clinical studies are given in Table 3. After entry into the clinical

Table 3. Minimal microbiological evaluation on entry into trials of sepsis

Blood cultures
20–30 ml of venous blood in at least 2 cultures from separate venupuncture sites[a]
Appropriate skin asepsis
Inoculated into a standard commercial isolation system[b]
Aerobic and anaerobic culture
Incubate at 37 °C for 7 days, preferably agitated
Routine subcultures only required for manual systems
Repeat blood cultures as clinically indicated
Sputum/lower respiratory tract specimens
Non-ventilated patients: Sputum of good quality (Murray and Washington criteria [56])
Ventilated patients: Qualitative culture of bronchial lavage or transtracheal aspirate (see Table 2)
Plus serology for Legionella etc. ... if clinically indicated
Central venous catheter
Line infection suspected:
– Remove line and culture tip[c] plus take 2 peripheral venous blood cultures
– Swab exit site only if pus is present
– Blood cultures taken through the line are of limited value
Arterial catheter
Culture tip and exit site if signs of infection are present, routine culture not indicated
Urine
Microscopy and quantitative culture on standard selective media (see Table 1)
Record whether specimen is catheter, mid-stream or suprapubic aspiration
Wounds
Gram-stain and culture of draining pus. Swabs of limited value.
Focal collections
All collections of pus should be aspirated or have open drainage
Culture pus on selective media appropriate for the site of infection
Intraoperative specimens
Such as peritoneal fluid, bile, pus, infected bone, etc. ...
Urgent transfer from the operating room to the laboratory for microscopy and selective culture
Other normally sterile body fluids
Culture CSF, joint fluid, pleural fluid as clinically indicated

[a] If possible cultures must be obtained before the administration of antibiotics
[b] The use of "antibiotic removal device" or similar methodologies is acceptable but not obligatory
[c] The use of quantitative or semi-quantitative methods are encouraged

trial, there is no consensus as to the frequency or extent of further assessment. However, careful follow-up investigation is required to document the outcome of the initial infection and the onset of any secondary infections. The ability to detect and diagnose specific infections may have a considerable impact on the interpretation and application of trial results. Thus, careful attention to the microbiological investigation of the patient and to the presentation of both the methods used and the results will improve the quality of trials and our ability to apply the results to clinical practice.

Recommendations

1. Clear protocols must be established for the collection and evaluation of microbiologic samples in clinical trials of sepsis. They should address the following points using the information given in this chapter:
   - Specimens to be collected upon entry to the trial and during follow-up.
   - Methodology for the collection, transport and culture of those specimens.
   - Definitions for the diagnosis of specific infections.
2. The study protocol must contain detailed methods regarding the collection and evaluation of microbiologic specimens.
3. In multicenter trials, each participating center must follow the same protocol for the collection of specimens and definitions of infection. As far as is practically possible, each center should also use the same microbiologic methods.
4. When presenting trial data, adequate details of the microbiologic samples and methods used must be included to allow evaluation and comparison of different studies.
5. Ideally, all trials of septic patients should be designed with the same, or very similar, criteria for microbiologic investigation of patients as outlined above.

References

1. Bone RC, Fisher CJ, Clemmer TP, Slotman GJ, Metz CA, Balk RA (1989) Sepsis syndrome: A valid clinical entity. Crit Care Med 17:389–393
2. Bone RC, Sprung CL, Sibbald WJ (1992) Definitions for sepsis and organ failure. Crit Care Med 20:724–725
3. American College of Chest Physicians/Society of Critical Care Medicine consensus conference committee (1992) Definitions for sepsis and organ failure and guidelines for the use of innovative therapies in sepsis. Crit Care Med 20:864–874
4. Baumgartner JD, Bula C, Vaney C, Wu MM, Eggimann P, Perret C (1992) A novel score for predicting the mortality of septic shock patients. Crit Care Med 20:953–960
5. Knaus WA, Draper EA, Wagner DP, Zimmerman JE (1985) APACHE II: A severity of disease classification system. Crit Care Med 20:818–829

6. van Deuren M, Santman FW, van Dalen R, Sauerwein RW, Span LF, van der Meer JW (1992) Plasma and whole blood exchange in meningococcal sepsis. Clin Infect Dis 15:424–430
7. Ziegler EJ, McCutchan JA, Fierer J, et al (1982) Treatment of gram-negative bacteremia and shock with human anti-serum to a mutant *Escherichia coli*. N Engl J Med 307:1225–1230
8. Ziegler EJ, Fisher CJ, Sprung CL, et al (1991) Treatment of gram-negative bacteremia and septic shock with HA-1A human monoclonal antibody against endotoxin. N Engl J Med 324:429–436
9. Greenman RL, Schein RMH, Martin MA, et al (1991) A controlled clinical trial of E5 murine monoclonal IgM antibody to endotoxin in the treatment of Gram-negative sepsis. JAMA 266:1097–1102
10. Wenzel R, Bone R, Fein A (1991) Results of a second double-blind, randomized, controlled trial of antiendotoxin antibody E5 in Gram-negative sepsis. In: 31st Intersciences Conferences on Antimicrobial Agents and Chemotherapy:294 (Abst)
11. Baselski V (1993) Laboratory diagnosis of infectious diseases: Microbiologic diagnosis of ventilator-associated pneumonia. Infect Dis Clin N Am 7:331–357
12. Bone RC, Fisher CJ, Clemmer TP, et al (1987) A controlled trial of high-dose methylprednisolone in the treatment of severe sepsis and septic shock. N Engl J Med 317:653–658
13. The Veterans Administration Systemic Sepsis Cooperative Study Group (1987) Effect of high-dose glucocorticoid therapy on mortality in patients with clinical signs of systemic sepsis. N Engl J Med 317:659–665
14. Hackshaw KV, Parker GA, Roberts JW (1990) Naloxone in septic shock. Crit Care Med 18:47–51
15. Fisher CJ, Opal SM, Dhainaut JF, et al (1993) Influence of an anti-tumor necrosis factor monoclonal antibody on cytokine levels in patients with sepsis. Crit Care Med 21:318–327
16. DeMaria AB, Craven DE, Heffernan JJ, McIntosh TK, Grindlinger GA, McCabe WR (1985) Naloxone versus placebo in treatment of septic shock. Lancet 1:1363–1365
17. The Intravenous Immunoglobulin Collaborative Study Group (1992) Prophylactic intravenous administration of standard immune globulin as compared with core-lipopolysaccharide immune globulin in patients at high risk of postsurgical infection. N Engl J Med 327:234–240
18. Thrupp LD, Cleeland R, Jones RN, et al (1992) General guidelines for clinical bacteriology. Clin Infect Dis 15 (Suppl 1):S339–S346
19. Garner JS, Jarvis WR, Emori TG, Horan TC, Hughes JM (1988) CDC definitions for nosocomial infections. Am J Infect Control 16:128–140
20. Spencer RC (1993) National prevalence survey of hospital-acquired infections: Definitions. J Hosp Infect 24:69–76
21. Bryant J, Strand C (1987) Reliability of blood culture collected from intravascular catheters versus venupuncture. Am J Clin Pathol 88:113–116
22. Washington II J (1975) Blood cultures: Principles and techniques. Mayo Clin Proc 50:91–97
23. Smith-Elekes S, Weinstein MP (1993) Laboratory diagnosis of infectious diseases. Blood cultures. Infect Dis Clin N Am 7:221–234
24. Reller LB, Murray P, Maclowery JD (1982) Cumitech 1A. Blood cultures II. American Society for Microbiology. Washington DC
25. Krumholz H, Cummings S, York M (1990) Blood culture phlebotomy: Switching needles does not prevent contamination. Ann Intern Med 113:290–292
26. Kreger BE, Craven DE, Carling PC, McCabe WR (1980) Gram-negative bacteremia III. Reassessment of etiology, epidemiology and ecology in 612 patients. Am J Med 68:332–343
27. Mermel LA, Maki DG (1993) Detection of bacteremia in adults: Consequences of culturing an inadequate volume of blood. Ann Intern Med 119:270–272

28. Hall MM, Ilstrup DM, Washington II JA (1976) Effect of volume of blood cultured on the detection of bacteremia. J Clin Microbiol 3:643–645
29. Arpi M, Bentzon MW, Jensen J, Frederiksen W (1989) Importance of blood volume cultured in the detection of bacteremia. Eur J Clin Micro Infect Dis 8:838–842
30. Brown DF, Warren RE (1990) Effect of sample volume on yield of positive blood cultures from adult patients with haematological malignancy. J Clin Pathol 43:777–779
31. Plorde JJ, Tenover FC, Carlson LG (1985) Specimen volume versus yield in the BACTEC blood culture system. J Clin Microbiol 22:292–295
32. Shanson DC, Thomas F, Wilson D (1984) Effect of volume of blood cultured on detection of *Streptococcus viridans* bacteraemia. J Clin Pathol 37:568–570
33. Kennaugh J, Gregory W, Powell K, et al (1984) The effect of dilution during culture on detection of low concentrations of bacteria in blood. Pediatr Infect Dis 3:317–318
34. Weinstein MP, Reller B, Murphy JR, Lichtenstein KA (1983) The clinical significance of positive blood cultures: A comprehensive analysis of 500 episodes of bacteremia and fungemia in adults. I. Laboratory and epidemiologic observations. Rev Infect Dis 5:35–53
35. Washington II J, Illstrup D (1986) Blood cultures: Issues and controversies. Rev Infect Dis 8:792–802
36. Weinstein M, Mirrett S, Wilson M, et al (1991) Controlled evaluation of BACTEC Plus 26 and Roche Septi-Chek blood culture bottles. J Clin Microbiol 29:879–882
37. Wilson M, Weinstein M, Reimer L (1992) Controlled comparison of the BacT/Alert and BACTEC 660/730 nonradiometric blood culture systems. J Clin Microbiol 30:323–329
38. Kim M, Gottshall R, Schwabe L, et al (1987) Effect of agitation and frequent subculturing on recovery of aerobic and facultative anaerobic pathogens by Roche Septi-Chek and BACTEC blood culture systems. J Clin Microbiol 25:312–315
39. Hawkins B, Peterson E, de la Maza L (1986) Improvement of positive blood culture detection by agitation. Diag Microbiol Infect Dis 5:207–213
40. Dorsher C, Rosenblatt J, Wilson W, et al (1991) Anaerobic bacteremia: Decreasing rate over a 15 year-period. Rev Infect Dis 13:633–636
41. Sharp S, Goodman J, Poppiti R (1991) Comparison of blood culture results after five and seven days of incubation using the BACTEC NR660. Diag Microbiol Infect Dis 14:177–179
42. Henry N, Grewel C, VanGrevenhof P, et al (1984) Comparison of lysis-centrifugation with a biphasic blood culture medium for the recovery of aerobic and facultatively anarobic bacteria. J Clin Microbiol 20:413–416
43. Brannon P, Kiehn TE (1985) Large scale clinical comparison of the lysis centrifugation and radiometric systems for blood culture. J Clin Microbiol 22:951–954
44. Murray P (1991) Comparison of the lysis-centrifugation and agitated biphasic blood culture systems for the detection of fungemia. J Clin Microbiol 29:96–98
45. Peterson L, Shanholtzer C, Mohn M, et al (1983) Improved recovery of microorganisms from patients receiving antibiotic with the antimicrobial removal device. Am J Clin Pathol 80:692–696
46. Wright AJ, Thompson RL, McLimans CA, et al (1982) The antimicrobial removal device: A microbiological and clinical evaluation. Am J Clin Pathol 78:173–177
47. Leanette EH, Balows A, Hausler WJ, Shadomy HJ (eds) (1991) Manual of Clinical Microbiology. American Society for Microbiology, Washington, DC, USA
48. Maki DG, Weise CE, Sarafin HW (1977) A semiquantitative method for identifying intravenous catheter-related infection. N Engl J Med 296:1305–1309
49. Cleri DJ, Corrado ML, Seligman SJ (1980) Quantitative culture of intravenous catheters and other intravascular inserts. J Infect Dis 141:781–786
50. Collignon P, Chan R, Munro R (1987) Rapid diagnosis of intravascular-related sepsis. Arch Intern Med 147:1609–1612
51. Zuffrey J, Rime B, Franciou P, et al (1988) Simple method for rapid diagnosis of catheter-associated infection by direct acridine orange staining of catheter tips. J Clin Microbiol 26:175–177

52. Felices FJ, Hernandez JL, Ruiz J (1979) Use of central venous catheter to obtain blood cultures. Crit Care Med 7:78–79
53. Tonnesen A, Peuler M, Lockwood WR (1976) Cultures of blood drawn by catheters vs venipuncture. JAMA 235:1877
54. MacFarlane JT, Finch RG, Ward MJ (1982) Hospital study of adult community-acquired pneumonia. Lancet 2:255–258
55. Donowitz GR, Mandell GL (1990) Acute pneumonia. In: Mandell GL, Douglas RG, Bennett JE (eds) Principles and practice of infectious diseases. Churchill Livingstone, New York, pp 540–554
56. Barrett-Connor E (1971) The non-value of sputum culture in the diagnosis of pneumococcal pneumonia. Am Rev Resp Dis 103:845–848
57. Murray PR, Washington II JA (1975) Microbiologic and bacteriologic analysis of expectorated sputum. Mayo Clinic Proc 50:339–344
58. Wimberly NW, Bass JB, Boyd BW, et al (1982) Use of a bronchoscopic protected catheter brush for the diagnosis of pulmonary infections. Chest 81:556–582
59. Palmer DL, Davidson M, Lusk R (1980) Needle aspiration of the lung in complex pneumonias. Chest 78:16–21
60. Geckeler RW, Gremillion DH, McAllister CK, et al (1977) Microscopic and bacteriological comparison of paired sputa and transtracheal aspirates. J Clin Microbiol 6:396–399
61. Bartlett JG, Rosenblatt JE, Finegold SM (1973) Percutaneous transtracheal aspiration in the diagnosis of anaerobic pulmonary infection. Ann Intern Med 79:535–540
62. Krook A, Homberg H (1987) Pneumococcal antigens in sputa. Diag Microbiol Infect Dis 7:73–75
63. Andrews CP, Coalson JJ, Smith JD, Johanson WG (1981) Diagnosis of nosocomial bacterial pneumonia in acute, diffuse lung injury. Chest 80:254–258
64. Meduri GU (1993) Laboratory diagnosis of infectious diseases: Diagnosis of ventilator-associated pneumonia. Infect Dis Clin N Am 7:295–329
65. Pollock HM, Hawkins EL, Bonner JR, et al (1983) Diagnosis of bacterial pulmonary infections with quantitative protected catheter cultures obtained during bronchoscopy. J Clin Microbiol 17:255–259
66. A'Court CHD, Gerard CS, Crook D, et al (1993) Microbiological lung surveillance in mechanically ventilated patients, using non-directed bronchial lavage and quantitative culture. Q J Med 86:635–648
67. Marquette CH, Georges H, Wallet F, et al (1993) Diagnostic efficiency of endotracheal aspirates with quantitative bacterial cultures in intubated patients with suspected pneumonia. Am Rev Resp Dis 148:138–144

Measurement of Inflammatory Mediators in Clinical Sepsis

S.F. Lowry, S.E. Calvano, and T. van der Poll

Introduction

The intensity of current interest in the clinical therapy of sepsis derives from advances in our understanding of pathologic mechanisms related to inflammatory mediators. Although clinical documentation that such mediators contribute to the pathophysiology of human sepsis remains limited, the availability of recombinantly derived, highly specific antagonists of their activity has engendered extensive clinical research in their application. While such efforts have, thus far, proven disappointing with respect to dramatic improvements in outcome, some populations do appear susceptible to improvements in both organ system dysfunction and mortality.

The ability to prospectively identify those populations susceptible to antimediator therapies remains perhaps the most vexing issue in such trials. To some extent, it has been anticipated that measurement of the purported mediators would serve to effectively identify these patients. Although such real-time utilization of this concept has yet to be undertaken, a growing body of literature attests to the interest in this approach. The current review will seek to discuss this literature and to define current and future issues related to the measurement of mediator activity (levels) within the context of prospective clinical trials and the mechanisms of human sepsis.

Clinical Evaluations of Cytokines, Endotoxin, and Natural Inhibitors

Several studies have documented the presence of detectable or elevated concentrations of cytokines or soluble cytokine inhibitors in the circulation of patients with sepsis. The following summarizes investigations on this issue published in peer reviewed literature.

Tumor Necrosis Factor α

Tumor necrosis factor α (TNF) was the first pro-inflammatory cytokine to be definitively detected in the circulation of patients with sepsis [1], shortly after this cytokine had been demonstrated to play a causal role in the development of sepsis-induced tissue injury in animal models (reviewed in [2]). Waage et al. [1] reported the serum levels of TNF activity, as measured with a cytotoxicity assay utilizing the WEHI 164 clone 13 fibrosarcoma cell line, in 79 patients with meningococcal disease. Of the 53 patients with meningococcal sepsis, 16 patients (30%) had detectable levels of TNF activity on admission to the hospital. A correlation between the detection of TNF activity and fatal outcome was also noted, as all patients with a TNF level above 440 U/mL (corresponding to approximately 100 pg/mL) died. Shortly thereafter, these findings were confirmed in a study in 35 children presenting with a clinical diagnosis of sepsis and purpuric lesions, the majority of whom had positive cultures for *Neisseria meningitidis* [3]. On admission, 30 of these children (86%) had immunoreactive TNF concentrations above the detection limit (150 pg/mL) of the radioimmunoassay (RIA) used. Again a correlation was found between TNF levels and outcome: the percentage of mortality was directly related to the serum concentrations of TNF.

Subsequently, numerous published studies have examined TNF levels in patients with other forms of (non-meningococcal) sepsis, including observations made upon admission as well as during subsequent hospitalization (Table 1). The circulating levels of TNF reported therein have demonstrated large interstudy variation. In most studies detection of immunoreactive TNF has largely been confined to a subset of septic patients (16–100%) on admission. This large variability relates, at least in part, to differences in assay technique. For example, in the two published studies in which TNF was found in all patients with sepsis, RIA techniques which also detected TNF in the serum of normal subjects were utilized. Such assays have additionally detected TNF consistently in the serum of normal subjects [4, 5]. By contrast, bioactive TNF is reported in a relatively low percentage of septic patients, and is almost never detectable in the circulation of healthy subjects. Using such a bioassay system (L929 lysis), Casey et al. [6] detected TNF activity in only 4 of 97 patients (4%), while 54 patients (54%) had detectable immunoreactive TNF, as assessed by ELISA. Employing the presumptively more sensitive WEHI bioassay, Van der Poll et al. [7] recently reported finding TNF activity in 9 of 20 septic patients (45%) on admission to the ICU. Eighteen of these patients also had immunoreactive TNF detected by an IRMA method.

Although several studies do comment upon a positive correlation between the serum or plasma concentration of TNF on admission and mortality [1, 3, 4, 8, 9–12], this association is by no means universal across all study populations. Indeed, in the study that included the largest number of patients (N=97), the mean plasma levels of TNF on admission did not differ between patients who survived and patients who died [6]. In this study, TNF levels were categorized according to a post-hoc analysis with resultant demonstration of an association between TNF levels and mortality.

Some data are available regarding TNF concentrations later in the course of sepsis. Such data suggest that TNF levels, when detectable, are usually

Table 1. Tumor necrosis factor concentrations in clinical sepsis

Author	Ref.	N	Sample	Assay	% positive	Correlation with mortality	Levels	Follow-up levels
Waage et al.	[1]	53	serum	Bioassay (WEHI)	30	Yes	10–1400 U/mL (one >100000)	No
Girardin et al.	[3]	35	serum	RIA	86	Yes	410 ± 50 pg/mL in survivors 830 ± 240 pg/mL in nonsurvivors	No
de Grootte et al.	[44]	38	heparin	ELISA	16	No	0–500 pg/mL	Yes (6 h intervals): variable
Debets et al.	[8]	43	EDTA	ELISA	26	Yes	0–122 pg/mL	No
Damas et al.	[4]	27	serum	RIA	100	Yes	100–>5000 pg/mL (median 250)	No
Calandra et al.	[9]	70	serum	RIA	79	Yes	<100–3500 pg/mL (median 180 in survivors, 330 in nonsurvivors)	Yes (day 1 and 10): decrease in survivors, remained elevated in nonsurvivors
Cannon et al.	[5]	15	EDTA/ Aprotinin	RIA	100	Not listed	119 ± 30 pg/mL	Yes (1 h): no important change
Offner et al.	[12]	34	serum	IRMA	Not listed	Yes	79 pg/mL (median) 329 (iqr)	Yes (daily for 6 days): levels relatively constant
Marano et al.	[10]	39	serum	ELISA	69	Yes	<34–1200 pg/mL (256 ± 40)	Yes (1 week): TNF appears transiently and repetitively
Marks et al.	[11]	74	EDTA	ELISA	37	Yes	181 ± 35 pg/mL	Yes (1 week): levels decrease

higher at the time of diagnosis than during subsequent sampling times, especially in survivors [9, 11, 13]. It is important to recognize that TNF concentrations can change substantially within hours in an individual patient [4, 10]. Further, the relationship between clearance of the free ligand or receptor/ligand complexes during conditions of organ dysfunction remains undefined.

Interleukin-1

Like TNF, IL-1 has been shown to occupy a pivotal and causal role in the pathogenesis of experimental sepsis (reviewed in [14]). Two forms of IL-1 exist (IL-1α and IL-1β), which bind to the same cellular receptors and exert essentially identical biological effects. In contrast to IL-1β, IL-1α is rarely found in body fluids in soluble form. Indeed, investigators who have tried to measure IL-1α in patients with septic shock have been unsuccessful [5, 15]. IL-1β has been found more frequently in patients with sepsis (Table 2). In 1988, Girardin et al. [3] were the first to describe the presence of immunoreactive IL-1β in the serum of septic patients. In 33 children with purpura fulminans they were able, utilizing an RIA with a detection limit of 200 pg/mL, to detect IL-1β in seven patients (21%) on admission. In addition, a positive correlation was found between the levels of IL-1β and mortality. Although several reports have since confirmed the detection of IL-1β in some patients presenting with sepsis, the relation of such observations to clinical outcome is unclear. The largest reported study found detectable IL-1β in 37% of 97 patients with sepsis using an ELISA with a detection limit of 20 pg/mL [6]. In that study IL-1β concentrations on admission did not differ between survivors and non-survivors. Although 70% of patients did not have detectable IL-1, for those patients with detectable levels, the authors suggested an association between increased IL-1β levels and a fatal outcome. Interestingly enough, other studies have reported an inverse relation between detection of circulating IL-1β and mortality [5, 15]. In those investigations, in which IL-1β concentrations on admission were higher in survivors than in non-survivors, the cytokine was measured with RIA's in samples that had undergone chloroform extraction [16]. However, this is an unlikely explanation for the discrepancy with, for example, the study by Casey et al. [6], since chloroform extraction is considered to have little effect on ELISA measurements [17].

Data on IL-1β concentrations in patients with sepsis later in the course of their disease are limited. In a study performed in 70 patients, IL-1β was found not to have changed significantly one and ten days after admission [9].

Interleukin-6

In comparison with other cytokines, IL-6 has been reported most consistently in the circulation of septic patients. IL-6 does not have the ability to

Table 2. Interleukin-1β concentrations in clinical sepsis

Author	Ref.	N	Sample	Assay	% positive	Correlation with mortality	Levels	Follow up levels
Girardin et al.	[3]	33	serum	RIA	21	Yes	220 ± 20 pg/mL in survivors; 1630 ± 70 pg/mL in nonsurvivors.	No
Damas et al.	[4]	27	serum	RIA	100	No	447 ± 60 pg/mL in survivors; 496 ± 34 pg/mL in nonsurvivors.	No
Calandra et al.	[9]	70	serum	RIA	Not listed	Yes	<150–3260 pg/mL (median 300 in survivors, 480 in nonsurvivors)	Yes (day 1 and 10): levels remained unchanged
Cannon et al.	[5]	15	EDTA/Aprotinin (chloroform extraction)	RIA	Not listed	No	120 ± 17 pg/mL (levels were higher in survivors!)	No
Munoz et al.	[15]	21	EDTA/Aprotinin (chloroform extraction)	RIA	48	No	Survivors: 275 ± 112 pg/mL Nonsurvivors: 121 ± 59 pg/mL	Yes (days): variable
Carey et al.	[6]	97	EDTA	ELISA	37	No (only if "categorized levels" were analyzed)	0–2850 pg/mL (median 20; mean 267)	No

cause a septic shock-like syndrome in animals, and passive immunization against IL-6 confers only limited protection in experimental endotoxemia. Therefore, it is now more widely assumed that IL-6 concentrations in patients with sepsis are less likely to reflect an offending agent than serving as a potential surrogate marker of disease severity.

The vast majority of published studies have utilized bioassays, based on IL-6 dependent proliferation of mouse hybridoma cells, to detect IL-6 in the circulation of septic patients (Table 3). Most such assays have employed either B.9 or 7TD1 hybridoma cells for this purpose. The first observations of IL-6 in the serum of patients with sepsis were independently reported by two groups [18, 19]. Waage et al. [18] measured IL-6 bioactivity in their population of patients with meningococcal disease (see also [1]). Of 53 patients with positive blood cultures, 83% had detectable IL-6 activity in their circulation, as measured by the B9 assay. The serum levels of IL-6 had a clear correlation with mortality. At approximately the same time, Helfgott et al. [19] reported the presence of IL-6 activity in serum of patients with various bacterial infections using a bioassay with the human hepatoma cell line Hep3B. Subsequent studies have confirmed both the high frequency of IL-6 detection in septic patients and, albeit to a lesser extent, the general positive correlation between IL-6 levels and mortality (Table 3).

It is important to note that the reported concentrations of IL-6 show considerable variation. For example, Waage et al. [18] found a median IL-6 level in patients with meningococcal sepsis of 189 ng/mL. Hack et al. [20], using the same (B9) assay, found median IL-6 levels of 0.039 ng/mL in survivors and 2.646 ng/mL in non-survivors in patients with sepsis caused by various microorganisms. This large variation cannot likely be explained by differences in the disease severity of the evaluated populations, as the mortality of the latter study was higher. Rather, other subtle clinical variables such as the timing of the samples in relation to the actual septic event must also be considered. It is also possible that other biologic factors may account for these differences. The issue that more severely ill patients might, in fact, exhibit a retardation of IL-6 production, although as yet clinically unproven, might also be considered. Additional factors to be considered include differences in the potency of internal standards utilized in such assays. IL-6, like several other cytokines, is polymorphic and assay sensitivity might be influenced by variations in the species of recombinant standard.

Several studies have measured IL-6 levels later in the course of sepsis [13, 18, 20, 21]. All found that IL-6 was generally at the highest level to be detected at the time of admission or diagnosis and the IL-6 concentrations consistently decrease at subsequent time points. This decrease in IL-6 levels is nearly always independent of outcome. The rate of decline in levels respective to outcome has not been adequately addressed.

Table 3. Interleukin-6 concentrations in clinical sepsis

Author	Ref.	N	Sample	Assay	% positive	Correlation with mortality	Levels	Follow up levels
Waage et al.	[18]	53	serum	Bioassay (B9)	83	Yes	Median 189 ng/mL	Yes (highest on admission)
Hack et al.	[20]	37	EDTA/polybrene	Bioassay (B9)	86	Yes	<20–150000 pg/mL (median 39 in survivors, 2646 in nonsurvivors)	Yes (highest on admission)
Calandra, et al.	[21]	70	serum	Bioassay (7TD1)	64	Yes	Median 0.5 (<0.1–135 ng/mL) in survivors; 3.5 (<0.1–305) in nonsurvivors	Yes (day 1 and 10): highest on admission
Munoz et al.	[15]	21	EDTA/Aprotinin	Bioassay (7TD1)	81	Yes	638 ± 158 U/mL in survivors; 15205 ± 6430 U/mL in nonsurvivors.	Yes
Girardin et al.	[45]	34	serum	Bioassay (7TD1)	Not listed	Yes	22.4 ± 5.4 ng/mL in survivors; 216.3 ± 84.2 ng/mL in nonsurvivors.	No
Wortel et al.	[13]	67	serum	Bioassay (B9)	100	Yes	1–57000 pg/mL (median 340)	Yes (1 and 24 h): highest on admission
Carey et al.	[6]	97	EDTA	ELISA	80	Yes	0–2380 pg/mL (median 415)	No
Munoz et al.	[15]	21	EDTA/Aprotinin	RIA	86	No	143 ± 25 pg/mL in survivors, 217 ± 41 in nonsurvivors (N.S.)	Yes (days): levels usually higher at later time points
Wortel et al.	[13]	65	serum	IRMA	Not listed	Not listed	5–2264 pg/mL (median 30)	Yes (1 and 24 h): decrease
vd Poll et al.	[7]	20	serum serum	IRMA Bioassay (WEHI)	95 45	No No	103 ± 26 pg/mL 45 ± 31 pg/mL	No No
Carey et al.	[6]	97	EDTA	ELISA Bioassay (L929)	54 4	No (only if "categorized levels" were analyzed)	0–1000 pg/mL (median 26)	No

Interleukin-8

The exact role of IL-8 in the pathophysiology of sepsis is poorly defined. IL-8 is considered to be an important activator of neutrophils. However, infusion of high doses of IL-8 into animals is not associated with significant tissue damage. To date, reports on IL-8 levels in clinical sepsis remain limited. Hack et al. [22] found elevated levels of IL-8 (i.e. >40 pg/mL as measured by ELISA) in 89% of 47 patients with sepsis. The concentrations measured varied widely between 7 and 66000 pg/mL (median 251 pg/mL in survivors and 335 pg/mL in non-survivors). Although IL-8 levels were higher in non-survivors than in survivors, there was no significant correlation between the initial IL-8 concentration and subsequent mortality. IL-8 levels were significantly correlated with the occurrence of shock. Sequential samples in 11 patients revealed that IL-8 values decreased later in the course of their disease. To our knowledge, the only other definitive report on IL-8 concentrations in septic patients is that from Friedland et al. [23]. They detected elevated IL-8 levels in 8 of 18 patients with localized or systemic *Pseudomonas pseudomallei* infection, and found IL-8 levels to be positively correlated with a fatal outcome. In contrast, in a preliminary report, Danner et al. [24] observed higher IL-8 levels in surviving septic patients when compared to non-survivors.

Interferons

The value of measurement of interferons in clinical sepsis is uncertain. Girardin et al. [3] reported detectable interferon-γ in six of 32 children with *purpura fulminans* (19%). The levels in non-survivors were significantly higher 2.65 ± 1.11 U/mL) than in survivors (0.09 ± 0.07 U/mL). Using the same assay (a commercially available RIA), Calandra et al. [8] found elevated interferon-γ concentrations in a small, not specified, number of 70 patients with sepsis, not correlating with the outcome. Finally, Waage et al. [18] were unable to detect interferon-γ in any of their patients with meningococcal sepsis.

Two of the above cited studies also attempted to measure interferon-α in their patients [3, 9]. In children with *purpura fulminans*, interferon-α levels, as measured by a RIA that also detected the cytokine in normal individuals, were within normal limits [3]. Remarkably, in the study by Calandra et al. [9] the same RIA was used and was reported to not detect interferon-α in normals. In that investigation, interferon-α was elevated in patients with sepsis, but showed a large variation and no correlation with outcome.

Endotoxin

Endotoxin is a lipopolysaccharide that is a major component of the outer membrane of gram-negative bacteria, and is considered to play a pivotal role in the pathogenesis of gram-negative sepsis (for review see [25]). The clinically most useful test to detect endotoxin is based on the fact that endotoxin is able to activate the coagulation system of the Limulus polyphemus, the horseshoe crab. In early clinical studies an *in vitro* test was used that depended upon the gelation of lysates derived from blood cells (amoebocytes) of the Limulus horseshoe crab secondary to endotoxin-induced coagulation [28–30]. More recent investigations utilized a modified Limulus amoebycate lysate (LAL) test, using an enzyme substrate that can be measured spectrophotometrically [6, 13, 18, 26–28]. Although this chromogenic LAL assay is more sensitive than its predecessor, detecting endotoxin levels as low as 0.50 pg/mL, it has no been standardized. Furthermore, a number of plasma proteins may interfere with the results of the chromogenic assay, and endotoxins from different bacterial species may differentially activate LAL. Test samples need to be handled with great care, since contamination with exogenous endotoxin can occur easily, resulting in false-positive results.

Four relatively large clinical studies utilizing a chromogenic LAL assay to detect endotoxin have been published [6, 13, 26, 28]. Van Deventer et al. [26] tried to measure endotoxin in 473 consecutive febrile patients to assess the value of endotoxemia for predicting development of sepsis. Endotoxemia was detected in 15 of the 19 patients who became septic, while 16 of 454 patients that did not develop sepsis had a positive LAL test. The sensitivity of the endotoxin test for sepsis was 79%, the specificity 96%, suggesting that the chromogenic LAL assay may be of use in febrile patients to identify those at risk to proceed to clinical sepsis [26]. Other studies differ fundamentally from the above in that patients had been admitted with sepsis [6, 13, 28]. Wortel et al. [13] detected endotoxinemia in 27 of 82 (33%) patients with suspected gram-negative sepsis. No association was found between endotoxemia and the presence of important clinical manifestations of sepsis such as acute respiratory distress syndrome (ARDS), disseminated intravascular coagulation (DIC), shock, renal or hepatic failure, and APACHE II scores, nor between endotoxemia and death [13]. Arguing that transient episodes of endotoxemia can go undetected when only a single endotoxin determination is performed, Danner et al. [26] determined endotoxin in 100 patients with septic shock every 4 h for the initial 24 h, every 12 h for the next 24 h, and then daily for 3 days. Detectable endotoxin was noted at one or more time points within the first 24 h in 43 of the patients (mean peak concentration 4.4 ± 1.2 EU/mL or 440 pg/mL of US standard endotoxin). It was shown that the majority of patients had intermittent endotoxemia during the study, the average number of specimens positive for endotoxin being over 4 per patient. In contrast to the study of Wortel et al., a number of clinical outcomes were associated with the presence of endotoxemia, including ARDS and renal failure. There was no correlation between endotoxemia and death, however [26]. Using the same chromogenic LAL assay, Casey et al. [6] found detectable endotoxin in 89% of 97 patients with sepsis (mean level 3.45 EU/mL). Hence, in this population the LAL test was positive in twice as many patients when compared with Danner's population, a remarkable difference, since only one sample, obtained on admission, was assayed. No correlation with mortality was found [6].

Although endotoxin is a moiety unique for gram-negative organisms, a positive LAL test has been found in pure gram-positive infections and fungal infections by virtually all investigators that have used this assay in clinical practice. For example, Danner et al. [26] found endotoxin in 8 of 14 patients with isolated gram-positive bacteremia and in 4 of 4 patients with *Candida* sepsis, while Casey et al. [6] measured similar endotoxin levels in patients with either gram-negative bacteremia, gram-negative infection without bacteremia, gram-positive bacteremia, or without a single positive bacterial culture. Possible explanations of this phenomenon could be translocation of endotoxin from the gut, or clinically undetected gram-negative bacteremia. Nonetheless, it is evident that a positive LAL test cannot be considered to be specific for gram-negative sepsis.

Endotoxin has been reported detected in 100% of patients with meningococcal sepsis [18, 27]. The levels of endotoxin were extremely high, ranging from 210 to 170000 ng/mL [27]. In these patients, endotoxemia significantly correlated with mortality [18, 27].

Multiple Determinants

Given the apparent lack of correlation to mortality that arises from individual cytokine levels, it has been proposed that concurrent examination of two or more cytokine levels might achieve improved risk prediction. This approach has recently been reported in a prospectively evaluated group of patients with severe sepsis [6]. This analysis utilized ELISA techniques for cytokine assay and revealed a similar incidence of individual cytokine detection to that noted in Table 1. The detection of any individual cytokine mediator, with the possible exception of IL-1, did not prove discriminatory for risk of mortality. This investigation also assayed for the presence of endotoxin, utilizing a standard chromogenic assay. Not surprisingly, neither the incidence of detection nor the categorical level of endotoxin were related to mortality.

The most discriminating aspect of such endotoxin and cytokine determinations was observed when a so-called LPS-cytokine score was derived. Utilizing a summed score derived from categorical levels of these mediators, an apparent relationship between these parameters and mortality was observed (Fig. 1). Although this report supports a correlation between such mediators and mortality, it should not, as discussed [29], be construed to establish causality. Further, the assay techniques utilized in this report may not necessarily quantify the biological active species of mediator. For example, the TNF determinations were more likely reflective of ligand/receptor complexes rather than bioassayable cytotoxicity. Clearly, this approach will require further investigation with precise immuno- and bioassays before the concept of a combined cytokine score can be validated.

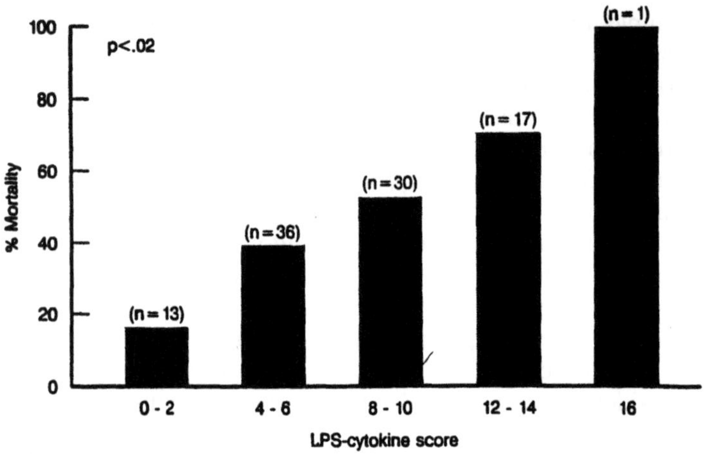

Fig. 1. Percentage mortality in patients with sepsis syndrome grouped according to categorical levels of endotoxin (LPS) plus cytokines (TNF, IL-1 and IL-6) measured at time of diagnosis. (n=number of patients at the defined level). (Adapted from [6])

Circulating Natural Antagonists

It has become increasingly evident that severe infection induces not only circulating levels of several pro-inflammatory cytokines, but also anti-inflammatory cytokine species, such as IL-10 [30] and other natural antagonist species, such as soluble receptors for TNF (sTNF-R, both Types I and II) and IL-1 receptor antagonist (IL-1ra). These endotoxin and inflammation inducible proteins do appear in the circulation in response to a variety of stressful stimulae and are regulated, at least in part, by the antecedent activity of pro-inflammatory cytokines [31]. Although endogenously derived TNF and IL-1 antagonist molecules have limited efficacy for attenuating activity of the pro-inflammatory ligands [32–34], it has been proposed that their presence in the circulation may partially serve as surrogate markers for the antecedent activity of pro-inflammatory cytokine species. The concept that natural cytokine antagonist levels may reflect the relative magnitude of preceding inflammatory insult is supported by observed incremental increases in their circulating levels along a spectrum from mild endotoxinemia [32, 34] to accidental injury [35] to severe infection [33, 36].

As with all mediator assays discussed above, several problems continue to limit the interpretation of sTNF-R and IL-1ra levels, including the specificity of currently available assays for free receptor or receptor ligand complexes. Additionally, acute or chronic organ dysfunction may significantly alter the clearance of both sTNF-R and IL-1ra and the potential impact of established immunologic dysfunction upon their production has not been clarified.

We have recently undertaken studies to assess levels of such antagonists in response to both controlled human endotoxinemia and severe clinical infection [36]. In critically ill patients who ultimately survived an episode of severe bacterial infection, the levels of sTNF-R (Type I) noted at initial diagnosis were similar to those achieved in response to mild endotoxin challenge in normal subjects (Table 2). However, patients who succumbed from the sequelae of sepsis, exhibited significantly higher levels of sTNF-R both at the time of diagnosis and for the duration of their hospital course. The initially elevated levels could not be ascribed to organ dysfunction as the degree of solid organ failure was similar to that observed in surviving patients.

By contrast, the initial levels of circulating IL-1ra noted in patients were not increased over those levels achieved during controlled endotoxinemia. Further, neither the initial levels of IL-1ra detected in septic patients nor those noted during subsequent testing discriminated between patients who would survive from those ultimately expiring. In contrast to other reports cited above, neither TNF (ELISA, bioassay) nor IL-1 (ELISA) were consistently detected at any point in these patients.

Thus far, there is limited published data upon which to assess the utility of such mediator antagonists for the ascribing initial disease severity. There is substantial overlap of levels between surviving and ultimately expiring patients. Given the apparent narrow range over which circulating levels are regulated in humans, it is unlikely that determination of these antagonists will prove more effective than their respective agonist cytokines in assessing risk. Rather, the addition of such antagonist levels to a categorical analysis with other inflammatory mediators may enhance the discriminating value of combined determinations. It will be of extreme interest to pursue such prospective analyses once some consensus as to appropriate assay techniques is achieved.

Alternative Assessments of the Host Response

The technical issues arising from analysis of endotoxin and cytokine mediators currently limit any impression that such levels can function as markers for the intensity of the infectious insult. Clearly, there is immediate need for such an analytical approach to assess not only the initial clinical severity of sepsis, but also to serve as a biologic marker for the efficacy of infection specific therapies.

Functional Assays

Unfortunately, approaches which address the functional defects of immune activity, like those which measure levels of single or multiple mediators, have yet to achieve widespread investigation in clinical trials. Initial efforts to relate functional components of immune response, such as LPS-induced cytokine production *in vitro* [15], have suggested that a relative diminution in such responses protends poorly for outcome. This approach has only recently been correlated with other clinical (physiologic) parameters of the septic response [37].

Some attention has been directed toward the regulation of immune cell receptor expression and activity [38, 39]. Such approaches demonstrate that severely septic patients exhibit abnormalities of cell surface cytokine or other receptor activities. Further, patients exhibiting such abnormalities may have increased risk of mortality. Unfortunately, these *in vitro* techniques are too cumbersome to permit anything other than a retrospective analysis of immune function. Hence, a specific and sensitive technique permitting a real time analysis of disordered immune function has great appeal as an adjunctive diagnostic and prognostic tool.

Given the growing body of evidence for disordered cytokine receptor function during clinical sepsis, we have undertaken recent studies to determine if circulating immune cells might exhibit similar abnormalities which could be assessed in a manner potentially useful to the clinical decision making process. To address this issue, we prospectively evaluated leukocyte surface expression of functional TNF receptors under conditions of overwhelming gram-negative bacteremia in primates [40] as well as in humans with experimental endotoxinemia and sepsis syndrome [42]. Utilizing flow microfluorometry techniques, we demonstrated that acute endotoxinemia in normal subjects was associated with a transient reduction of monocyte surface TNF binding of biotinylated TNF and simultaneous appearance of soluble TNF receptor species. The duration of this downregulation of monocyte TNF receptors occurred within one hour after endotoxin exposure and was associated with full recovery of binding capacity within five hours. Interestingly, the apparent reduction in TNF receptor activity preceded the evolution of systemic symptoms associated with endotoxin administration and also persisted beyond the brief period of measurable TNF activity.

These observations suggested that such an assay might be capable of assessing the immune response induced by endotoxin (or other mediator activities) under clinical conditions. Consequently, a group of critically ill patients meeting standard criteria for sepsis syndrome were prospectively evaluated [41]. While all other clinical parameters failed to effectively discriminate patient risk, prospectively determined monocyte surface TNF receptors identified two distinct patient populations (Fig. 2) at the time of initial diagnosis. Those patients destined to ultimately expire of their disease (over ensuing several days to weeks) exhibited a significant reduction in cell surface TNF receptor activity. By contrast, those patients who would survive their septic event exhibited a normal level of cell TNF receptor activity both at diagnosis and at the time of recovery several weeks later. Of interest is that determinations of cell TNF receptor activity during intermediate points yield similar results to those obtained at diagnosis. This suggests that the alterations of cell TNF receptor activity are not random events but rather are identifiable throughout the period of risk.

Functional immunologic testing such as that outlined above may serve as a means of discriminating patients with increased risk of mortality from sepsis.

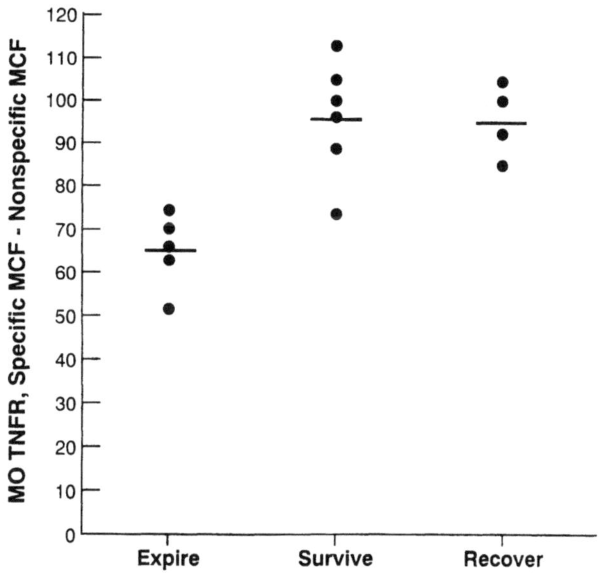

Fig. 2. Circulating monocyte (MO) TNF-receptor activity in 11 patients with sepsis syndrome. Initial values in non-surviving (Expire) and surviving (Survive) patients were obtained at the time of clinical diagnosis. Subsequent samples in surviving patients (Recover) were obtained where feasible 21–28 days later. MCF=mean channel fluorescence. (Adapted from [41])

Current assessment techniques are predictive of risk on an individual basis only in extreme cases. By contrast, a single functional assessment or combination of methods addressing the severity of mediator signalling may prove useful, in conjunction with other clinical information, for assignment of treatment modalities. To be clinically acceptable, these methods must exhibit sufficient sensitivity and specificity for the septic disease process. Further, such techniques must be available for bedside or clinical laboratory utilization, readily standardized, and cost-effective. Such approaches must also be sensitive, and relatively selectively so, to effective clinical intervention. If the intensity (and cost) of resource allocation for management of severe infection expands, techniques similar to, or perhaps variations of, those discussed above will be actively investigated as adjuncts to the clinical decision making process.

Clinical Perspectives in Cytokine Measurements for Assessing the Host Response

Any discussion of the practicality for determination of cytokines in critical illness must address several issues inherent in the therapeutic decision process. Initially, one might question the sensitivity and specificity of such determinants as markers of the severity of the septic insult. The most obvious criteria for such an analysis is by ultimate mortality. Approaching this issue seeks, in essence, to define the mediator-induced attributable risk of the sepsis process reflected by such markers. This approach requires, at a minimum, the assumption that the pro-inflammatory mediator(s) in question contributes significantly to the pathophysiology of the septic process. The tenet that the above discussed mediators are significant participants in the sepsis process, and therefore drive associated morbidity and mortality, is beyond the scope of the current discussion. Pending the outcome of current and future clinical trials, this issue must be considered speculative.

It is clinically germane to address the concept that circulating levels of these mediators may reflect the underlying severity of infectious insult and, hence, lend more specificity of risk. As noted earlier, a growing body of literature has begun to address this issue in a prospective manner. While some preliminary data suggests that analysis of selected mediators might prove useful in this regard, major obstacles such as assay standardization are likely to preclude the utility of this method for the immediate future. It is also unclear to what extent such changes are specific to infectious challenge as opposed to other inflammatory states and how such responses are influenced by other clinical conditions, such as malignancy or chronic steroid administration.

Several additional issues will need clarification, including the concept that the measurable mediator milieu established at the time of diagnosis accurately depicts the functionally relevant host response to a given infectious challenge. This concept is supported by controlled pre-clinical data in which healthy animals are exposed to such challenges. It is evident that healthy animals exhibit a temporally reproducible pattern of pro-inflammatory mediators in response to graded infectious challenges [42]. Importantly, such pre-clinical studies also demonstrate that the response magnitude of most such mediators as well as of their actual detection frequency are sensitive to the intensity of challenge. For instance, studies performed in adult primates have demonstrated the uniform temporal relationship between endotoxin/bacterial challenge and the appearance of several circulating cytokines (Fig. 3) [32]. Such studies also demonstrate a correlation between the challenge and the magnitude of antigen exposure. These relationships are also substantiated in studies of controlled human endotoxinemia although some mediators, such as IL-1, are detected with less frequency than is observed in animal models [48].

Unfortunately, evidence to substantiate such a well-defined mediator cascade relationship in clinical sepsis is generally lacking. For example, the levels of pro-inflammatory cytokines measured in relatively uniform disease processes may vary considerably. It is also unclear whether traditional clinical therapies alter this responsiveness. There is evidence to suggest that exogenous steroids alter many aspects of non-specific and specific immune function. Recent information also demonstrates that such therapy may dramatically influence the generation of both pro-inflammatory cytokines as well as

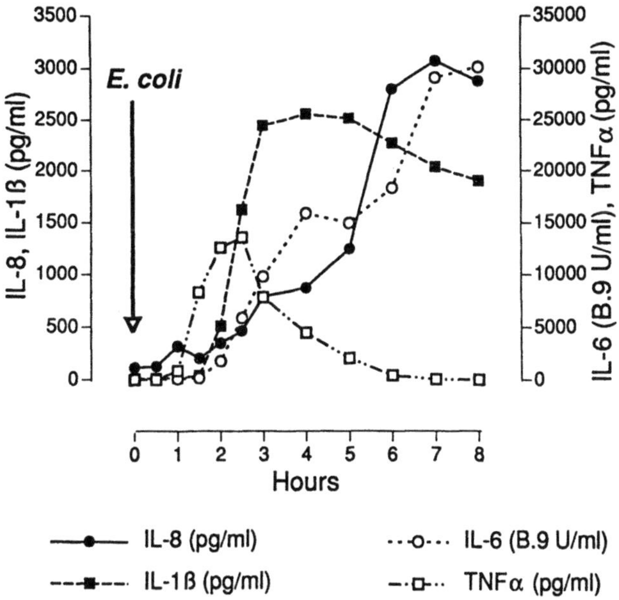

Fig. 3. Blood samples were obtained every 30 to 60 min from baboons that had received a lethal dose of live *E. coli.* Mean cytokine levels for each timepoint are shown for TNFα (□), IL-1β (■), IL-6 (○), and IL-8 (●) and were determined by ELISA (TNFα, IL-1β, and IL-8) and by B.9 hybridoma proliferation assay (IL-6)

of their natural antagonists (Barber and Lowry, unpublished observations) [43]. It is also possible that other commonly utilized therapies, such as those which increase cellular cAMP, may alter the host mediator responses in complex ways.

We have recently evaluated the relationship between initial cytokine/natural antagonist levels in a prospectively identified group of adult patients with documented gram-negative bacteremia/sepsis syndrome. The results of this analysis, obtained from a prospective evaluation of 29 patients are shown in Table 4. All subjects were defined as septic by current clinical criteria and assessed over the initial 72 h. This interval was selected as reflective of a period of sufficient duration for all appropriate clinical interventions to be instituted in the management of the septic focus and the practical reason that the half-lives or therapy period of currently available biologic response modifying agents would permit maximal therapeutic influences over this time frame. Selected aspects of this data are shown, including IL-6 levels (B.9 assay) and soluble TNF receptor, type I (ELISA) at the time of clinical diagnosis (0 h) and 72 h later.

At the time of diagnosis, when pro-inflammatory cytokines are not detectable, IL-6 and sTNF-R levels are clearly elevated. While IL-6 did not discriminate between ultimate survivors and non-survivors, there is some evidence that sTNF-R was more reflective of this clinical component.

Table 4. IL-6 and sTNF-R levels as a function of outcome and change in APACHE III

		IL-6 (U/mL)		sTNF-R (ng/mL)	
Outcome		0 h	72 h	0 h	72 h
Survivors (n=15)		327±132	44±15[a]	20.6±7.9	16.7±8.4
Non-survivors (n=14)		364±104	201±67	41.1±7.7	43.9±8.5[b]
as percent Δ→72 h	%Δ APACHE	%Δ IL-6		%Δ sTNF-R	
Δ APACHE III (<20%) (n=13)	6±9	−38±14		23±13	
Δ APACHE III (>20%) (n=16)	−42±3[c]	−67±9		−28±8[c]	

[a] $p<0.05$ vs. respective 0 h; [b] $p<0.05$ vs. respective 72 h; [c] $p<0.01$ vs Δ APACHE (<20%)

In addition, it should be established whether such measurements correlate with clinical parameters both at the outset of the sepsis process and respond in an appropriate direction to the subsequent clinical course of the patient. Such an analysis assumes that some component(s) of the measurable mediator cascade is reflective of the integrated clinical response to infection. It is also of interest to determine whether such parameters correlate to commonly applied physiologic aspects of sepsis, as reflected for instance in a logistic risk model. We have sought to address this issue in the above mentioned population. To do so, an arbitrary reduction in APACHE III score (20%) was selected as reflecting physiologic improvements in these septic patients. The data in Table 4 also demonstrate the relative changes in IL-6 and sTNF-R in relation to this 72 h change in risk score.

Conclusions

1. Measurement of endotoxin and cytokine mediators has thus far been confined to small investigator initiated or therapeutic trials.
2. The reported levels of such mediators (with the possible exception of IL-6) at the time of diagnosis and/or meeting entry criteria provide little insight into the magnitude of host response or risk. Level of Evidence: II/III
3. Measurements of mediator-induced species, such as soluble, natural antagonists, or biochemical/hormone markers may provide a better correlate (surrogate) for estimating the initial magnitude of host response or risk. Level of Evidence: III
4. Although not discriminatory for risk at the time of diagnosis, current data suggest that some mediator levels are responsive to the short term clinical response to therapy. Level of Evidence: II/III
5. Additional risk discrimination may be provided by functional immunologic parameters. This is evident during the later course of sepsis, but may also be of importance at the outset. Level of Evidence: III

Recommendations

1. Efforts to standardize mediator assays among centers and across studies is mandatory. Grade A.
2. In several cases (TNF, IL-1), it is also equally necessary to clarify the correlation of such assays with *relevant* biologic functions. Grade B.
3. Such assays should be performed and analyzed, at least in placebo patients, for those completed/anticipated clinical trials in sepsis. Grade A.
4. Interactions with treatment effects and organ dysfunction should be established. Grade B.
5. Correlations of single and multiple determinants to current predictive (initial and dynamic) models should be undertaken. Grade C.

References

1. Waage A, Halstensen A, Espevik T (1987) Association between tumour necrosis factor in serum and fatal outcome in patients with meningococcal disease. Lancet 1:355–357
2. Fong Y, Lowry SF (1990) Tumor necrosis factor in the pathophysiology of infection and sepsis. Clin Immunol Immunopathol 55:157–170
3. Girardin E, Grau GE, Dayer JM, Roux-Lombard P, the J5 study group, Lambert PH (1988) Tumor necrosis factor and interleukin-1 in the serum of children with severe infectious purpura. N Engl J Med 319:397–400
4. Damas P, Reuter A, Gysen P, Demonty J, Lamy M, Franchimont P (1989) Tumor necrosis factor and interleukin-1 serum levels during severe sepsis in humans. Crit Care Med 17:975–978
5. Cannon JG, Tompkins RG, Gelfand JA, et al (1990) Circulating interleukin-1 and tumor necrosis factor in septic shock and experimental endotoxin fever. J Infect Dis 161:79–84
6. Casey LC, Balk RA, Bone RC (1993) Plasma cytokine and endotoxin levels correlate with survival in patients with the sepsis syndrome. Ann Intern Med 119:771–778
7. Van der Poll T, Jansen J, van Leenen D, et al (1993) Release of soluble receptors for tumor necrosis factor in clinical sepsis and experimental endotoxemia. J Infect Dis 168:955–960
8. Debets JMH, Kampmeijer R, van der Linden MPMH, Buurman WA, van der Linden CJ (1989) Plasma tumor necrosis factor and mortality in critically ill patients. Crit Care Med 17:489–494
9. Calandra T, Baumgartner JD, Grau GE, et al (1990) Prognostic values of tumor necrosis factor/cachectin, interleukin-1, interferon-α, and interferon-γ in the serum of patients with septic shock. J Infect Dis 161:982–987
10. Marano MA, Fong Y, Moldawer LL, et al (1990) Serum cachectin/tumor necrosis factor in critically ill patients with burns correlates with infection and mortality. Surg Gynecol Obstet 170:32–38
11. Marks JD, Marks CB, Luce JM, et al (1990) Plasma tumor necrosis factor in patients with septic shock. Am Rev Respir Dis 141:94–97
12. Offner F, Philippé J, Vogelaers D, et al (1990) Serum tumor necrosis factor levels in patients with infectious disease and septic shock. J Lab Clin Med 116:100–105
13. Wortel CH, von der Möhlen MAM, van Deventer SJH, et al (1992) Effectiveness of a human monoclonal anti-endotoxin antibody (HA-1A) in gram-negative sepsis: Relation to endotoxin and cytokine levels. J Infect Dis 166:1367–1374
14. Dinarello CA (1991) Interleukin-1 and interleukin-1 antagonism. Blood 77:1627–1652

15. Munoz C, Misset B, Fitting C, Blériot JP, Carlet J, Cavaillon JM (1991) Dissociation between plasma and monocyte-associated cytokines during sepsis. Eur J Immunol 21:2177–2184
16. Cannon JG, van der Meer JWM, Kwiatkowski D, et al (1988) Interleukin-1β in human plasma: Optimization of blood collection, plasma extraction and radioimmunoassay methods. Lymphokine Res 7:457–467
17. Cannon JG, Nerad JL, Poutsiaka DD, Dinarello CA (1993) Measuring circulating cytokines. J Appl Physiol 75:1897–1902
18. Waage A, Brandtzaeg P, Halstensen A, Kierulf P, Espevik T (1989) The complex pattern of cytokines in serum from patients with meningococcal septic shock. J Exp Med 169:333–338
19. Helfgott DC, Tatter SB, Santhanam U, et al (1989) Multiple forms of IFN-β_2/IL-6 in serum and body fluids during acute bacterial infection. J Immunol 142:948–953
20. Hack CE, de Groot ER, Felt-Bersma RJF, et al (1989) Increased plasma levels of interleukin-6 in sepsis. Blood 74:1704–1710
21. Calandra T, Gérain J, Heumann D, Baumgartner JD, Glauser MP, the Swiss-Dutch J5 Immunoglobulin Study Group (1991) High circulating levels of interleukin-6 in patients with septic shock: Evolution during sepsis, prognostic value, and interplay with other cytokines. Am J Med 91:23–29
22. Hack CE, Hart M, Strack van Schijndel RJM, et al (1992) Interleukin-8 in sepsis: Relation to shock and inflammatory mediators. Infect Immunol 60:2835–2842
23. Friedland JS, Suputtamongkol Y, Remick DG, et al (1992) Prolonged elevation of interleukin-8 and interleukin-6 concentrations in plasma and of leukocyte interleukin-8 mRNA levels during septicemic and localized Pseudomonas pseudomallei infection. Infect Immunol 60:2402–2408
24. Danner RL, Suffredini AF, Van Dervort AL, et al (1990) Detection of interleukin 6 (IL-6) and interleukin 8 (IL-8) during septic shock in humans. Clin Res 38:352a (Abst)
25. Hoffmann WD, Natanson C (1993) Endotoxin in spetic shock. Anesth Analg 77:613–624
26. Van Deventer SJH, Büller HR, ten Cate JW, Sturk A, Pauw W (1988) Endotoxaemia: An early predictor of septicaemia in febrile patients. Lancet 1:605–609
27. Brandtzaeg P, Kierulf P, Gaustad J, et al (1988) Plasma endotoxin as a predictor of multiple organ failure and death in systemic meningococcal disease. J Infect Dis 159:195–204
28. Danner RL, Elin RJ, Hosseini JM, Wesley RA, Reilly JM, Parillo JE (1991) Endotoxemia in human septic shock. Chest 99:169–175
29. Dinarello CA, Cannon JG (1993) Cytokine measurements in septic shock. Ann Intern Med 119:853–854
30. Coyle SM, Van Zee KJ, Trousdale RK, et al (1993) Circulating cytokine antagonists in endotoxemia and sepsis. Clin Nutr 12 (Suppl 2):29
31. van der Poll T, van Deventer SJH, ten Cate H, Levi M, ten Cate JW (1994) Tumor necrosis factor is involved in the appearance of interleukin-1 receptor antagonist in endotoxemia. J Infect Dis 169:665–667
32. Van Zee KJ, Kohno T, Fischer E, Rock CS, Moldawer LL, Lowry SF (1992) Tumor necrosis factor soluble receptors circulate during experimental and clinical inflammation and can protect against excessive Tumor Necrosis Factor α *in vitro* and *in vivo*. Proc Natl Acad Sci 89:4845–4849
33. Lowry SF, Moldawer LL (1992) Cytokines and cytokine antagonists in sepsis and critical illness. In: Vincent JL (ed) Yearbook of Intensive Care and Emergency Medicine 1992. Springer-Verlag, Berlin, pp 36–43
34. Fischer E, Van Zee KJ, Marano MA, et al (1992) Interleukin-1 receptor antagonist circulates in experimental inflammation and in human disease. Blood 79:2196–2200
35. Cinat ME, Waxman K, Granger GA, Pearce W, Annas C, Daughters K (1993) Trauma causes sustained elevation of soluble tumor necrosis factor receptors. Surg Gynecol Obstet (in press)

36. Rogy MA, Coyle SM, Rock CS, et al (1993) Persistently elevated soluble tumor necrosis factor receptor and interleukin-1 receptor antagonist levels in critically ill patients. J Am Coll Surg 178:132–138, 1994
37. Rogy MA, Oldenburg HSA, Trousdale RK, Coyle SM, Moldawer LL, Lowry SF (1993) Correlation between physiological and immunological parameters in critically ill septic patients. Intensive Care Med 20 (Suppl 1):S109
38. Simms HH, D'Amico R (1992) Intra-abdominal sepsis alters tumor necrosis factor-alpha and interleukin-1 beta binding to human neutrophils. Crit Care Med 20:11–16
39. McCall CE, Grosso-Wilmoth LM, LaRue K, Guzman RN, Cousart SL (1993) Tolerance to endotoxin-induced expression of the interleukin-1β gene in blood neutrophils of humans with the sepsis syndrome. J Clin Invest 91:853–861
40. Rogy MA, Oldenburg HSA, Calvano SE, et al (1993) Impact of anti-endotoxin therapy utilizing bacterial/permeability-increasing protein during primate bacteremia. Surg Forum 44:111–114
41. Calvano SE, Thompson WA, Coyle SM, et al (1993) Changes in monocyte and soluble TNF receptors during endotoxemia or sepsis. Surg Forum 44:114–116
42. Fischer E, Marano MA, Van Zee KJ, et al (1992) Interleukin-1 receptor blockade improves survival and hemodynamic performance in *E. coli* septic shock, but fails to alter host responses to sublethal endotoxemia. J Clin Invest 89:1551–1557
43. Barber AE, Coyle SM, Marano MA, et al (1993) Glucocorticoid therapy alters hormonal and cytokine responses to endotoxin in man. J Immunol 150:1999–2006
44. de Groote MA, Martin MA, Densen P, Pfaller MA, Wenzel RP (1989) Plasma tumor necrosis factor levels in patients with presumed sepsis. JAMA 262:249–251
45. Girardin E, Roux-Lombard P, Grau GE, et al (1992) Imbalance between tumour necrosis factor-alpha and soluble TNF receptor concentrations in severe meningococcaemia. Immunology 76:20–23
46. van der Poll T, van Deventer SJH, ten Cate H, Levi M, ten Cate JW (1994) Tumor necrosis factor is involved in the appearance of interleukin-1 receptor antagonist in endotoxemia. J Infect Dis 169:665–667
47. Cinat ME, Waxman K, Granger GA, Pearce W, Annas C, Daughters K (1994) Trauma causes sustained elevation of soluble tumor necrosis factor receptors. J Am Coll Surg (in press)
48. Rogy MA, Oldenburg HSA, Trousdale RK, Coyle SM, Moldawer LL, Lowry SF (1994) Correlation between physiological and immunological parameters in critically ill septic patients. Inten Care Med 20 (Suppl 1):S109

Whole Body and Organ Measures of O_2 Availability

M. P. Fink

Introduction

It is generally accepted that maintaining an "adequate" (or "optimal") level of oxygen delivery is an important therapeutic goal in the management of patients with sepsis or septic shock. There is much controversy, however, about the proper way to define and monitor the adequacy of oxygen delivery (DO_2) in sepsis. This controversy reflects our poor understanding – despite more that thirty years of intensive research – of the effects of sepsis on cellular oxygen utilization (VO_2) and energy metabolism. Indeed, the very notion that organ dysfunction in sepsis occurs as a result of cellular energy starvation remains an attractive, but poorly substantiated, hypothesis.

Current Concepts of Energy and Oxygen Metabolism in Sepsis

Several lines of evidence support the idea that sepsis leads to tissue hypoxia and/or depletion of energy stores in cells. However, in most cases, other observations, or contradictory findings, can be cited, which call into question the assertion that sepsis leads to derangements in energy metabolism at the cellular level. Some of the arguments for and against the notion that sepsis impairs cellular oxygenation and/or energy stores are reviewed here.

Direct Measurements of Cellular Concentrations of High-Energy Phosphates

In some studies, direct measurements, using ^{31}P-nuclear magnetic resonance spectroscopy (NMR) or conventional biochemical assays, have documented that cellular levels of adenosine triphosphate (ATP) are depleted in septic patients [1] or animals with sepsis or endotoxemia [2–6]. Other studies have determined that tissue levels of ATP are within the normal range in various organs, including liver [7], heart [8–11], brain [12], and skeletal muscle [13], obtained from septic or endotoxic animals. Although levels of phosphocreatine (PCr), another high-energy phosphate compound, have been shown to be slightly diminished in skeletal muscle in some studies of sepsis in rats, the observed changes in PCr concentration have not been associated with a decrement in ATP concentration [14, 15], and it is ATP rather PCr, which is thought to be the primary energy "currency" of the cell. The lack of agreement among studies regarding the effect of sepsis on cellular ATP concentrations may reflect differences in the response to sepsis among various organs [2, 16] or differences among the models employed; for example, some data suggest that renal and hepatic ATP levels are depleted in "late" but not "early" sepsis [17–20].

Increased Circulating and Tissue Concentrations of Lactate as a Marker of Anaerobiosis in Sepsis

Sepsis is frequently associated with the development of metabolic acidosis and increased circulating concentrations of lactate [21]. These findings have been interpreted as evidence of increased anaerobic metabolism due to cellular hypoxia in patients with sepsis [22–25]. Since ATP is generated much less efficiently by anaerobic as compared to aerobic metabolism, the presence of high circulating lactate levels in sepsis has been viewed as indirect evidence of energy starvation at the cellular level.

It is increasingly apparent, however, that increased cellular and/or circulating lactate concentrations in sepsis do not necessarily indicate the presence of tissue hypoxia or depletion of cellular stores of high-energy phosphates. Perhaps the most direct data in this regard comes from a recent study by Hurtado et al. [26], which compared a number of parameters in two groups of rabbits. In the first group of rabbits (called "LOQ"), cardiac output was decreased by inflating a balloon in the right ventricle. In the other group (called "SEP"), cardiac output was diminished to a similar extent by infusing a bolus dose of lipopolysaccharide (LPS). In both groups, systemic DO_2 and VO_2, decreased by about the same amount, but arterial lactate concentrations were significantly higher in the SEP group. Moreover, skeletal muscle lactate concentrations were much higher in the SEP group than LOQ group, although skeletal muscle pO2 values, ATP concentrations, and PCr concentrations were similar in the two groups. In another study, we compared blood lactate concentrations in several groups of pigs, two of which are of particular interest in the context of this discussion [27]. One group was challenged with LPS and infused with crystalloid solution at a rate sufficient to keep cardiac output at approximately the baseline (i.e. normal) level. Another group was challenged with the same dose of LPS, but, in addition to receiving crystalloid solution, also was resuscitated with colloid solution and dobutamine so that cardiac output was increased to approximately twice the baseline value. Blood lactate concentrations increased progressively in both endotoxic groups despite the large difference in systemic DO_2 in the group which received colloid and dobutamine resuscitation. Similar results recently were reported by Rudinsky and Meadow [28].

Work by Vary and colleagues [30] suggests that an important mechanism responsible for hyperlactatemia in sepsis is inactivation of the enzyme complex, pyruvate dehydrogenase (PDH). This enzyme, which catalyzes the first irreversible step in the mitochondrial oxidative pathway for pyruvate, exists in both active (dephosphorylated) and inactive (phosphorylated) forms. If the relative proportion of inactive PDH were to increase in sepsis, then flux of substrate through the tricarboxylic acid (Krebs) cycle would decrease and maintenance of intracellular levels of ATP would require an increased rate of substrate level phosphorylation, i.e. the rate of pyruvate (and lactate) production via glycolysis would increase. Vary et al. [2] have demonstrated that sepsis does not affect total PDH activity, but increases the proportion in the inactive form in skeletal muscle. Treatment of septic or endotoxemic animals with dichloroacetate, an agent which activates the PDH complex, has been shown to decrease tissue and circulating lactate levels [29, 30].

Another mechanism that may be responsible for hyperlactatemia in sepsis is an increase in the rate glycolysis independent of the flux of substrate through the Krebs cycle; i.e. accelerated aerobic glycolysis [31]. Lang and colleagues have established that glucose utilization is increased in septic or endotoxic animals [32, 33]. Moreover, recent data suggest that one mechanism for this phenomenon may be increased availability of glucose transporters on the surface of cells, either due to translocation of "spare" transporters from the cytosol to the plasma membrane [34] or transcription of new message for the transporter protein [35].

The etiology of "metabolic" acidosis in sepsis remains incompletely understood. Excess hydrolysis of ATP to adenosine diphosphate (ADP) plus inorganic phosphate plus protons might explain the development of some of the acidosis of sepsis [36], although as noted above, many studies suggest that ATP levels are normal in tissues obtained from septic animals. If ATP levels are preserved in sepsis by increased fermentation of glucose to lactate (i.e. increased substrate level phosphorylation of ADP), then metabolic acidosis would be a consequence, since the stoichiometry of anaerobiosis necessitates the production of protons [37]. Data exist, however, to suggest that lactate is not the only anion associated with metabolic acidosis in sepsis, and other, poorly defined, anions may be important as well. In a study of 30 septic patients, Mecher et al. [38] calculated a "corrected ion gap" as the conventional anion gap minus the anionic contributions of lactate, phosphate, urate, and total serum proteins. In this study, the mean (uncorrected) anion gap was 21.8 ± 1.4 mM and the mean "corrected anion gap" was 3.7 ± 0.8 mM, suggesting the presence of an unidentified anion (or anions) in patients with metabolic acidosis secondary to sepsis. This same group of investigators conducted a similar study in a rat model of peritonitis [39], and found that only 15% of the increase in the anion gap in septic animals could be accounted for by an increase in lactate concentration. Moreover, the widened anion gap in this animal model of severe sepsis could not be explained by changes in the circulating concentrations of several other anionic metabolic intermediates, including citrate, β-hydroxybutyrate, acetoacetate, creatinine, albumin, or anionic amino acidis.

Pathological Supply-Dependency of Oxygen Uptake

In mammals, different organs and tissues display differing metabolic responses to variations in DO_2 [40]. In many tissues, which have been termed "O_2 regulators", VO_2 is maintained or *regulated* by the cells at a nearly constant rate, unless oxygen availability falls to very low levels. Thus, a plot of VO_2 versus DO_2 is biphasic, being characterized by a flat availability-independent region and a sloped availability-dependent region. The point of transition between these two regions has been termed the "critical DO_2" or DO_{2crit}.

In some tissues, called "O_2 conformers", VO_2 is a function of oxygen availability over a wide range of values [40]. For example, some studies suggest that skeletal muscle exhibits an O_2 conforming pattern, at least under certain conditions [41–43]. Liver expresses an intermediate pattern. This organ displays evidence of O_2 regulation at relatively high rates of DO_2, but shifts to a conforming pattern with even modest reductions in oxygen availability [44].

In anesthetized animals, the normal relationship between systemic DO_2 and systemic VO_2 is one of O_2 regulation [45–48]. In anesthetized dogs, DO_{2crit} occurs at about 8 mL/min/kg [48]. Using data points pooled over multiple patients, Shibutani et al. [49] and Komatsu et al. [50] have estimated that DO_{2crit} occurs at about 300–330 mL/min/M^2 (8 mL/min/kg) in anesthetized humans. Recently, Ronco et al. [51] reported the results of an elegant and important clinical study, which was designed to determine DO_{2crit} in critically ill patients in whom the decision to discontinue life support had been made by the patients' families and attending physicians. In this study, systemic DO_2 and VO_2 were repetitively determined at 5 to 20 min intervals as life support was progressively withdrawn, first by discontinuing vasoactive drugs, then decreasing fractional inspired oxygen concentration to 0.21, and then removing mechanical ventilatory support. In this way, DO_{2crit} could be determined on a subject-by-subject basis, rather than by pooling data obtained by studying multiple patients. The eight nonseptic subjects in this study tended to display a pattern of O_2 regulation; the mean DO_{2crit} was 4.5 ± 1.3 mL/min/kg.

In 1978, in a study of 11 patients with the acute respiratory distress syndrome (ARDS), Rhodes et al. [52] examined the effects on systemic oxygen metabolism of acutely expanding circulating volume with an IV infusion of mannitol solution. Sepsis was the underlying cause of ARDS in 6 of the patients studied. Although cardiac output and systemic DO_2 were already supranormal prior to the volume challenge in these patients, infusing mannitol significantly increased both systemic DO_2 and systemic VO_2. Thus, the patients manifested an O_2 conforming pattern; i.e. supply-dependency of VO_2 even at high rates of DO_2. Numerous subsequent studies, using a variety of means for manipulating systemic DO_2, have replicated this observation in patients with sepsis and/or ARDS [53–57].

This phenomenon, which Cain has termed "pathological supply-dependency" of oxygen uptake [58], has two key features:

1. dependency of (systemic or regional) VO_2 and DO_2 even at normal or supranormal levels of DO_2; and
2. impaired O_2 extraction by tissues, manifested by a flattening of the slope of the dependent region on a plot of VO_2 as a function of DO_2.

In studies using septic or endotoxic dogs, which seem to confirm the findings in patients cited above, Schumacker and colleagues have obtained evidence of impaired systemic and transmesenteric O_2 extraction [25, 59, 60].

Dependence of VO_2 on DO_2 implies that utilization of oxygen is being determined by availability rather than metabolic demand. Thus, it has been suggested that the demonstration of "pathological" supply-dependency of systemic VO_2 in patients with sepsis is evidence of an oxygen deficit at the tissue level [61], a notion that seems (at least at first glance) to be supported by studies showing that supply-dependency in septic patients is demonstrable only in those with elevated circulating concentrations of lactate [23, 24, 62, 63].

Few topics in critical care medicine have generated as much controversy as the notion that systemic or regional VO_2 is "pathologically" supply-dependent in septic patients. In contrast to the data just cited, there now exist numerous studies which support the following conclusions:

1. systemic VO_2 are independent of DO_2 in patients with sepsis and/or ARDS, irrespective of whether circulating lactate concentrations are normal or elevated [51, 64–70];
2. DO_{2crit} and maximal systemic oxygen extraction are similar in septic and nonseptic patients [51]; and
3. systemic and mesenteric oxygen extraction ratios at DO_{2crit} are similar in endotoxic and nonendotoxic pigs [71].

Many reasons have been proposed to account for the discrepant findings among the numerous studies, which have investigated the relationship between oxygen availability and utilization in sepsis. A full review of this issue is beyond the scope of the present chapter. There are multiple confounding factors which may have clouded the data in this area, including: "mathematical coupling" of DO_2 and VO_2, when both parameters are calculated using data obtained by pulmonary arterial catheterization; the effects of spontaneous changes in VO_2 (acting as the independent variable) on DO_2; inappropriate "pooling" of data obtained over multiple patients; and, the direct thermogenic (i.e. VO_2-increasing) effects of inotropic agents, like dopamine, dobutamine, and norepinephrine. It is sufficient to say here that the question of "pathological" supply-dependency of VO_2 in sepsis remains controversial, but, in my opinion, the weight of evidence currently favors the view that the ability of tissues to extract oxygen is *not* deranged in sepsis.

Mitochondrial Dysfunction

Another very controversial area is the effect of sepsis, LPS, or cytokines on mitochondrial respiration. Over the years, widely divergent results in this area have been obtained by different investigators. For example, in 1975, Greer and Milazzo [72] showed that adding *Pseudomonas aeruginosa* LPS to mitochondria isolated from rat livers resulted in increased utilization of oxygen in the presence of substrate and the absence of ADP (State 4 respiration) and a decreased respiratory response to the addition of ADP (State 3 respiration). These findings are indicative of uncoupling of respiration from phosphorylation; i.e. an effect similar to that induced by the classic uncoupling agent, 2,4-dinithrophenol. Evidence of uncoupled oxidative phosphorylation also was obtained by Mela et al. [73], who harvested hepatic mitochondria after *in vivo* exposure to LPS. In contrast to these findings, Decker et al. [74] found no evidence of dysfunction of mitochondria harvested from rats with gram-negative bacterial peritonitis. Similarly, negative findings have been reported by many other groups as well, including Tanaka et al. [75] Clemens et al. [76], and Spitzer and Deaciuc [77].

Recently, the Pittsburgh group led by Simmons and Billiar [78, 79] reopened the question of mitochondrial dysfunction in sepsis. These workers demonstrated that two mediators implicated in the pathophysiology of sepsis, namely, tumor necrosis factor α (TNF) and nitric oxide (NO), inhibit mitochondrial State 3 respiration; i. e. these mediators induce changes in mitochondrial function reminiscent of those observed by Mela et al. and others. The mechanism, at least in part, seems to be inhibition of key mitochondrial enzymes, including aconitase, NADH-ubiquinone oxidoreductase, and succinate-ubiquinone oxidoreductase [78].

The Rationale for Monitoring Oxygen Availability, Oxygen Utilization, and Cellular Bioenergetics in Patients with Sepsis

From the preceding discussion, one is tempted to conclude that although tissue oxygenation and/or cellular bioenergetics may be deranged in sepsis, the data supporting the existence of such phenomena must be considered, at best, controversial. Accordingly, one might conclude that monitoring (and, attempting to manipulate) DO_2, VO_2 or cellular energy status in patients with sepsis is not a strategy that is likely to improve outcome. This conclusion, however, is unwarranted for two reasons.

First, patients with sepsis often have other problems (e.g. hypovolemia, anemia, hypoxemia, myocardial dysfunction) that clearly *can* cause hypoperfusion and/or inadequate delivery of oxygen tissues; awareness and correction of these problems undoubtedly can improve outcome irrespective of whether sepsis *per se* leads to disruption of energy homeostasis at the cellular level.

Second, hints are starting to appear in the experimental and clinical literature that organ system function and/or survival can be improved when septic subjects are resuscitated to supranormal levels of cardiac output and systemic DO_2. Consider:

- We have shown that infusing pigs with LPS leads to mesenteric hypoperfusion and gut mucosal hyperpermeability to hydrophilic solutes [80]. If mesenteric hypoperfusion is prevented by infusing endotoxic animals with a colloid solution and dobutamine, a regimen that leads an approximate doubling of cardiac output with respect to normal values, then LPS-induced ileal mucosal hyperpermeability is abrogated [27].
- Tuchschmidt et al. [81] enrolled 51 patients with septic shock in prospective clinical trial, which was designed to test the hypothesis that resuscitation to supranormal indices of DO_2 can improve outcome. Twenty-five were randomized to receive normal treatment (i.e. colloid solution, dopamine, and/or dobutamine titrated to maintain cardiac output at ≥ 3 L/min/M^2 and systolic blood pressure ≥ 90 mm Hg). Twenty-six patients were randomized to receive treatment (colloid solution, dopamine, and/or dobutamine) titrated to maintain cardiac output at ≥ 6 L/min/M^2. When the results were analyzed on an intent-to-treat basis, mortality was 72% in the control arm as compared to 50% in the ("optimal treatment") group receiving therapy titrated to a supranormal cardiac output ($p=0.14$); i.e. there was a trend toward improved outcome, which did not achieve statistical significance, when septic patients were managed with the "optimal treatment" strategy. However, when results were analyzed by stratifying the patients into low (<4.5 L/min/M^2) and high (≥ 4.5 L/min/M^2) cardiac output groups, both survival and systemic DO_2 were significantly ($p<0.05$) higher in the high cardiac output group than in the low Q_T group (60 vs 26% and 13.8 mL/min/kg vs 10.9 mL/min/kg, respectively). Thus, it is unclear whether high cardiac output and DO_2 are direct determinants of survival, or whether the ability to increase cardiac output is a marker for greater "physiologic reserve" which portends a better outcome.
- Yu et al. [82] recently reported the results of a randomized trial which was similar in design to the one just described by Tuchschmidt and colleagues. The study by Yu et al. enrolled 67 patients with sepsis or ARDS. Patients were randomly allocated to treatment or control groups. In the treatment group, resuscitation (intravenous fluids, blood products, inotropic agents, and/or vasodilators) were titrated to achive a systemic DO_2 of 600 mL/min/M^2, whereas in the control group, the hemodynamic endpoint of therapy was a systemic DO_2 of "450 to 550" mL/min/M^2. The protocol sought to achieve the desired DO_2 goal within the first 24 h of therapy. The interventions were continued until death or removal of the pulmonary artery catheter. Because some patients in treatment group failed to achieve the desired DO_2 goal of 600 mL/min/M^2, and some patients in the control group increased DO_2 to greater than 600 mL/min/M^2 on their own, the

actual mean DO_2 values measured at 24 h were quite similar in the two arms of trial (604 ± 169 ml/min/M^2 in controls, 617 ± 202 mL/min/M^2 in the experimental group). When results were analyzed on an intent-to-treat basis, mortality (34%) was the same in both treatment groups. However, when patients were stratified according to measured DO_2 at 24 h, mortality was 5/35 (14%) in those achieving a DO_2 greater than 600 mL/min/M^2 as compared to 15/27 (56%) in those failing to achieve a DO_2 greater than 600 mL/min/M^2 ($p < 0.001$). Further subset analyses suggested that mortality was similarly low in patients who achieved a high DO_2 on their own and patients who achieved a high DO_2 as a result of active intervention. Unfortunately, the sizes of these subsets were small, and the analytical plan for the trial was designed to look at the effect of the intervention. Thus, it is premature that "pushing" DO_2 to high levels prevents mortality in septic patients. The data, however, suggest that another trial, designed specifically to compare mortality in patients "pushed" to high DO_2 with those achieving this outcome on their own, is warranted.

From the preceding, it seems prudent to monitor cardiac output and arterial oxygen content in septic patients, with the objective of using intravenous fluids and inotropic agents to keep systemic DO_2 at or above 600 mL/min/M^2. While unequivocal data are lacking to show that such a strategy is beneficial, the findings reported by Tuchschmidt et al. [81] and Yu et al. [82] suggest that resuscitation of septic patients to supranormal levels of DO_2 may improve outcome. Certainly, the data obtained in these two studies makes it clear that this therapeutic approach is by no means harmful.

Gut Mucosal Acidosis as an Endpoint

In the past few years, tonometric estimation of gastrointestinal (particularly, gastric) mucosal pH ("pHi") has been extensively investigated as a means for assessing the adequacy of "delivery of oxygen" to a key visceral bed (the gut) in critically ill patients [83]. In this technique, muscosal PCO_2 is measured tonometrically, as originally described by Bergofsky [84] and Dawson et al. [85]. The assumption is then made that tissue and arterial bicarbonate concentrations are similar. By substituting mucosal PCO_2 and arterial bicarbonate into the Henderson-Hasselbach equation, it is possible to back-calculate pHi. Our group has compared tonometric estimation of ileal pHi to direct measurements made with micro-electrodes, and shown that, in pigs with endotoxicosis or mesenteric hypoperfusion (but not complete ischemia), the two methods agree reasonably well [86].

We [87] and others [88] have shown that ileal mucosal acidosis is reproducibly elicited when pigs are subjected to an endotoxic or septic challenge. Moreover, we have shown that a portion of the LPS-induced decrease in muscosal pH reflects the development of systemic acidosis, but the remainder is caused by a local (i.c. mucosa-specific) increase in hydrogen ion concentration [89]. Since we [87, 90] and others [91], have demonstrated that endotoxemia and sepsis are associated with decreases in mesenteric and gut mucosal blood flow, one mechanism contributing to mucosal acidosis in sepsis or endotoxemia might be cellular hypoxia due to ischemia. However, recent data obtained by our group suggest that mucosal PO_2 actually *increases* to supranormal levels in endotoxemic pigs [unpublished observations]. Furthermore, transmesenteric VO_2 is well-preserved in septic [88] or endotoxemic [27] pigs. Thus, cellular hypoxia probably is not a major factor contributing to sepsis-induced mucosal acidosis, at least in animal models.

Another factor, which may account for the development of gut mucosal acidosis in sepsis, is the effect of mucosal hypoperfusion on the clearance of carbon dioxide generated by normal cellular respiration. As Johnson and Weil have pointed out [92], organ and tissue hypercarbia are an inevitable consequence of hypoperfusion, simply on the basis of the Fick relationship. Thus, in contradistinction to some stratements which have been made in the literature [83], tonometric evidence of gut mucosal acidosis in critically ill patients (including those with sepsis) is not necessarily indicative of tissue hypoxia, but may simply reflect tissue hypoperfusion.

Irrespective of the pathophysiological basis for gut mucosal acidosis in critical illness, there can be little doubt that this finding portends a bad prognosis [93–95]. Indeed, recent data obtained by Marik et al. suggest that gastric pHi is a better predictor of outcome in septic patients than are a number of other commonly measured parameters, including blood lactate concentration, systemic DO_2, cardiac output, and systemic VO_2. In a multi-institutional trial conducted in Argentina, Gutierrez et al. [96] showed that titrating therapy to achieve a normal gastric pHi can improve survival in critically ill patients. Although sepsis was not specifically addressed in this study, the results obtained by Gutierrez and colleagues suggest that preventing (or limiting the duration of) gut mucosal acidosis may be important in the management of patients with this diagnosis.

Recent results from our group may provide a hint of at least one reason for the association of gastrointestinal mucosal acidosis with a bad outcome in critically ill patients [90]. In an extensive series of studies in pigs, we showed that ileal mucosal permeability is linearly related to the degree of mucosal acidosis in pigs subjected to graded degrees of mechanically-induced mesenteric ischemia or injected with graded doses of LPS (Fig. 1). In a second series of experiments, we induced ileal mucosal acidosis in normal pigs by mechanical ventilation with either a hypoxic or a hypercarbic gas mixture. In the hypoxic group, tissue acidosis occurred as a direct consequence of anaerobiosis. However, in the hypercarbic group, mesenteric DO_2 and mucosal blood flow were well preserved. Nevertheless, in both groups, ileal mucosal permeability to a macromolecular hydrophilic solute (dextran with an average molecular weight of 4000 D) increased dramatically (Fig. 2). These data suggest that gut mucosal acidosis (whether on the basis of anaerobic metabolism or hypoperfusion or both), may lead to functional derangements in the integrity of the mucosal barrier.

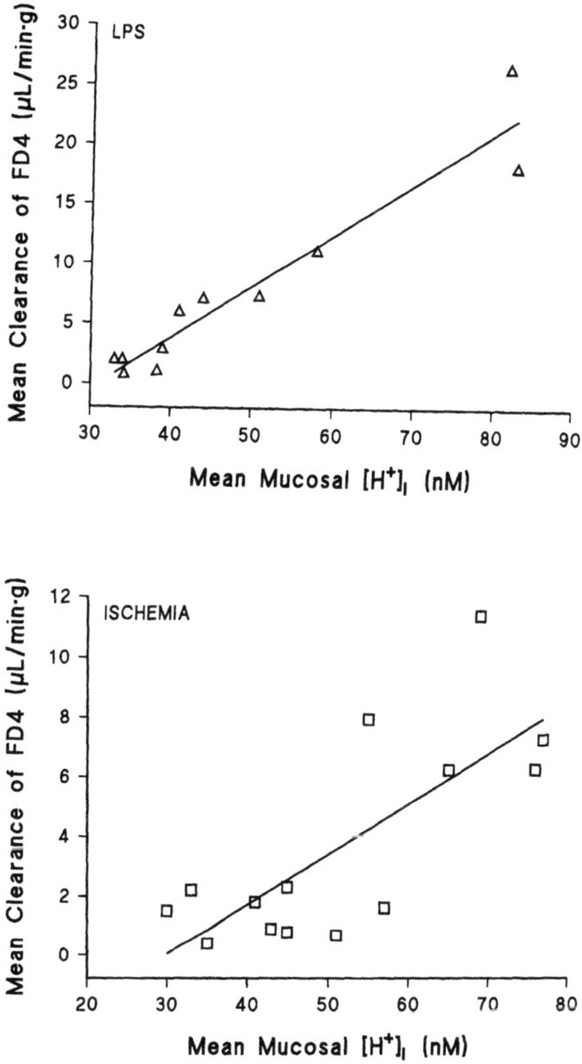

Fig. 1. Relationship of mean mucosal hydrogen ion concentration, $[H^+]_I$, to the mean plasma-to-lumen clearance (a measure of ileal mucosal permeability) of fluorescein-labelled dextran (avg molecular weight = 4000 D) over a 4-hour-period of observation in pigs infused with graded doses of LPS (top panel) or subjected to graded degrees of mechanically-induced partial mesenteric ischemia (bottom panel). Mean $[H^+]_I$ and mean dextran clearance (i. e. permeability) were well correlated in animals subjected to either endotoxicosis ($R^2=0.93$, $p<0.001$) or mechanically-induced partial mesenteric ischemia ($R^2=0.58$, $p<0.002$). (From [90] with permission)

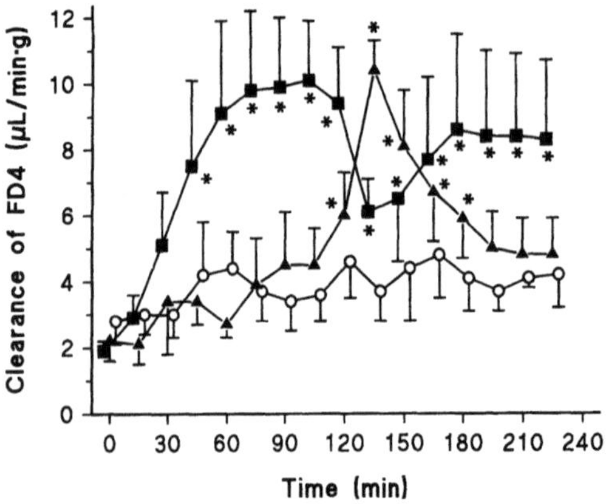

Fig. 2. Plasma-to-lumen clearance of fluorescein-labelled dextran (avg molecular weight = 4000 D) in pigs subjected to hypoxemia (0–120 min; ■), hypercarbia (0–120 min; ▲), or only to general anesthesia and surgical preparation (○). * indicates $p<0.05$ by analysis of variance and Dunnett's test. (From [90] with permission)

Speculations

A number of investigational means for monitoring tissue oxygenation, perfusion, and/or energetics are currently being evaluated. Among these are near-infrared spectroscopy (to monitor the redox state of the terminal cytochrome in the mitochondrial electron transport chain, cytochrome a, a_3), NMR spectroscopy (to monitor intracellular concentrations of ATP, Pi, and hydrogen ion), and subcutaneous oxygen tension monitors. However, until more is learned about cellular energetics in spesis, the use of such sophisticated monitoring in patients with sepsis or septic shock probably is premature. Given currently available information, monitoring conventional markers of oxygen availability (especially cardiac output and systemic DO_2) makes some sense, although the final word on this issue has yet to be written. Interestingly, improving cardiac output may improve outcome not by increasing oxygen availability at the tissue level, but by augmenting clearance of carbon dioxide. Increasingly, it seems likely that monitoring gastrointestinal pHi (or maybe simply the tissue-arterial PCO_2 gap) will play an important role in the management of patients with sepsis. Improvements in the technology for monitoring mucosal PCO_2 [97], which decrease the cost and increase the ease of obtaining the data, will further spur needed research in this area.

Conclusions

1. The following parameters consistently have been shown to have prognostic significance in patients with sepsis: systemic DO_2, blood lactate concentration, and gastric mucosal pH (Grades A to B).
2. The degree of metabolic acidosis (i.e. base deficit) also has prognostic significance (Grade B).
3. To date, solid data are lacking to support the notion that titrating therapy to specific goals for these parameters improves (or affects) outcome.

Recommendations

1. The monitoring of indices of oxygen metabolism (or related variables such as blood lactate concentration or gastric mucosal pH) may be of value in the conduct of clinical trials of new agents for sepsis in order to:
   a) detect imbalances in randomization, and
   b) track the biological effects of therapeutic intervention (Grade A to B).
2. In designing trials of new agents for the adjuvant treatment of sepsis, it is not necessary or warranted to specify target values for indices of oxygen transport (Grade B).

References

1. Bergstrom J, Bostrom H, Furst P, Hultman E, Vinnars E (1976) Preliminary studies of energy-rich phosphagens in muscle from severely ill patients. Crit Care Med 4:197–204
2. Vary TC, Siegel JH, Nakatani T, Sato T, Aoyama H (1986) Effect of sepsis on activity of pyruvate dehydrogenase complex in skeletal muscle and liver. Am J Physiol 250:E634–E640
3. Astiz M, Rackow EC, Weil MH, Schumer W (1988) Early impairment of oxidative metabolism and energy production in severe sepsis. Circ Shock 26:311–320
4. Pelias ME, Townsend MC (1992) *In vivo* [^{31}P]NMR assessment of early hepatocellular dysfunction during endotoxemia. J Surg Res 52:505–509
5. Burns AH, Giaimo ME, Summer WR (1986) Dichloroacetic acid improves in vitro myocardial function following in vivo endotoxin administration. J Crit Care 1:11–17
6. Mori E, Hasebe M, Kobayashi K, Lijima N (1987) Alterations in metabolite levels in carbohydrate and energy metabolism of rat in hemorrhagic shock and sepsis. Metabolism 36:14–20
7. Pedersen P, Saljo A, Hasselgren PO (1987) Protein and energy metabolism in liver tissue following intravenous infusion of live *E. coli* bacteria in rats. Circ Shock 21:59–64
8. Hotchkiss RS, Song SK, Neil JJ, et al (1991) Sepsis does not impair tricarboxylic cycle in the heart. Am J Physiol 260:C50–C57
9. McDonough KH, Henry JJ, Lang CH, Spitzer JJ (1986) Substrate utilization and high energy phosphate levels of hearts from hyperdynamic septic rats. Circ Shock 18:161–170
10. Laughlin MH, Smyk-Randall EM, Novotny MJ, Brown OR, Adams HR (1988) Coronary blood flow and cardiac adenine nucleotides in *E. coli* endotoxemia in dogs: Effects of oxygen radical scavengers. Circ Shock 25:173–185
11. Pasque MK, Murphy CE, Van Trigt P, Pellom GL, Currie WD, Wechsler AS (1983) Myocardial adenosine triphosphate levels during early sepsis. Arch Surg 118:1437–1440
12. Hotchkiss RS, Rust RS, Song SK, Ackerman JJH (1993) Effect of sepsis on brain energy metabolism in normoxic and hypoxic rats. Circ Shock 40:303–310
13. Jepson MM, Cox M, Bates PC, et al (1987) Regional blood flow and skeletal muscle energy status in endotoxemic rats. Am J Physiol 252:E581–E587
14. Song SK, Hotchkiss RS, Karl IE, Ackerman JJH (1992) Concurrent quantification of tissue metabolism and blood flow via $^{2}H/^{31}P$ NMR in vivo, III: Alterations in muscle blood flow and metabolism during sepsis. Magn Reson Med 25:67–77
15. Jacobs DO, Kobayashi T, Imagire J, Grant C, Kesselly B, Wilmore DW (1991) Sepsis alters skeletal muscle energetics and membrane function. Surgery 110:318–326

16. Zager RA (1991) Adenine nucleotide changes in kidney, liver, and small intestine during different forms of ischemic injury. Circ Res 68:185–196
17. Haybron DM, Townsend MC, Hampton WW, Schirmer WJ, Schirmer JM, Fry DE (1987) Alterations in renal perfusion and renal energy charge in murine peritonitis. Arch Surg 122:328–331
18. Chaudry IH, Wichterman KA, Baue AE (1979) Effect of sepsis on tissue adenine nucleotide levels. Surgery 85:205–211
19. Shimahara Y, Kono Y, Tanaka J, et al (1987) Pathophysiology of acute renal failure following living *Escherichia coli* injection in rats: High-energy metabolism and renal functions. Circ Shock 21:197–205
20. Hampton WA, Townsend MC, Haybron DM, Shirmer WJ, Fry DE (1987) Effective hepatic blood flow and hepatic bioenergy status in murine peritonitis. J Surg Res 42:33–38
21. Blair E (1971) Acid-base balance in bacteremic shock. Arch Intern Med 127:731–739
22. Groeneveld ABJ, Kester ADM, Nauta JJP, Thijs LG (1987) Relation of arterial blood lactate to oxygen delivery and hemodynamic variables in human shock states. Circ Shock 22:35–53
23. Kruse JA, Haupt MT, Puri VK, Carlson RW (1990) Lactate levels as predictors of the relationship between oxygen delivery and consumption in ARDS. Chest 98:959–962
24. Haupt MT, Gilbert EM, Carlson RW (1985) Fluid loading increases oxygen consumption in septic patients with lactic acidosis. Am Rev Respir Dis 131:912–916
25. Nelson DP, Beyer C, Samsel RW, Wood LDH, Schumacker PT (1987) Pathological supply dependence of O_2 uptake during bacteremia in dogs. J Appl Physiol 63:1487–1492
26. Hurtado FJ, Gutierrez AM, Silva N, Fernandez E, Khan AE, Gutierrez G (1992) Role of tissue hypoxia as the mechanism of lactic acidosis during *E. coli* endotoxemia. J Appl Physiol 72:1895–1901
27. Fink MP, Kaups KL, Wang H, Rothschild HR (1991) Maintenance of superior mesenteric arterial perfusion prevents increased intestinal mucosal permeability in endotoxic pigs. Surgery 110:154–161
28. Rudinsky BF, Meadow WL (1992) Relationship between oxygen delivery and metabolic acidosis during sepsis in piglets. Crit Care Med 20:831–839
29. Curtis SE, Cain SM (1992) Regional and systemic oxygen delivery/uptake relations and lactate flux in hyperdynamic, endotoxin-treated dogs. Am Rev Respir Dis 145:348–354
30. Vary TC, Siegel JH, Tall BD, Morris JG (1988) Metabolic effects of partial reversal of pyruvate dehydrogenase activity by dichloroacetate in sepsis. Circ Shock 24:3–18
31. Hotchkiss RS, Karl IE (1992) Reevaluation of the role of cellular hypoxia and bioenergetic failure in sepsis. J Am Med Assoc 267:1503–1509
32. Lang CH, Bagby GJ, Dobrescu C, Ottlakan A, Spitzer JJ (1992) Sepsis- and endotoxin-induced increase in organ glucose uptake in leukocyte-depleted rats. Am J Physiol 263:R1324–R1332
33. Lang CH, Obih JCA, Bagby GJ, Bagwell JN, Spitzer JJ (1991) Increased glucose uptake by intestinal mucosa and muscularis in hypermetabolic sepsis. Am J Physiol 261:G287–G294
34. Windell CC, Baldwin SA, Davies A, Martin S, Pasternak CA (1990) Cellular stress induces a redistribution of the glucose transporter. FASEB J 4:1634–1637
35. Zeller WP, The SM, Sweet M, et al (1991) Altered glucose transporter mRNA abundance in a rat model of endotoxic shock. Biochem Biophys Res Commun 176:535–540
36. Gores GJ, Nieminen AL, Wray BE, Herman B, Lemasters JJ (1989) Intracellular pH during "chemical hypoxia" in cultured rat hepatocytes: Protection by intracellular acidosis against the onset of cell death. J Clin Invest 83:386–396
37. Mommsen TP, Hochachka PW (1983) Protons and anaerobiasis. Science 219:1391–1397
38. Mecher C, Rackow EC, Astiz ME, Weil MH (1991) Unaccounted for anion in metabolic acidosis during severe sepsis in humans. Crit Care Med 19:705–711

39. Rackow EC, Mecher C, Astiz ME, Goldstein C, McKee D, Weil MH (1990) Unmeasured anion during severe sepsis with metabolic acidosis. Circ Shock 30:107–115
40. Hochachka PW (1987) Metabolic suppression and oxygen availability. Can J Zool 66:152–158
41. Gutierrez G, Pohil RJ, Strong R (1989) Skeletal muscle oxygen consumption and energy metabolism during hypoxemia. J Appl Physiol 66:2117–2123
42. Duran WN, Renkin EM (1974) Oxygen consumption and blood flow in resting mammalian skeletal muscle. Am J Physiol 226:173–177
43. Whalen DF, Buerk D, Thuning CA (1973) Blood flow-limited oxygen consumption in resting cat skeletal muscle. Am J Physiol 224:763–768
44. Edelstone DI, Paulone ME, Holzman IR (1984) Hepatic oxygenation during arterial hypoxemia in neonatal lambs. Am J Obstet Gynecol 150:513–518
45. Cain SM (1975) Oxygen delivery and utilization in dogs with a sublethal dose of cobalt chloride. J Appl Physiol 38:20–25
46. Cain SM (1977) Oxygen delivery and uptake in dogs during anemic and hypoxic hypoxia. J Appl Physiol 42:228–234
47. Adams RP, Dieleman LA, Cain SM (1982) A critical value for O_2 transport in the rat. J Appl Physiol 53:660–664
48. Cilley RE, Polley TZ Jr, Zwischenberger JB, Toomasian JM, Bartlett RH (1989) Independent measurement of oxygen consumption and oxygen delivery. J Surg Res 472:242–247
49. Shibutani K, Komatsu T, Kubal K, Sanchala V, Kuman V, Bizzari D (1983) Critical level of oxygen delivery in anesthetized man. Crit Care Med 11:640–643
50. Komatsu T, Shibutani K, Okamoto K, et al (1987) Critical level of oxygen delivery after cardiopulmonary bypass. Crit Care Med 15:194–197
51. Ronco JJ, Fenwick JC, Tweeddale MG, et al (1993) Identification of the critical oxygen delivery for anaerobic metabolism in critically ill septic and nonseptic humans. J Am Med Assoc 270:1724–1730
52. Rhodes GR, Newell JC, Shah D, et al (1978) Increased oxygen consumption accompanying increased oxygen delivery with hypertonic mannitol in adult respiratory distress syndrome. Surgery 84:490–497
53. Danek SJ, Lynch JP, Weg JG, Dantzker DR (1980) The dependence of oxygen uptake on oxygen delivery in the adult respiratory distress syndrome. Am Rev Respir Dis 122:387–395
54. Mohsenifar Z, Goldbach P, Tashkin DP, Campisi DJ (1983) Relationship between O_2 delivery and O_2 consumption in the adult respiratory distress syndrome. Chest 84:267–271
55. Clarke C, Edwards JD, Nightingale P, Mortimer AJ, Morris J (1991) Persistence of supply dependency of oxygen uptake at high levels of delivery in adult respiratory distress syndrome. Crit Care Med 19:497–502
56. Lorente JA, Renes E, Gomez-Aguinaga MA, Landin L, de la Morena JL, Liste D (1991) Oxygen delivery-dependent oxygen consumption in acute respiratory failure. Crit Care Med 19:770–775
57. Wolf YG, Cotev S, Perel A, Manny J (1987) Dependence of oxygen consumption on cardiac output in sepsis. Crit Care Med 15:198–203
58. Cain SM (1984) Supply dependency of oxygen uptake in ARDS: Myth or reality? Am J Med Sci 288:119–124
59. Nelson DP, Samsel RW, Wood LDH, Schumacker PT (1988) Pathological supply dependence of systemic and intestinal O_2 uptake during endotoxemia. J Appl Physiol 64:2410–2419
60. Samsel RW, Nelson DP, Sanders WM, Wood LDH, Schumacker PT (1988) Effect of endotoxin on systemic and skeletal muscle O_2 extraction. J Appl Physiol 65:1377–1382
61. Bihari D, Smithies M, Gimson A, Tinker J (1987) The effects of vasodilation with prostacyclin on oxygen delivery and uptake in critically ill patients. N Engl J Med 317:397–403

62. Fenwick JC, Dodek PM, Ronco JJ, Phang PT, Wiggs BR, Russell JA (1990) Increased concentrations of plasma lactate predict pathologic dependence of oxygen consumption on oxygen delivery in patients with adult respiratory distress syndrome. J Crit Care 5:81–86
63. Vincent JL, Roman A, De Backer D, Kahn RJ (1990) Oxygen uptake/supply dependency. Effects of short-term dobutamine infusion. Am Rev Respir Dis 142:2–7
64. Ronco JJ, Fenwick JC, Wiggs BR, Phang PT, Russell JA, Tweedale MG (1993) Oxygen consumption is independent of increases in oxygen delivery by dobutamine in septic patients who have normal or increased plasma lactate. Am Rev Respir Dis 147:25–31
65. Ronco JJ, Phang PT, Walley KR, Wiggs B, Fenwick JC, Russell JA (1991) Oxygen consumption is independent of changes in oxygen delivery in severe adult respiratory distress syndrome. Am Rev Respir Dis 143:1267–1273
66. Vermeij CG, Feenstra BWA, Adrichem WJ, Bruining HA (1991) Independent oxygen uptake and oxygen delivery in septic and postoperative patients. Chest 99:1438–1443
67. Carlile PV, Gray BA (1989) Effect of opposite changes in cardiac output and arterial PO_2 on the relationship between mixed venous PO_2 and oxygen transport. Am Rev Respir Dis 140:891–898
68. Vermeij CG, Feenstra BWA, Bruining HA (1990) Oxygen delivery and oxygen uptake in postoperative and septic patients. Chest 98:415–420
69. Dietrich KA, Conrad SA, Hebert CA, Levy GL, Romero MD (1990) Cardiovascular and metabolic response to red blood cell transfusion in critically ill volume-resuscitated nonsurgical patients. Crit Care Med 18:940–944
70. Mink RB, Pollack MM (1990) Effect of blood transfusion on oxygen consumption in pediatric septic shock. Crit Care Med 18:1087–1091
71. Heard SO, Baum TD, Wang H, Rothschild HR, Fink MP (1991) Systemic and mesenteric O_2 metabolism in endotoxic pigs: Effect of graded hemorrhage. Circ Shock 35:44–52
72. Greer GG, Milazzo FH (1975) *Pseudomonas aeruginosa* lipopolysaccharide: An uncouple of mitochondrial oxidative phosphorylation. Can J Microbiol 21:877–883
73. Mela L, Bacalco LV Jr, Miller LD (1971) Defective oxidative metabolism of rat liver mitochondria in hemorrhagic and endotoxin shock. Am J Physiol 220:571–577
74. Decker GAG, Daniel AM, Blevings S, Maclean LD (1971) Effect of peritonitis on mitochondrial respiration. J Surg Res 11:528–532
75. Tanaka J, Kono Y, Shimahara Y, et al (1982) A study of oxidative phosphorylative activity and calcium-induced respiration of rat liver mitochondria following living Escherichia coli injection. Adv Shock Res 7:77–90
76. Clemens M, Chaudry IH, Baue AE (1981) Oxidative capability of hepatic tissue in late sepsis. Adv Shock Res 6:55–64
77. Spitzer JA, Deaciuc IV (1986) Effect of endotoxicosis and sepsis on intracellular calcium homeostasis in rat liver. Mitochondrial and microsomal calcium uptake. Circ Shock 18:81–93
78. Stadler J, Billiar TR, Curran RD, Stuehr DJ, Ochoa JB, Simmons RL (1991) Effect of exogenous and endogenous nitric oxide on mitochondrial respiration rat hepatocytes. J Appl Physiol 260:C910–C916
79. Stadler J, Bentz BG, Harbrecht BG, et al (1992) Tumor necrosis factor alpha inhibits hepatocyte mitochondrial respiration. Ann Surg 216:539–546
80. Fink MP, Antonsson JB, Wang H, Rothschild HR (1991) Increased intestinal permeability in endotoxic pigs: Mesenteric hypoperfusion as an etiologic factor. Arch Surg 126:211–218
81. Tuchschmidt J, Fried J, Astiz M, Rackow E (1992) Elevation of cardiac output and oxygen improves outcome in septic shock. Chest 102:216–220
82. Yu M, Levy MH, Smith P, Takiguchi SA, Miyasaki A, Myers SA (1993) Effect of maximizing oxygen delivery on morbidity and mortality rates in critically ill patients: A prospective, randomized, controlled study. Crit Care Med 21:830–838
83. Dantker DR (1993) The gastrointestinal tract: The canary of the body? J Am Med Assoc 270:1247–1248

84. Bergofsky EH (1964) Determination of tissue O_2 tensions by hollow visceral tonometers: Effect of breathing enriched O_2 mixtures. J Clin Invest 43:193–200
85. Dawson AM, Trenchard D, Guz A (1965) Small bowel tonometry: Assessment of small gut mucosal oxygen tension in dog and man. Nature 206:943–944
86. Antonsson JB, Boyle CC, Kruithoff KL, et al (1990) Validation of tonometric measurement of gut intramural pH during endotoxemia and mesenteric occlusion in pigs. Am J Physiol 259:G519–G523
87. Fink MP, Cohn SM, Lee PC, et al (1989) Effect of lipopolysaccharide on intestinal intramucosal hydrogen ion concentration in pigs: Evidence of gut ischemia in a normodynamic model of septic shock. Crit Care Med 17:641–646
88. Antonsson JB, Kuttila K, Niinikoski J, Haglund UH (1993) Subcutaneous and gut tissue perfusion and oxygenation changes as related to oxygen transport in experimental peritonitis. Circ Shock 41:261–267
89. Fink MP, Rothschild HR, Deniz YF, Wang H, Lee PC, Cohn SM (1989) Systemic and mesenteric O_2 metabolism in endotoxic pigs: Effect of ibuprofen and meclofenamate. J Appl Physiol 67:1950–1957
90. Salzman AL, Wang H, Wollert PS, et al (1994) Endotoxin-induced ileal mucosal hyperpermeability in pigs: Role of tissue acidosis. Am J Physiol (in press)
91. Whitworth PW, Cryer HM, Garrison RN, Baumgarten TE, Harris PD (1989) Hypoperfusion of the intestinal microcirculation with increased cardiac output during live *Escherichia coli* sepsis in rats. Circ Shock 27:111–122
92. Johnson BA, Weil MH (1991) Refefining ischemia due to circulatory failure as dual defects of oxygen deficits and carbon dioxide excesses. Crit Care Med 19:1432–1438
93. Maynard N, Bihari D, Beale R, et al (1993) Assessment of splanchnic oxygenation by gastric tonometry in patients with acute circulatory failure. J Am Med Assoc 270:1203–1210
94. Gys T, Hubens A, Neels H, Lauwers LF, Peeters R (1988) Prognostic value of gastric intramural pH in surgical intensive care patients. Crit Care Med 16:122–124
95. Doglio GR, Pusajo JF, Egurrola MA, et al (1991) Gastric mucosal pH as a prognostic index of mortality in critically ill patients. Crit Care Med 19:1037–1040
96. Gutierrez G, Palizas F, Doglio G, et al (1992) Gastric intramucosal pH as a therapeutic index of tissue oxygenation in critically ill patients. Lancet 339:195–199
97. Salzman AL, Strong KE, Wang H, Wollert PS, Vander Meer T, Fink MP (1994) Intraluminal "baloonless" air tonometry: A new method for determination of gastrointestinal mucosal PCO_2. Crit Care Med 22:126–134

Multiple Organ Dysfunction Syndrome (MODS)

J. C. Marshall

Introduction

The emergence of organ system failure as the defining challenge in the management of the critically ill mirrors the origins of the discipline of intensive care itself. Intensive care units (ICU) were first organized in the late 1950's as a geographic locale that brought together new technology for the monitoring and support of physiologic organ system function through the use of mechanical ventilation, invasive hemodynamic monitoring and vasoactive therapy, dialysis, and parenteral nutrition [1]. It was natural, therefore, that organ system failure became the metaphor for the challenges encountered in the management of the most complex critically ill patients [2–4], and ultimately, the dominant paradigm for the limitations to the survival of the critically ill [5].

However the development of organ dysfunction represents more than simply the protracted process of dying despite maximal supportive care. Organ system dysfunction in the critically ill is potentially reversible and arises following a definable group of insults including infection, ischemia, and tissue injury. The introduction of the term, Multiple Organ Dysfunction Syndrome (MODS) reflects an emerging consensus that organ dysfunction comprises a clinical syndrome that, although variable in expression, has a common pathophysiologic basis that is potentially amenable to specific therapeutic intervention through strategies designed to modulate the host septic response [6].

Yet there is at present no explicit consensus on the functional definition of MODS: the organ systems whose function is altered, the nature of those alterations and how best to describe them, and the level of abnormality that establishes the presence of the syndrome. Characterization of the epidemiology and clinical course of MODS has been largely studied on the basis of retrospective studies that employ widely differing criteria to define the systems comprising the syndrome and the markers of abnormal function within any given system [8–16]. This chapter undertakes a systematic review of existing criteria for the description of organ system dysfunction in the critically ill, as a necessary prerequisite to the development of consensus on clinical criteria for MODS.

Methodologic Considerations

The objective of this review is to evaluate specific descriptors of organ dysfunction as a background to the development of a valid definition of MODS that can be used in the context of clinical trials in the ICU. **Validity** as a methodologic concept is concerned with the use of a measurement for a particular purpose (prognostication, stratification, description, evaluation, etc.) and can be evaluated on the basis of three types of evidence [7]:

1. *Construct-related Evidence:* How well a particular variable is a meaningful measure of the characteristic or quality of interest;
2. *Content-related Evidence:* How well a variable derived from a sample of measures represents the domain of all possible cases; and
3. *Criterion-related Evidence:* How well a specific variable predicts outcome or estimates current status as measured by a separate instrument.

The selection of valid criteria for the description of organ dysfunction in critical illness thus requires:

1. that the criteria reflect the clinical phenomenon that the intensivist perceives to be MODS;
2. that they be generalizable to an heterogeneous group of patients and to differing manifestations of dysfunction within a given organ system; and
3. that they provide diagnostic or prognostic information as measured by an independent criterion.

Construct-related Evidence

Construct-related evidence considers the syndrome as it is perceived by the intensivist. To define the spectrum of clinical definitions of MODS (both the systems considered to define the syndrome and the criteria used to define organ dysfunction or failure), we undertook a systematic Medline review of all clinical studies indexed under the keyword "multiple organ failure" between 1976 and 1993. Additional articles were identified through the references of these publications. We required that articles selected for inclusion in the present review provide adequate documentation of the diagnostic criteria employed to define MODS, and be based on an evaluation of at least 20 subjects. In cases where an author had published more than one study using a given set of criteria, only one publication was selected for inclusion in the review. This process identified 30 papers providing criteria for the clinical description of MODS [3, 4, 8–35].

Content-related Evidence

Content-related evidence considers the extent to which a given descriptor of organ dysfunction is an accurate reflection of the entire spectrum of abnormality in the system of interest. To evaluate content validity, we generated a list of characteristics of the "ideal" descriptor of organ system dysfunction in MODS (Table 1), and measured criteria identified through the literature review against these.

Criterion-related Evidence

Although it has been hypothesized that circulation levels of inflammatory cell products such as neopterin or elastase [36] or the magnitude of biochemical alterations such as the ketone body ratio [37] reflect the biologic severity of MODS, there is at present no biochemical or pathologic marker that can be considered to define the syndrome. Since the severity of MODS has, in virtually all published reports, been quantitated by its associated mortality, we consider mortality to be the appropriate independent standard against which to evaluate descriptors of organ dysfunction. The need for exogenous life support is intrinsic to the concept of MODS (see below), therefore ICU mortality rather than hospital mortality is the better indicator of unsuccessful resolution of organ dysfunction, since ICU discharge implies the potential for survival in the absence of intensive organ system support.

Organ Function Descriptors: General Considerations

Dysfunction or Failure?

Multiple organ failure was originally defined as a syndrome characterized by the development of physiologic derangement in two or more organ systems such that organ function was inadequate to meet the needs of the host with-

Table 1. Characteristics of the ideal descriptor of organ dysfunction

The ideal variable to describe organ system dysfunction in MODS should be:

1. Simple
2. Readily, routinely, and reliably measured
3. Objective and independent of clinical evaluation
4. A comprehensive reflection of function in a given organ system
5. Specific for the function of that organ system
6. Unaffected by transient abnormalities associated with resuscitation or acute, reversible complications of therapy
7. Minimally altered by specific patterns of therapeutic intervention
8. Maximally abnormal after resuscitation and well before the time of death
9. A reflection, not of chronic primary disease in the organ system of interest, but of the sequelae of an acute homeostatic insult
10. Reproducible in heterogeneous groups of critically ill patients
11. Abnormal in one direction only
12. A continuous rather than a dichotomous variable

out exogenous support [5]. The implicit diagnostic criterion for its presence was the need for exogenous support and therefore descriptors of dysfunction in individual organ system were dichotomous variables: the need for mechanical ventilation, the need for transfusion to treat stress-induced bleeding, a creatinine level greater than an arbitrary value or the need for dialysis, a serum bilirubin level above a certain value, etc. It has become apparent, however, that these dichotomous criteria represent only arbitrary cut-off points on a continuum of organ dysfunction, and that outcome (measured independently as ICU mortality) is a function of both the number of failing systems, and the severity of dysfunction within a system [16, 24]. If MODS is not a dichotomous event, but a continuous process, there are two implications for the selection of descriptors for the syndrome:

1. continuous variables are preferable to dichotomous variables; and
2. the magnitude of the global organ system dysfunction can be appropriately expressed by a score or scale.

Models for the Description of Organ Dysfunction

The dysfunction or failure of a given organ system can be described in one of three ways:

1. by the degree of abnormality of a single parameter of function;
2. by the presence of a combination of variables that defines a syndrome of abnormality; and
3. by the clinical intervention employed to support organ system function.

For example, respiratory dysfunction can be characterized by the PO_2/FiO_2 ratio, as ARDS defined by an abnormal PO_2/FiO_2 ratio in combination with a wedge pressure of less than 18 mm Hg and a characteristic radiographic appearance, or by the duration of ventilatory support or the level of PEEP used to obtain maximal PO_2. There are advantages and disadvantages to each of these approaches.

The use of a single parameter such as the PO_2/FiO_2 ratio or the platelet count has the great advantage of simplicity, and provides a measure that can be very sensitive to graded degrees of organ system dysfunction. Such an approach suffers, however, from lack of specificity. Moreover individual variables can be significantly affected by random extreme values resulting from measurement error or therapeutic intervention. An elevated serum bilirubin, for example, may reflect hemolysis and be largely unrelated to liver dysfunction, while increases in the prothrombin time or International Normalized Ratio may reflect therapeutic anticoagulation. Specific conditions or limitations can be attached to the use of a variable, however to do so introduces an element of subjectivity, and complicates the determination of the appropriate value for the variable.

The use of a combination of two or more variables to characterize dysfunction in a particular organ system improves specificity but at the potential cost of sensitivity. More importantly, the incorporation of two or more variables into a criterion converts it from a continuous to a categorical measure (the presence or absence of the component criteria). Finally, since it is more likely that at least one of the components of the criterion will not be available for evaluation, combined criteria provide a more conservative estimate that is potentially biased between centers by local patterns of data collection and test usage.

The use of descriptors of therapeutic intervention to characterize the severity of organ dysfunction mirrors the clinical origins of MODS and therefore has construct validity. It also permits the measurement of organ dysfunction to be used as a direct measure of the intensity of resource usage. Patterns of therapy, and indications for the use of particular modalities differ considerably from one center to the next, and from one era to the next, therefore the use of therapy-based descriptors diminishes the generalizability of the criteria. Moreover therapy-based variables are usually categorical, rather than continuous in nature (for example, the need for hemodialysis, the use of non-conventional forms of ventilatory support, the use of inotropes, or the use of parenteral nutrition).

Because of considerations of simplicity, objectivity, and the desirability of employing continuous descriptors, we favor the use of single physiologic variables to reflect function in any given organ system.

Descriptors of Dysfunction in Specific Organ Systems

A review of 30 published clinical studies of MODS demonstrated considerable heterogeneity in the definitions employed, both in the systems whose dysfunction comprises the syndrome and in the criteria used to define dysfunction. Seven systems (respiratory, renal, gastrointestinal, hepatic, central nervous system, hematologic, and cardiovascular) were included in more than half of the published reports. Table 2 summarizes the organ systems considered in these studies.

Construct-related Evidence

Construct validity describes the extent to which specific descriptors of organ dysfunction reflect the clinical entity that the intensivist perceives MODS, and was evaluated by tabulating the organ systems and descriptive variables that have been used in published studies of MODS. For each system, we attempted to determine both the specific physiologic abnormalities and the nature of the therapeutic intervention that are seen to define the organ dysfunction characteristic of MODS.

Table 2. Organ systems included in published studies of MODS

Organ System	# of Studies	References
Respiratory	29	[3, 4, 8–35]
Renal	28	[4, 8–35]
Hepatic	26	[3, 4, 8–12, 14–16, 18–35]
Cardiovascular	24	[3, 4, 10–17, 19–21, 23–32, 34, 35]
Hematologic	22	[8, 10, 11, 14–19, 21, 23–35]
Gastrointestinal	21	[3, 4, 8–11, 14–16, 18–21, 23, 25–29, 32, 33, 35]
Central Nervous System	17	[4, 10, 12, 14, 16, 17, 19–21, 23–25, 27–29, 32, 34, 35]
Endocrine/Metabolic	5	[10, 14, 20, 21, 24]
Immunologic	4	[13, 21, 28, 31]
Other:		
Pancreas	2	[4, 10]
Pleura	1	[10]

Respiratory Dysfunction: All 30 published papers considered respiratory dysfunction to be a cardinal manifestation of MODS. The need for mechanical ventilation was the most common criterion for determining the presence of respiratory failure and was a component of the definition of respiratory failure in 23 studies. Impaired oxygenation reflected in a raised FiO_2, an elevated A-a gradient, or a decreased PO_2/FiO_2 ratio was cited in 22 papers, while the duration of mechanical ventilation was considered relevant in 9 reports. The level of PEEP was cited as a criterion for respiratory failure by 4 authors. Other variables employed included ventilatory rate (3 studies), evidence of ARDS by X-ray criteria (3 studies), and hypercarbia and an increase in V_D/V_T (1 study each).

Construct-related criteria therefore show that respiratory failure is uniformly considered a manifestation of MODS. The essential physiologic abnormality is perceived to be impaired oxygen uptake and the therapeutic intervention, the provision of mechanical ventilation.

Renal Dysfunction: Renal dysfunction is considered to be a component of MODS in all but one of the published studies [3]. In 25 of these 29 papers, an increased serum creatinine level defines the presence of renal dysfunction, while the need for dialysis is cited in 8 studies. A falling urine output is a criterion for renal failure in 6 studies, while elevation of the serum BUN level is employed in 3 reports; reduced creatinine clearance is cited in two reports, hypervolemia, and azotemia in one report each.

There appears to be general consensus that renal dysfunction as a component of MODS is best reflected physiologically in an increasing serum creatinine level, and therapeutically in the need for dialysis.

Hepatic Dysfunction: Hepatic dysfunction appears as a component of MODS in all but 3 published reports [13, 17, 32]. There is, however, considerable heterogeneity in the criteria used to define liver dysfunction. Hyperbilirubinemia or the presence of clinical jaundice is a feature of hepatic dysfunction in all 25 reports that specify specific criteria. Other criteria include elevation of serum transaminases (12 papers), of alkaline phosphatase (6 papers), of LDH (4 papers) and of the prothrombin time (1 paper). A low serum albumin is a component of the definition in 2 reports, while one author each considers cirrhosis or abnormal histology to define liver failure in MODS. In two reports, liver failure is defined on the basis of biochemical abnormalities that are not explicitly outlined. No paper alluded to liver specific supportive measures in the form of dietary alterations, oral lactulose or neomycin, therapy for portal hypertension, the administration of plasma factors in the definition of liver dysfunction, or the use of a bioartificial liver support device.

Jaundice and hyperbilirubinemia, therefore, define liver dysfunction in MODS as it is seen by the intensivist; abnormalities in other biochemical parameters vary widely from one report to the next. There is no specific therapeutic intervention that defines the liver dysfunction of MODS.

Cardiovascular Dysfunction: Impaired cardiovascular function is cited in 25 of the 30 studies of MODS, and omitted in 5 [8, 9, 18, 22, 33]. Considerable variability in the criteria defining MODS is apparent. Hypotension or the need for inotropic support is the most commonly used criterion, occurring in 11 reports each. Seven authors consider myocardial dysfunction to be defined by the development of arrhythmias, both atrial and ventricular, while 7 incorporate elevation of right atrial and pulmonary capillary wedge pressures in the definition. Five authors consider myocardial infarction to be a manifestation of MODS, and two define cardiac arrest as a diagnostic criterion. Bidirectional alterations in heart rate (bradycardia or tachycardia, one paper each) or cardiac output (decreased in four reports, elevated in one) are cited by several authors. Cardiac tamponade, endocarditis, acidosis, and unspecified EKG changes are mentioned by one author each. No author considered alterations in peripheral vascular resistance or vascular permeability to be a manifestation of cardiovascular dysfunction in MODS.

Construct-related criteria define cardiac dysfunction in MODS by inadequate pump function reflected physiologically in hypotension and increased filling pressures, and therapeutically in the need for inotropic support.

Hematologic Dysfunction: Abnormalities of hematologic function are considered to be a manifestation of MODS in 23 reports. Thrombocytopenia is the most commonly employed criterion for hematologic dysfunction (21 studies). Nine authors consider leukopenia to be a manifestation of MODS while 2 authors cite leukocytosis as a criterion. Other criteria include abnormalities of coagulation manifested in elevations of the prothrombin time (7 studies) or partial thromboplastin time (6 studies) or the need for clotting factors (1 study). Five authors cite the presence of DIC as a criterion, while another 4 use evidence of fibrin degradation products. Other criteria include a reduction in hematocrit (4 reports), visible bleeding or ecchymosis (2 reports), and underlying hematologic disease (1 report).

Construct-related evidence shows hematologic dysfunction in MODS to be defined physiologically by abnormalities in the clotting system, primarily by thrombocytopenia, but also by abnormalities of the coagulation cascade, DIC being the most extreme form. Abnormalities of the white blood cell response (both leukopenia and leukocytosis) are less commonly employed criteria. Therapy-based definitions are not commonly used to describe hematologic dysfunction.

Gastrointestinal Dysfunction: Variables reflecting GI dysfunction are included in 22 published reports. All of these reports consider GI bleeding from stress ulceration to be the cardinal feature of GI dysfunction in MODS. Other manifestations cited include acalculous cholecystitis (4 reports), pancreatitis (4 reports), persistent ileus (3 reports), intolerance of enteral feeding (2 reports), GI perforation (2 reports), and ischemia, obstruction, and mesenteric venous thrombosis (one report each).

Stress-induced GI bleeding is perceived to be the defining characteristic of GI dysfunction; criteria to define lesser degrees of dysfunction such as intolerance to feeding or reduced peristalsis are highly subjective. Therapeutic intervention in the form of transfusion is widely used as a marker of the severity of stress bleeding.

Neurologic Dysfunction: Neurologic dysfunction appears as a component of MODS in 18 of the reports reviewed. Alterations in level on consciousness are the predominant manifestations of neurologic dysfunction, whether measured quantitatively by the Glasgow Coma Score (9 papers), or qualitatively using such descriptors as coma (7 reports), obtundation (3 reports), or confusion or psychosis (3 reports). One author considers meningitis or intracranial hemorrhage to be a manifestation of MODS.

Construct-related evidence indicates that alterations in consciousness are the defining features of neurologic dysfunction in MODS; therapy-based definitions are not employed.

Endocrine/Metabolic: Endocrine or metabolic dysfunction is considered a component of MODS in 5 reports. Criteria include diabetes or insulin resistance [10, 24, 27], hypertriglyceridemia [27], hypermetabolism [22], and weight loss or hypoalbuminemia [14].

Immunologic: Four reports consider immunologic dysfunction to be a component of MODS, and employ as descriptive criteria the presence of bacteremia or other invasive infection [13, 32, 34], pyrexia and leukocytosis [32], unspecified clinical manifestations of sepsis [13], and impaired delayed type hypersensitivity reactivity [24].

Other Systems: Pancreatic dysfunction is cited as a manifestation of MODS in two reports [4, 10], and infection within the pleural space in one [10].

In summary, although there is variability from one report to the next, 7 systems (respiratory, renal, hepatic, cardiovascular, hematologic, gastrointestinal, and central nervous system) appear in more than half of the published studies, and by construct-related criteria are the defining systems of MODS. All are defined primarily by physiologic abnormalities; definition on the basis of therapeutic intervention is also employed by some authors to describe respiratory, renal, cardiovascular, and gastrointestinal dysfunction.

Content-related Evidence

Content validity concerns the extent to which a particular variable is representative of the entire domain of abnormality that it is used to measure. To evaluate the content validity of existing descriptors of individual organ system dysfunction in the critically ill, we developed a series of criteria that would define the "ideal" descriptor of organ system dysfunction (Table 1).

These criteria, in turn, address several discrete aspects of content validity as the concept is applied to a candidate descriptor of organ system dysfunction in MODS:

- the extent to which the given variable reflects the entire spectrum of MODS-related abnormality for a given organ system;
- the ability of the variable to differentiate abnormalities associated with inadequate or incomplete resuscitation on the one hand, and pre-existing chronic disease on the other, from those arising in the maximally-resuscitated and supported patient;
- the independence of the variable from manipulation by observer bias or therapeutic approach;
- the generalizability of the variable across heterogeneous patient groups or geographic locales; and
- the ease of use of the variable.

Respiratory Dysfunction: Respiratory dysfunction as a component of MODS is defined primarily by impaired oxygen uptake. Although this physiologic state can be quantitated in a number of ways (FiO_2, PO_2, A-a gradient, level of PEEP, etc.), the use of the ratio of PO_2 to FiO_2 [38] satisfies all but one of the criteria outlined in Table 1 (its value can be altered by such therapeutic interventions as the institution of mechanical ventilation or PEEP, in the absence of change in intrinsic lung pathology), and is the best available measure of the severity of respiratory dysfunction. Other commonly used measures of respiratory dysfunction such as the FiO_2, duration of mechanical ventilation, or level of PEEP reflect clinical practices that may differ significantly from one center to the next, and suffer from their lack of independence from therapy, as well as from their susceptibility to alteration by transient changes associated with readily reversible complications of therapy. Criteria such as pulmonary compliance or dead space have not been evaluated, and are neither readily nor routinely evaluated in most ICU settings.

Renal Dysfunction: Impaired excretory function defines renal dysfunction in MODS. The serum creatinine level is the most widely used measure of altered renal function, and meets all but 2 of the 12 criteria for the ideal descriptor of organ dysfunction. Elevation of the serum creatinine may reflect the presence of pre-existing chronic disease, and can be reduced by therapeutic intervention (dialysis) in the absence of improvement in intrinsic renal function. Calculation of creatinine clearance is a more sensitive marker of altered function and correlates with adverse outcome in the ICU setting [39], but is not generally performed on a routine basis. Moreover, the creatinine clearance provides good discrimination in the presence of mild degrees of functional impairment, but is less able to differentiate abnormality with more severe degrees of dysfunction. Serum BUN levels, although inexpensive and easy to obtain, have not been widely used as a marker of renal dysfunction, perhaps because they are more susceptible to the influence of non-renal factors. Urinary output is a suboptimal marker of renal dysfunction. It may be reduced as a result of pre-renal factors (it lacks specificity), and may be adequate even in the setting of advanced renal dysfunction as evaluated by elevation of the serum creatinine (it lacks sensitivity). Moreover, it is influenced by therapeutic decisions such as the administration of fluids or diuretics. Similarly the need for dialysis, although specific for renal failure, is both insensitive to minor functional alterations, and represents a therapeutic decision, rather than a physiologic alteration.

Hepatic Dysfunction: Hyperbilirubinemia is the most widely employed criterion used to define hepatic dysfunction. The serum bilirubin concentration as a marker of hepatic dysfunction meets only 9 of the criteria established for the ideal variable. Hyperbilirubinemia lacks specificity for hepatic dysfunction and can occur as a result of hemolysis or extrahepatic biliary obstruction, does not reflect the entire spectrum of liver dysfunction in MODS, and may be a result of pre-existing chronic disease. Published reports have incorporated other biochemical markers of hepatic function including those reflecting hepatocellular injury (transaminases), synthetic function (albumin and prothrombin time), and cholestasis (alkaline phosphatase). Each of these individually is subject to the same shortcomings as the serum bilirubin level. There is no convincing evidence that a particular combination of variables would circumvent these limitations, indeed it remains to be proven that there truly is a characteristic constellation of biochemical abnormalities that defines the hepatic dysfunction of MODS.

Cardiovascular Dysfunction: Criteria for the description of cardiovascular dysfunction in MODS are both variable and unsatisfactory from the perspective of content validity. Hypotension is the physiologic variable most commonly employed, however it satisfies only 8 of the prerequisites of an ideal descriptor of organ system dysfunction. It is readily affected by transient abnormalities associated with resuscitation and therapy, and commonly the greatest degree of abnormality reflects events early in the course of resuscitation or immediately prior to death. Blood pressure can be readily manipulated by therapeutic intervention (both volume infusion and the use of inotropic agents) and hypotension may not be specific for intrinsic cardiovascular dysfunction. The use of inotropes, on the other hand, while specific for cardiovascular dysfunction in the critically ill, reflects a therapeutic decision, and there is considerable variability between centers in the indications for the use of inotropic or vasoconstrictive medications, and in the particular agents and dosages used. Alterations in heart rate and rhythm are neither specific for MODS, nor widely used in published reports, and it is not intuitively evident that a particular type of dysrhythmia is characteristic of MODS. Invasive measures of right and left sided filling pressures or of myocardial contractility show a spectrum of abnormalities including impaired right and left ventricular contractility and altered myocardial oxygen extraction [40, 41], however documentation of these changes requires the presence of a pulmonary artery catheter, and a conceptually and technologically simple paradigm for their description does not yet exist. Alterations in regional blood flow, in peripheral vascular tone, and in capillary permeability are also features of cardiovascular dysfunction in MODS, but suffer as markers from the lack of simple instruments to quantitate the degree of their abnormality. Elevations of the serum lactate level reflect the sequelae of impaired cardiovascular dysfunction with inadequate oxygen delivery and anaerobic metabolism, and correlate well with outcome [42]. However lactate levels have not been widely cited in published studies of MODS, are costly, not routinely performed in most centers, and may be relatively insensitive to early and subtle degrees of dysfunction. Myocardial infarction, endocarditis, cardiac tamponade, or the presence of EKG abnormalities are cited as manifestations of MODS in several reports, but are more commonly manifestations of primary myocardial pathology.

Hematologic Dysfunction: Hematologic dysfunction is most commonly defined by thrombocytopenia, and less commonly by leukopenia. Coagulation abnormalities reflected in increases in prothrombin or partial thromboplastin times were cited in a minority of reports. Thrombocytopenia satisfies all the requirements outlined in Table 1. It is readily measured, objective, and relatively specific for the clinical abnormalities associated with MODS [43]. Coagulation profiles are altered by therapeutic anticoagulation, while alterations in numbers of circulating leukocytes more typically reflect the transient response to an acute stress-infectious or non-infectious episode.

Gastrointestinal Dysfunction: Stress-related upper GI bleeding is uniformly employed as a criterion to define GI dysfunction in MODS. As a descriptor, however, bleeding satisfies only 8 of the criteria outlined in Table 1. The evaluation of stress bleeding relies on clinical evaluation to establish its significance and degree and yields a dichotomous rather than a continuous variable. Bleeding is poorly reflective of the scope of GI dysfunction in critical illness, and may reflect primary pathology such as a bleeding ulcer, esophageal varices, or an aorto-enteric fistula. Its utility is further diminished by the fact that significant bleeding in the contemporary ICU occurs in fewer than 4% of patients and often arises from non-gastric sites [44]. Other descriptors are cited infrequently. Acalculous cholecystitis shares the drawbacks of stress bleeding as a descriptor. The presence of ileus or the intolerance of enteral feeding are difficult parameters to quantitate objectively.

Neurologic Dysfunction: The Glasgow Coma Score is the most frequently cited measure of neurologic dysfunction in MODS; it satisfies 9 of the 12 criteria for an ideal descriptor of organ system dysfunction. Its calculation requires clinical evaluation (although the resulting bias may be minimized by having this calculation done by the patient's nurse) and is readily affected by therapy in the form of sedation, paralysis, or anesthesia (although this bias can be minimized through the use of conservative estimates of Glasgow Coma Score). Its level may, in the head-injured patient, be a reflection of primary disease.

Other variables reflecting neurologic dysfunction that have been used to date are highly subjective, and less producible than the Glasgow Coma Score. Meningitis or intracranial hemorrhage is cited as a manifestation of MODS in one report, but both processes are much more likely to reflect primary intracranial disease, than the secondary sequelae of a major insult.

Because of the paucity of reports that consider the dysfunction of organ systems other than those listed to be a component of MODS, the variables employed will not be further considered here.

Criterion-related Evidence

Criterion validity describes the performance of a test or measure relative to an independent gold standard. As discussed earlier, criterion validity was assessed by the ability of a given variable to predict ICU mortality in a dose-dependent manner. MODS is not the only process resulting in ICU mortality, and the use of mortality is not therefore specific for the process of MODS. On the other hand, in a non-coronary ICU, the majority of deaths occur in association with multiple organ dysfunction, rather than as a result of single system disease [15, 24, 25]. It is also a truism of contemporary critical care practice that the probability of an adverse outcome increases with increasing degrees of abnormality of almost any variable, whether it is a single biochemical variable such as lactate [42], a composite variable such as APACHE II score [45], an aggregate clinical variable reflecting the severity of the host septic response [46], an aggregate biochemical variable reflecting levels of mediators of that response [47], or even a non-specific marker of illness severity such as the number of infusion pumps by the bedside.

The global severity of organ dysfunction during an ICU stay shows a strong correlation with ICU mortality [24], as well as with susceptibility to ICU-acquired infection and the expression of a clinical septic response [48]. Similarly, graded degrees of dysfunction within given organ systems can readily be shown to correlate with incremental increases in ICU mortality [24]. Adequate evaluation of the specific individual variables used to characterize organ dysfunction is not possible using the information sources employed for this review, however a correlation between mortality and increasing abnormality has been shown for the PO_2/FiO_2 ratio [38], serum creatinine level [24], serum bilirubin level [49], platelet count [24], and Glasgow Coma Score [24].

MODS: a State, a Process, or an Outcome?

Organ dysfunction in the critically ill can be viewed in one of three ways: as a state, as a process, or as an outcome. The description of MODS as a state implies that the defining variables coexist at a single point in time, and can change from one day to the next. The severity of the syndrome is quantitated by the degree of organ dysfunction on a given day, typically the day of ICU admission [34, 35]. The description of MODS as a process implies that the syndrome evolves over a finite time period, and predicts a subsequent outcome. The report of Knaus and colleagues [17], in which the most severe manifestations of organ dysfunction over the first three days of ICU admission is used to predict subsequent ICU mortality is such a model. Most papers, however, consider MODS as an outcome, incorporating into the assessment of the severity of the process, the worst manifestations of individual organ dysfunction during the ICU stay. These models are not mutually exclusive. Point descriptions of MODS reflect the intensity of resource utilization at a given time, while cumulative evaluations of evolving organ dysfunction can provide information of prognostic significance. Systems that determine the severity of MODS during an entire ICU stay may be useful as outcome measures for purposes of both research and quality assurance.

Conclusions and Recommendations

The evaluation of descriptors of organ system dysfunction in MODS does not readily lend itself to a classical evidence-based analysis, since criteria must of necessity be defined in advance, rather than through the mechanism of a randomized clinical trial. Therefore, we have used a modified approach based on consideration of **construct**-related evidence, **content-**related evidence, and **criterion**-related evidence. These 3 areas characterize validity as the concept is employed by educators in the evaluation of tests [7], and a similar approach appears rational for the analysis of a clinical evaluative tool.

Construct-related evidence considers the extent to which a descriptive variable reflects the process as it is perceived by the clinician, and was evaluated here by a systematic literature review to ascertain *which* systems and descriptors have been used to characterize organ dysfunction in MODS. **Content**-related evidence reflects the ability of a single descriptor to reflect the entire domain of abnormalities in a given organ system, and was evaluated here by determining the extent to which a given descriptor satisfied the conditions of an "ideal" descriptor (Table 1). Finally, **criterion**-related evidence evaluates a variable against an independent gold standard; in the case of organ dysfunction, the appropriate outcome gold standard, in the absence of validated biochemical markers, is mortality.

Conclusions

1. Seven organ systems define MODS, and each is included in more than half of the published descriptions of MODS: the respiratory, renal, hepatic, hematologic, cardiovascular, gastrointestinal, and central nervous systems.
2. Organ system dysfunction within each of these systems is best characterized by the use of single variables reflecting physiologic dysfunction (the PO_2/FiO_2 ratio, for example), rather than by variables reflecting the nature of the therapeutic intervention (such as the need for mechanical ventilation or the level of PEEP) or by composite variables (such as the presence of ARDS defined by hypoxemia and bilateral chest X-ray infiltrates in the absence of elevation of the pulmonary capillary wedge pressure).
3. Physiologic descriptors satisfying criteria for construct-related validity and content-related validity are available for 5 of these systems – the PO_2/FiO_2 ratio for the respiratory system, the serum creatinine level for the renal system, the serum bilirubin level for the hepatic system, the platelet count for the hematologic system, and the Glasgow Coma Score for the central nervous system. Descriptors of dysfunction for the cardiovascular system and the gastrointestinal system are suboptimal.
4. Each of the 5 descriptors listed in 2 demonstrates criterion-related validity in correlating with ICU mortality in a dose-dependent fashion. Hypotension demonstrates similar validity; quantitation of GI dysfunction using a continuous descriptor has not yet been accomplished.
5. In aggregate, combinations of these variables have increased power to predict ICU mortality.
6. The development of an organ dysfunction score based on validated physiologic variables can be readily accomplished. Such an aggregate measure can serve as a surrogate outcome measure in Phase II and Phase III clinical trials, and may shed light on the physiologic mechanisms of action of novel therapies.

Recommendations

1. There is sufficient consensus on the systems comprising MODS and the variables describing dysfunction within each of these to justify the more widespread use of organ dysfunction as a means of stratifying patients for entry into clinical trials, and of quantitating ICU morbidity as an outcome in these studies.
2. Development of an organ dysfunction score as an aggregate measure of the severity of organ dysfunction is feasible and intuitively appealing as a method of describing the severity of MODS.
3. Although reliable variables for the description of organ system function currently exist for 5 systems, optimal cut-offs for a scoring system need to be determined by evaluating the mortality of a large and heterogeneous group of ICU patients at differing levels of abnormality for each variable.

References

1. Safar P, DeKornfeld TJ, Pearson JW, Redding JS (1961) The intensive care unit. A three year experience at Baltimore city hospitals. Anesthesia 16:275–284
2. MacLean LD, Mulligan WG, McLean APH, Duff JH (1967) Patterns of septic shock in man. A detailed study of 56 patients. Ann Surg 166:543–562
3. Skillman JJ, Bushnell LS, Goldman H, Silen W (1969) Respiratory failure, hypotension, sepsis, and jaundice. A clinical syndrome associated with lethal hemorrhage from acute stress ulceration of the stomach. Am J Surg 117:523–530
4. Tilney NL, Bailey GL, Morgan AP (1973) Sequential system failure after rupture of abdominal aortic aneurysms: An unsolved problem in postoperative care. Ann Surg 178:117–122
5. Baue AE (1975) Multiple, progressive or sequential systems failure. A syndrome of the 1970's. Arch Surg 110:779–781
6. ACCP/SCCM Consensus Conference (1992) Definitions of sepsis and multiple organ failure. Crit Care Med 20:864–874
7. Gronlund NE (1985) Measurement and Evaluation in Teaching. (5th Ed) MacMillan Publishing Co, New York. pp 55–85
8. Eiseman B, Beart R, Norton L (1977) Multiple organ failure. Surg Gynecol Obstet 144:323–326
9. Fry DE, Pearlstein L, Fulton RL, Polk HC (1980) Multiple system organ failure. The role of uncontrolled infection. Arch Surg 115:136–140
10. Bell RC, Coalson JJ, Smith JD, Johanson WG (1983) Multiple organ system failure and infection in adult respiratory distress syndrome. Ann Intern Med 99:293–298
11. Faist E, Baue AE, Dittmer H, Heberer G (1983) Multiple organ failure in polytrauma patients. J Trauma 23:775–786
12. Pine RW, Wertz MJ, Lennard ES, Dellinger EP, Carrico CJ, Minshew BH (1983) Determinants of organ malfunction or death in patients with intra-abdominal sepsis. Arch Surg 118:242–249
13. Marshall WG, Dimick AR (1983) The natural history of major burns with multiple subsystem failure. J Trauma 23:102–105
14. Stevens LE (1983) Gauging the severity of surgical sepsis. Arch Surg 118:1190–1192
15. Manship L, McMillin RD, Brown JJ (1984) The influence of sepsis and multiorgan failure on mortality in the surgical intensive care unit. Am Surg 50:94–101
16. Goris RJA, te Boekhurts TPA, Nuytinck JKS, Gimbrere JSF (1985) Multiple-organ failure. Generalized autodestructive inflammation? Arch Surg 120:1109–1115

17. Knaus WA, Draper EA, Wagner DP, Zimmerman JE (1985) Prognosis in acute organ system failure. Ann Surg 202:685–692
18. Maetani S, Nishikawa T, Hirakawa A, Tobe T (1986) Role of blood transfusion in organ system failure following major abdominal surgery. Ann Surg 203:275–281
19. Bihari D, Smithies M, Gimson A, Tinker J (1987) The effects of vasodilation with prostacyclin on oxygen delivery and uptake in critically ill patients. N Engl J Med 317:397–403
20. Shen PF, Zhang SC (1987) Acute renal failure and multiple organ system failure. Arch Surg 122:1131–1133
21. Bumaschny E, Doglio G, Pusajo J, et al (1988) Postoperative acute gastrointestinal tract hemorrhage and multiple organ failure. Arch Surg 123:722–726
22. Cerra FB, McPherson JP, Konstantinides FN, Konstantinides NN, Teasley KM (1988) Enteral nutrition does not prevent multiple organ failure syndrome (MOFS) after sepsis. Surgery 104:727–733
23. Darling GE, Duff JH, Mustard RA, Finley RJ (1988) Multiorgan failure in critically ill patients. Can J Surg 31:172–176
24. Marshall JC, Christou NV, Horn H, Meakins JL (1988) The microbiology of multiple organ failure. The proximal GI tract as an occult reservoir of pathogens. Arch Surg 123:309-315
25. Tran DD, Groeneveld ABJ, van der Meulen J, Nauta JJP, Strack van Schijndel RJM, Thijs LG (1990) Age, chronic disease, sepsis, organ system failure, and mortality in a medical intensive care unit. Crit Care Med 18:474–479
26. Henao FJ, Daes JE, Dennis RJ (1991) Risk factors for multiorgan failure: A case-control study. J Trauma 31:74–80
27. Moore FA, Moore EE, Poggetti R, et al (1991) Gut bacterial translocation via the portal vein: A clinical perspective with major torso trauma. J Trauma 31:629–638
28. Ruokonen E, Takala J, Kari A, Alhava E (1991) Septic shock and multiple organ failure. Crit Care Med 19:1146–1151
29. Villar J, Manzano JJ, Blazquez MA, Quintana J, Lubillo S (1991) Multiple system organ failure in acute respiratory failure. J Crit Care 6:75–80
30. Bone RC, Balk R, Slotman G, et al and the Prostaglandin E_1 Study Group (1992) Adult respiratory distress syndrome. Sequence and importance of development of multiple organ failure. Chest 101:320–326
31. Martin LF, Booth FVMcL, Reines HD, et al (1992) Stress ulcers and organ failure in intubated patients in surgical intensive care units. Ann Surg 215:332–337
32. Shoemaker WC, Appel PL, Kram HB (1992) Role of oxygen debt in the development of organ failure, sepsis, and death in high risk surgical patients. Chest 102:208–215
33. Waydhas C, Nats-Kolb D, Jochum M, et al (1992) Inflammatory mediators, infection, sepsis, and multiple organ failure after sever trauma. Arch Surg 127:460–467
34. Fagon JY, Chastre J, Novara A, Medioni P, Gibert C (1993) Characterization of intensive care unit patients using a model based on the presence or absence of organ dysfunctions and/or infection: the ODIN model. Intensive Care Med 19:137–144
35. Hebert PC, Drummond AJ, Singer J, Bernard GR, Russell JA (1993) A simple multiple system organ failure scoring system predicts mortality of patients who have sepsis syndrome. Chest 104:230–235
36. Pachter R, Redl H, Frass M, Petzl DH, Schuster E, Woloszczuk W (1989) Relationship between neopterin and granulocyte elastase plasma levels and the severity of multiple organ failure. Crit Care Med 17:221–226
37. Ozawa K, Aoyama H, Yasuda K, et al (1983) Metabolic abnormalities associated with postoperative organ failure. A redox theory. Arch Surg 118:1245–1251
38. Murray JF, Matthay MA, Luce JM, Flick MR (1988) An expanded definition of the adult respiratory distress syndrome. Am Rev Respir Dis 138:720–723
39. Wilson RF, Soullier G, Antonenko D (1979) Creatinine clearance in critically ill surgical patients. Arch Surg 114:461–467
40. Bersten A, Sibbald WJ (1989) Circulatory disturbances in multiple systems organ failure. Crit Care Clin 5:233–254

41. Vincent JL, Gris P, Coffernils M, et al (1992) Myocardial depression characterizes the fatal course of septic shock. Surgery 111:660–667
42. Bakker J, Coffernils M, Leon M, Gris P, Vincent JL (1991) Blood lactate levels are superior to oxygen-derived variables in predicting outcome in human septic shock. Chest 99:856–962
43. Baughman RP, Lower EE, Flessa HC, Tollerud DJ (1993) Thrombocytopenia in the intensive care unit. Chest 104:1243–1247
44. Cook DJ, Fuller H, Guyatt GH, et al and the Canadian Critical Care Trials Group (1994) Risk factors for gastrointestinal bleeding in critically ill patients. N Engl J Med 330:377–381
45. Knaus WA, Draper EA, Wagner DP, Zimmerman JE (1985) APACHE II: A severity of disease classification system. Crit Care Med 13:818–829
46. Marshall JC, Sweeney D (1990) Microbial infection and the septic response in critical surgical illness. Sepsis, not infection, determines outcome. Arch Surg 125:17–25
47. Casey LC, Balk RA, Bone RC (1993) Plasma cytokine and endotoxin levels correlate with survival in patients with sepsis syndrome. Ann Intern Med 119:771–778
48. Marshall JC (1992) Multiple organ failure and infection: Cause, consequence or coincidence? In: Vincent JL (ed) Update in Intensive Care and Emergency Medicine. Volume 17. Springer-Verlag, Heidelberg, pp 1–13
49. Schwartz DB, Bone RC, Balk RA, Szidon JP (1989) Hepatic dysfunction in the adult respiratory distress syndrome. Chest 95:871–875

Monitoring Illness Severity

What Determines Prognosis in Sepsis?

W. A. Knaus, D. P. Wagner, and F. E. Harrell

Introduction

Patients presenting with sepsis are complexly ill with multiple risk factors for short-term mortality. In order to fully represent this complexity, an accurate comprehensive individual patient risk mortality based on reliable risk factors available at the time of treatment can be constructed from large, contemporary, clinically-accurate databases. The individual patient risk assessments produced by this approach can be used within clinical evaluations to insure that baseline risks for mortality were equally distributed among treatment groups and to investigate whether there is a relationship between baseline risk and efficacy of new therapeutic compounds.

If clinical evaluations performed in this manner use common definitions and data collection procedures, then the results of such assessment can further refine and revise the risk predictions, and describe the relative benefit of new compounds or combinations of such compounds for individual patients.

In order to properly evaluate new therapeutic approaches to sepsis, we will have to provide a baseline estimate of a patient's short-term mortality risk based on patient characteristics available and reliably measured prior to treatment. This estimate should be uniform in regard of risk assessment and clinical definitions, but specific to the particular inclusion and exclusion criteria used in the clinical evaluations, and should be updated as new information becomes available regarding prognostic factors or the efficacy of specific new compounds.

Background and Rationale

No "Typical" Septic Patient

One of the major reasons infection and sepsis have increased as a cause of morbidity and mortality in hospitalized patients is that we are treating more severely ill patients at more advanced stages of disease [1]. The majority of patients who develop sepsis in our acute care hospitals have chronic illnesses such as cancer, cirrhosis, or other conditions that decrease their immunologic function and leave them vulnerable to infection. We are also providing more intensive care services to severely ill patients in the initial stages of illness, such as trauma and shock, and after complex operations, making it possible to survive previously fatal conditions. This progress comes at the cost of prolonged invasive life support that also increases the risk of acquiring infection.

As a result of these changes, there really is not any "typical" patient with sepsis. Potential candidates range from a young previously healthy individual with the sudden onset of urinary tract infection to a patient with cirrhosis, suffering from multiple organ system failure on prolonged ventilatory support in an intensive care unit (ICU) following emergency surgery for a leaking abdominal aneurysm who develops a sudden episode of septic shock. The term sepsis is not sufficient to describe either patient, and reliance on such terms alone are unlikely to assist in the value and indications of new therapeutic approaches.

Categorical Definitions and Patient Risk

Recognizing this problem, new categorical definitions such as sepsis syndrome or sepsis syndrome with shock were developed [2] that improved patient identification and refined entry criteria for clinical investigations. More recently, these categorical definitions have been refined to acknowledge that it is not only infection but systemic inflammation that is the underlying disorder, hence the new term "systemic inflammatory response syndrome" (SIRS) and "Severe Sepsis" to replace the former septic syndrome [3].

It has also been recently discovered that these categorical definitions both new and old have three important limitations [4]. First, they identify patients at a wide variety of baseline or pre-treatment risk. This can be seen in Fig. 1–3 which provide the risk distributions for 519 ICU patients admitted with a primary diagnosis of sepsis and classified according to the categorical definitions for sepsis syndrome (severe sepsis) (Fig. 1), sepsis syndrome with shock (Fig. 2), and the new definition SIRS (Fig. 3). Regardless of the definition chosen, there is a wide distribution of patient risks for hospital mortality from less than 10 to over 90%. The risk predictions used in these analyses were based on the general APACHE III hospital mortality equation [4], and the relative advantages of this approach, compared to a disease-specific assessment, will be discussed shortly.

Second, depending on the manner in which these screening definitions are applied, the group mortality risk can also vary widely (Fig. 1–3). The overall group mortality risk will be a function of the proportion of patients selected for inclusion in the trial who fall at a specific risk level.

Third, it has been recognized that many patients with clinical evidence of sepsis may not fulfill the exact criteria for a categorical definition like sepsis syndrome, and yet have risks similar to those patients included. This can be seen in Fig. 1 where, of the 519 patients admitted to an ICU with a primary

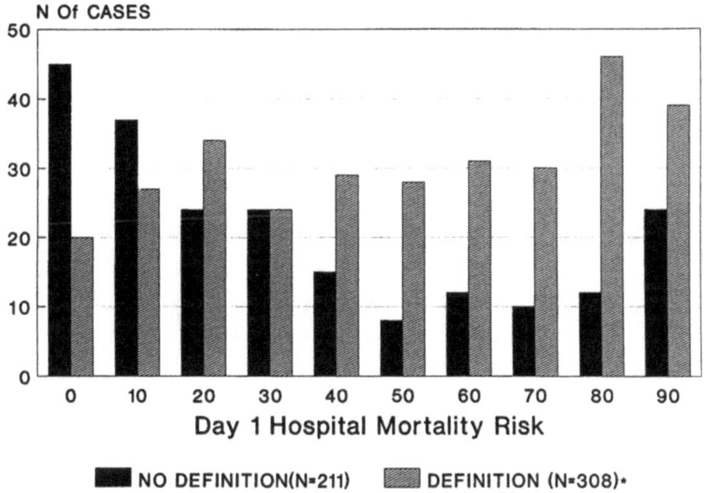

Fig. 1. Risk distribution of 519 ICU admissions with a primary clinical diagnosis of sepsis divided into patients who met categorical criteria for septic syndrome (n=308; hatched) and those who did not (n=211; black). Risk predictions are calculated from the APACHE III first day hospital mortality risk equation [44]. (From [4] with permission)

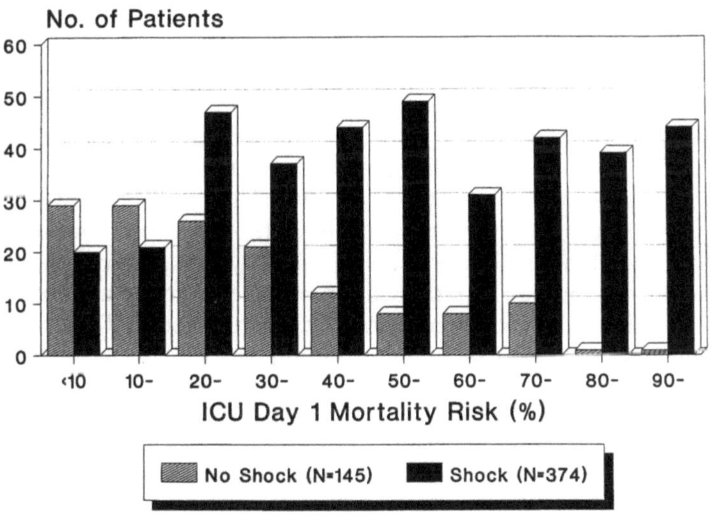

Fig. 2. Risk distribution of 519 ICU admissions with a primary clinical diagnosis of sepsis, divided into patients who met categorical criteria for shock (n=374; black) and those who did not (n=145; hatched). Risk predictions are calculated from the APACHE III first day hospital mortality risk equation [44]. (From [4] with permission)

diagnosis of sepsis, only 308 fulfill the definition for sepsis syndrome, and in Fig. 2 where only 374 of 519 met criteria for another categorical definition: septic shock.

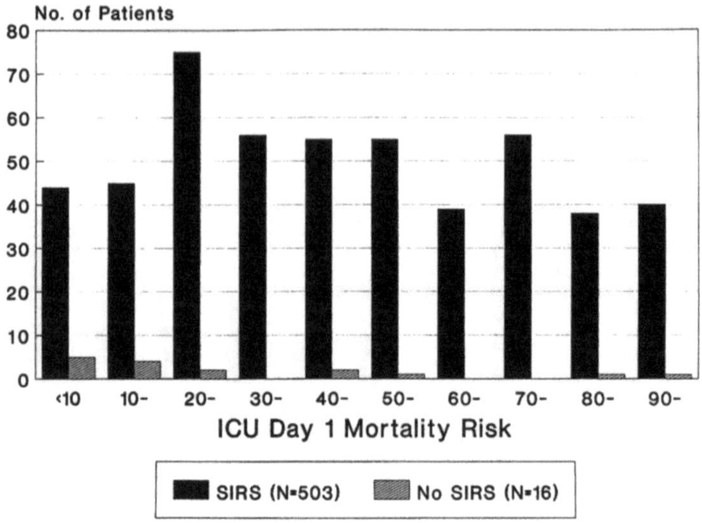

Fig. 3. Risk distribution of 519 ICU admissions with a primary clinical diagnosis of sepsis, divided into patients who met categorical criteria for SIRS (n = 503; black) and those who did not (n = 16; hatched). Risk prediction are calculated from the APACHE III first day hospital mortality risk equation [44]. (From [3] with permission)

Recognition of these limitations, in part, encouraged the development of more general and inclusive definitions for the inflammatory cascade, e.g. SIRS. For example, in Fig. 3, it can be seen that virtually all (503) of the 519 patients with a clinical diagnosis of sepsis meet SIRS criteria. This is substantially more than the 308 who qualified for the more restrictive definition: sepsis syndrome. Regardless of the definition chosen, however, it is now recognized that in all future clinical trials, these definitions should be combined with appropriate risk stratification or risk prediction methods [3]. The rational behind this recommendation are summarized in Table 1. The overall advantages for risk assessment are summarized in Table 2.

Table 1. Rationale for baseline risk assessment

- Using categorical definitions, e.g. severe sepsis, sepsis with shock, patients have a wide range of mortality risks
- Efficacy of new therapies may be related directly to mortality risk
- Risk factors cannot be identified and weighted from trial data

Table 2. Advantages of baseline risk assessment

- Confirm equal risk distribution in placebo and treatment groups
- Reduce reliance on and enhance subgroup analyses
- Quantities benefit relative to individual patient's risk

Risk Assessment and Drug Efficacy?

These advantages and their underlying rationales were made even more compelling by the recent provocative evidence that variations in estimated patient risk may be related directly to variations in therapeutic efficacy of one major new anticytokine, Interleukin-1ra (IL-1ra) [5]. This Phase III double-blind study involving 893 patients randomized at 63 medical centers suggested that patients above a specific risk level (24% risk of 28-day mortality) received benefit from IL-1ra, while patients whose risk was below 24% did not.

These results suggesting a relationship between patient risk and efficacy of IL-1ra are consistent with animal and recent clinical trial data evaluating the efficacy of another anticytokine, tumor necrosis factor (TNF) antagonists. A 1989 study of mice unable to produce TNF in response to infection demonstrated a 1000-fold greater susceptibility to lethal infection with *Escherichia coli* than TNF-responsive mice [6]. This suggested that certain levels of TNF may be involved in host protection, presumably patients with low risk may have low levels of TNF. A recent clinical trial of the influence of anti-TNF monoclonal antibody on cytokine levels also demonstrated a positive relationship between the efficacy of a murine anti-TNF and serum levels of TNF in a limited sample of 20 patients receiving a 10 mg/kg dose [7].

In that study, patients with a pre-treatment TNF level less than 50 pg/mL had a 62% 28-day mortality (8/13), while patients with high pre-treatment TNF levels (>50 pg/mL) appeared to receive benefit from blocking TNF having a 14% (1/7) 28-day mortality ($p=0.07$). The findings from these evaluations relate directly to one of the major rationales for a comprehensive approach to risk assessment, the possibility that a patient's pretreatment risk may be directly related to drug efficacy (Table 1).

By the mid 1980's, it was widely recognized that a lack of efficacy of traditional antimicrobial therapy against infection was not the primary reason for therapeutic failure [1]. Rather there was concern that prolonged life support was creating the opportunity for normally protective biological responses to be magnified, and to create irreversible organ system damage. Basic investigation turned to agents that might modify these responses. This lead to the development of compounds aimed at antagonizing components of the inflammatory cascade, e.g. IL-1, TNF, that are stimulated when infection occurs [8].

Each of these new therapeutic compounds vary widely in their presumed mechanism of action. One aspect common to all, however, is the presumption that the normal biologic responses designed to create a defense against infection can create untoward effects if they persist because of failure to entirely eliminate the infectious focus, and the continued application of life support. For example, the ability of IL-1 to mediate neutrophil emigration can also produce distant organ system damage if the mediator persists at high levels following the initial inflammatory cascade. The optimal role of new compounds, therefore, would be to allow the protective aspects of the inflammatory cascade to continue while blocking its potentially damaging influences. Such an action assumes that blocking the inflammatory response may be a life-saving strategy but total or premature blockade may leave the patient with a less than optimal response [9]. Presumable, this is the reason the preliminary results from the Phase III evaluation of IL-1ra suggested a relationship between efficacy and patient severity or risk of death [5]. If we accept this hypothesis, the question then becomes whether predicted risk is the best way to measure the level or stage of the inflammatory response so that compounds may be appropriately targeted to block its persistent untoward effects while permitting its benefit.

One response would be to use the actual levels of the mediators, for example IL-1, to determine the appropriateness of therapy. Several investigators have attempted to correlate serum concentrations of mediators including key mediators, such as IL-1 and TNF, with patient outcome and risk but the results have been disappointing [7, 10–21]. The frequency of detection is generally less than 50%. A short circulating half-life is partially responsible for these results, along with the compartmentalization of these mediators within tissues. This can result in a significant amount of cytokine activity but low to absent circulatory concentrations [16]. It is unlikely that these measurement problems will be resolved without substantial additional investigation.

Physiology as Major Risk Factor

Anticipating that the complex biologic and measurement challenges involved in cytokine assays will not be easily or shortly resolved, attention has focused on identifying other more reliable and accurate identifiers of patient risk that could be linked to the therapeutic activity of new anticytokine and other therapies. For example, Calandra et al. [21] performed a logistic regression analysis of various risk factors for mortality from sepsis. While serum levels of IL-1 and TNF were independently associated with a poor outcome, stepwise regression analysis failed to confirm the associations. Instead, the severity of the patient's underlying disease, their age, urine output and arterial pH were found to be the major determinants of outcome.

These extremely important findings confirm numerous studies published during the past two decades that have pointed toward the importance of physiology and patient characteristics in determining outcome from sepsis. Some of these efforts have been designed at predicting mortality for ICU admissions while others have been specifically designed for outcome prediction in sepsis. A comprehensive review of these efforts is beyond the scope of this chapter, but an overview summarized in Table 3 suggests that a combination of patient factors, most importantly the acute severity of the patient's condition, were influential in determining outcome. What was not resolved from these efforts, however, was the exact weighting and optimal combination of these various risk factors and the relative influence of the type of infection or nature of infecting organism when compared to patient factors. The latter is a critical point. While type of organism has been linked

Table 3. Major current pretreatment prognostic variables in sepsis

	Ref.
Severity of sepsis	
– General physiologic abnormalities	[4, 21, 37–41, 44–46]
– Shock	[22–25, 28–30, 36, 42, 43]
– Organ system failure	[22–24, 27, 28, 30]
– Neutropenia	[25, 27, 29]
Underlying acute disease	[4, 22, 23, 25, 26, 28–30, 34–36, 40, 41, 44]
Patient's chronic health condition	[4, 41, 44]
Timing of onset of sepsis	[4, 41, 44, 46]

in many studies to risk and patient outcome [22–30], exact identification of type of organism is not widely available when treatment decisions are being considered making this a problematic risk factor at this time.

More important, however, than the question of whether a particular prognostic variable should be included is how should the multiple risk factors in Table 3 be combined? It is not possible for every clinical trial to identify and determine the appropriate weight for each risk factor. First, the placebo arms of these clinical trials are not large enough to identify stable, reliable weighting schemes for each factor. Second, the data search or multiple comparisons inherent in such model-building are not appropriate when evaluating the potential efficacy of new compounds. Third, the patients selected for these trials may not be representative of the larger population of patients with sepsis.

Furthermore, what previous efforts at evaluation have taught us, however, and what the articles in Table 3 confirm is that there are *multiple* risk factors for death from sepsis, and unless we recognize and account for this complexity, we may continue to be limited in our ability to properly evaluate new therapeutic approaches. Relying on one or two risk factors, e.g. shock or a combination of these factors in categorical definitions, may also not improve our ability to discriminate because, as illustrated in Figures 1–3, categorical definitions contain patients at multiple levels of risk.

In view of these findings, we are proposing the development of a comprehensive individual patient baseline risk assessment that would take into consideration all the key variables listed in Table 3 that have been demonstrated to influence the risk of any seriously ill patient with sepsis [1]. Such assessments and analyses are now possible using large clinical databases and multivariate statistical techniques [31]. These capabilities can be used to create an estimate for short-term mortality that would reduce the ambiguity of current attempts at case mix control and risk prediction. Such an effort might not only lead to a better understanding of risk in sepsis, but could also lead to indications of the potential value of these new drugs for individual patients. Because our knowledge in this field is expanding rapidly and because many new compounds are undergoing clinical evaluation, it will be important to create a uniform approach to risk assessment, so the results of such analyses can be combined for comparative purposes. It is also important that this be a dynamic process that can incorporate new insights rapidly.

Methods for a Comprehensive Baseline Risk Assessment in Sepsis

Recent advances in the storage and retrieval of clinically-accurate patient data has resulted in the development of large contemporary databases. Simultaneous advances in the ability to analyze and model risk factors for outcome from an acute illness, like sepsis, have created a new technical and intellectual basis for risk adjustment in clinical evaluations of new therapeutic compounds. Using the steps outlined in Table 4, these databases can be used as large contemporary "control" groups. The groups can be used to investigate, confirm, and compile risk factors for outcome. As the size and representativeness of these databases expand, these efforts at risk prediction can be revisited and improved. If similar data collection procedures are followed then, as indicated in Table 4, the risk prediction may also involve comparison of the efficacy of combinations of new therapeutic compounds. For our current purposes, however, we will begin with the development of an initial sepsis-specific risk model.

While there have been many candidates for prognostic factors in sepsis, the overwhelming evidence is that because of their reliability and availability, a combination of physiologic and other patient-related risk variables, offer the most promising current approach. Each of the specific components in Table 3 is supported by studies that have examined its relationship with outcome, usually hospital or other short-term mortality outcomes. For example,

Table 4. Methods for developing a comprehensive risk assessment approach for patients with sepsis

Step 1. Apply exact study selection criteria, e.g. sepsis syndrome, severe sepsis, SIRS to large clinically-accurate database of severely ill hospitalized patients to select cohort of patients for risk assessment.

Step 2. Analyze cohort of patients meeting exact study entry criteria to create comprehensive risk assessment model. Investigate various approaches to modelling and risk assessment.

Step 3. Develop and validate risk model prior to analysis of clinical trial data.

Step 4. Apply independent risk prediction on patients at time of study qualification. Use risk assessment to check for imbalances in risk between treatment and control groups, and to investigate relationship between risk and drug efficacy.

Step 5. Use results from clinical trial to refine entry criteria for next trial, or to develop indications for use.

Note: As clinical trials are performed and the clinical databases described in Step 1 expand, steps 2 to 4 can be repeated to improve risk prediction, and to investigate indications for specific compounds or combinations of compounds.

a number of studies (see specific references in Table 3) have linked the developments of physiologic changes such as shock and multible organ system failure to mortality. As previously emphasized, what has not been done is to combine these factors into a single comprehensive model.

A preliminary step in this regard, however, was begun with the risk predictions used in Fig. 1–3 [44]. These risk predictions were produced using most of the components listed in Table 3 and represent an early attempt to provide a comprehensive risk adjustment. Specifically, a logistic regression equation was developed on 519 patients with sepsis as their primary reason for admission to the ICU. Hospital mortality was the dependent variable. The predictive variables were the first ICU day APACHE III score (the acute physiology score along with age and chronic health points), the etiology of sepsis defined as urosepsis or other sources, and the patient's treatment location prior to ICU admission (ward, emergency department, operating room, etc) [44]. All three of these independent variables were significantly related to the hospital mortality risk. The APACHE III score was the most important with a partial Wald chi-square of 100 compared to 16 for etiology and 12 for prior treatment location. This supports the many studies listed in Table 3 that have associated physiologic abnormalities with outcome in sepsis. The model also acknowledges, however, that the etiology of the sepsis and the state of the patient prior to development of the septic episode are also important prognostically.

The overall explanatory power of the predictive system was good with the receiver-operator-characteristics (ROC) curve = 0.82. The accuracy of this approach to risk prediction can be seen in Fig. 4 where the model is applied to the 503 patients from the original 519 who were admitted to an ICU with the primary diagnosis of sepsis and who also met criteria for SIRS.

In a more recent study, and in keeping with the objective of constantly improving the risk adjustment, we have taken this approach the next logical step and created a sepsis specific comprehensive risk predictive model [32]. This was done by analyzing a larger group of 1195 patients with a variety of indications of sepsis. Each of these patients had to meet entry criteria for clinical evaluations of septic drugs, e.g. sepsis syndrome or severe sepsis, to use the more recently proposed definition.

Using this database, we refined our predictive model for sepsis by discovering that in addition to the acute physiologic abnormalities as measured by the acute physiology score of APACHE III, additional weight provided to two physiologic variables, white blood cell count and serum pH, improved explanatory power. These findings are compatible with previous investigations suggesting the importance of very low white counts and metabolic acidosis in sepsis. We also were able to take this opportunity to further refine two of the other constructs listed in Table 3: acute disease and timing of onset of sepsis. This was done by refining the use of diagnoses and by incorporating as predictive variables the number of days the patient was in the hospital and the ICU prior to meeting the criteria for sepsis

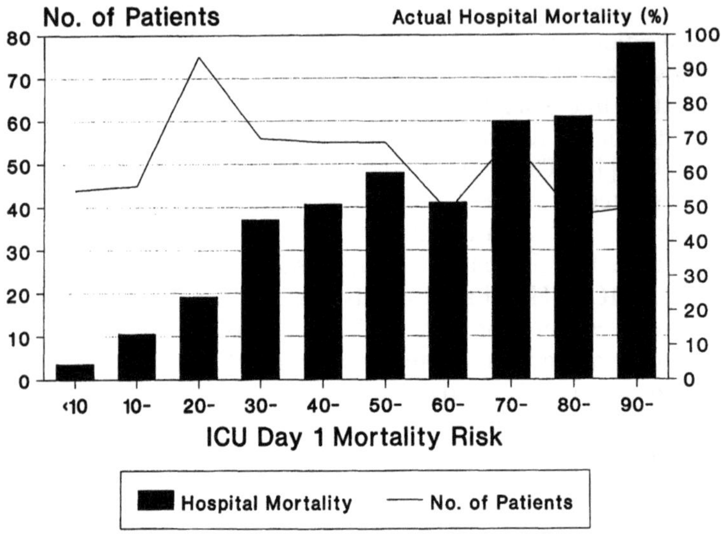

Fig. 4. Risk distribution of 503 patients with a primary clinical diagnosis of sepsis who met the criteria for SIRS, demonstrating the relationship between risk of hospital mortality, calculated on the first of the ICU day, and actual hospital mortality rates. Risk prediction are calculated from the APACHE III first day hospital mortality risk equation [44]. (From [3] with permission)

syndrome. All of these factors were combined in a comprehensive model that would provide an estimate of the patient's risk of 28-day mortality at the time they were entered into a clinical trial [Table 4]. The exact details of this modelling effort can be found in the acticle [32], but the results support the conclusions of previous efforts that the severity of the illness, the etiology of the septic episode, the prior health of the patient, and the duration of illness prior to treatment are all independent and complementary risk factors for mortality by 28 days. Evidence from validation efforts within the original 1195 patient database, an independent validation sample of 295 [32], and recent application to a large scale clinical evaluation all support the accuracy of this approach in predicting 28-day mortality risk [5].

But demonstrating that a comprehensive risk model based on the construct listed in Table 3 can accurately predict risk in sepsis does not entirely address the question of whether this is the optimal approach to determining outcome. Ideally, one would also want to know that the approach was superior to other efforts and that it corresponded to the underlying severity of the septic or inflammatory cascade.

In regard to previous risk prediction efforts in sepsis, the comprehensive approach we have taken using a sepsis specific modification of a general prognostic scoring system, APACHE III, can be demonstrated to be superior to the use of the scoring system alone or earlier approaches to sepsis scoring [32].

It can also be demonstrated that, once a comprehensive measure of patient is available, it is superior in identifying patients who may benefit from new therapy than a variety of categorical definitions of infection or specific organ system failures such as shock or ARDS. The latter finding is most likely because, as seen in Figure 3, patients with the septic syndrome and shock still have a wide variety of baseline predicted risk.

But what evidence do we have that this comprehensive risk estimate is related to the underlying severity of the inflammatory cascade? One potential source of evidence would be to relate the risk predictions produced by this approach to circulating cytokine levels. Considering the aforementioned difficulties with cytokine measurements, however, such determinations may not be possible or may only be possible with less specific determinations of inflammation, such as IL-6 [13, 17]. Another still indirect but important consideration is how does the pre-treatment risk estimate relate to the time of the patient's death? If some of the new approaches to therapy, such as anticytokine therapy, is effective, it should be reducing deaths because it reduces the untoward effects of circulating cytokines. This can only occur during the time of infusion. This implies that the severity of the inflammatory cascade at the time of the infusion may be influential in determining the benefit of the compound. The more active the septic cascade the more likely the patient will be to die from sepsis.

In Figure 5, we have plotted the relationship between the predicted risk of 28-day mortality from sepsis and the mean time to death. The risk prediction is drawn from the above-mentioned comprehensive individual risk assessment [32], and the time to death is the mean time to death of all deaths (424) within the original 1195 patients upon which the risk prediction was based. It can be seen that patients at low predicted risk of death take almost twice as long to die as those at high risk. Among the 95 patients with a baseline predicted mortality risk, less than 30% mean survival time was 10.3 days. For the 245 patients in the 30 to 70% predicted mortality range, mean survival time was 9.4 days; but for the 84 patients who died and had a predicted risk over 70%, mean survival time was only 5.2 days. This suggests that patients at a predicted high risk are not only at high risk of dying but at high risk of dying in the next few days. If this high risk of death in the short-term is from the effects of biologic mediators creating unstable hemodynamic and other acute end-organ damage, then the association between the risk estimate and drug efficacy would be further established. It would suggest that the patients for whom anticytokine therapy are most useful are those patients with sepsis that are at substantial risk of short-term death.

Future Investigations

The sepsis-specific risk model referred to above must be considered dynamic. If a uniform data collection strategy encompassing the data elements included in Table 3 is adopted in most clinical evaluations, we will have

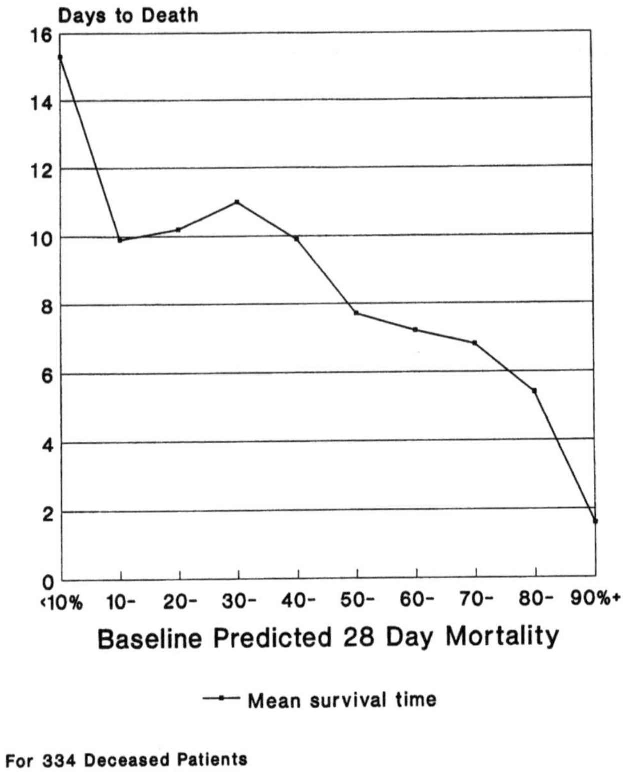

Fig. 5. Distribution of mean time to death of all 424 patients who died by 28 days within cohort of 1195 patients according to baseline predicted risk at the time they met criteria for septic syndrome (severe sepsis). Patients at low baseline risk of death demonstrate longer survival time. Baseline predicted risk of 28-day mortality calculated from a sepsis-specific risk model. (From [32] with permission)

larger and more comprehensive databases from which to build and refine predictive models. Included in Table 5 for future consideration is the nature of the infecting organism and the level of the circulating mediators. If our current measurement difficulties with these variables are overcome, they could be incorporated into future predictive efforts.

Table 5. Future possible prognostic factors in sepsis (Assuming accurate pre-treatment measurement)

- Cytokine levels
  e.g. IL-1, TNF, IL-6
- Type of organism
  e.g. gram-negative/pseudomonas
- Factors related to efficacy of specific compounds
  e.g. low platelet counts, IL-1ra, myocardial depression, TNF

As we learn more about the contribution of various pre-treatment patient elements we can refine the model to incorporate this new knowledge. For example, the risk model referred to above did not, because of data availability, contain information on platelet count or coagulation abnormalities. Since these elements have been related to patient risk in sepsis, they may contribute incrementally to the model's accuracy. As databases expand, we will also be able to explore the most appropriate statistical techniques for combining the predictive elements. In our recent sepsis-specific model, we found that an accelerated failure time statistical model log-normal provided the best fit between the predictive elements and patient outcome [32]. Specifically, we found that patients who were severely ill with substantial acute physiologic abnormalities dies within a few days. The relative influence of these same acute physiologic abnormalities was substantially less two or three weeks later. This relationship is in violation of the Cox proportional hazards model and other commonly used statistical approaches to recent larger scale clinical trial evaluations [47, 48]. It is also becoming apparent from these and other recent trials [5] that determining the incremental value of new therapies, the magnitude of their mortality reduction, and their indications for use is a complex process. Large, independent data files and risk prediction can assist in this effort.

The risk prediction can be useful, for example, to investigate the influence of other treatment factors, such as the adequacy of antibiotic therapy, and the type of affecting organism on outcome. Both of these factors have been demonstrated to relate to outcome, but the exact role each plays, when considered along with a comprehensive measure of patient risk requires further investigation. It is possible, for example, that the prognostic influence of infection with particular organism, such as *Pseudomonas* [25–27], is related to the type of patients that acquire such infections or the organism itself may have independent value. Likewise, the important influence of the adequacy of antibiotic therapy must be continually scrutinized as a potential confounding factor [33, 34].

The availability of a comprehensive pre-treatment risk assessment will also be useful in investigating the potential efficacy of new therapeutic compounds in regard to their most appropriate use. While current preliminary evidence suggests that a comprehensive physiologic-based risk assessment may be a valid indicator of the incremental benefit of new compounds, additional work is needed to reinforce and refine that assessment. These efforts must await the availability of larger databases containing substantial number of patients treated with these new compounds. When such databases are available, we can examine the interaction among the risk estimate, use of the new compound, and patient benefit taking into consideration other potentially useful patient descriptors such as type of organ system failure or individual physiologic measures. These efforts could then lead not only to improve clinical evaluations, but to refinements in development of exact indications for use.

Conclusions

1. Patients with sepsis have multiple risk factors mortality. This is a grade "A" conclusion. It is supported by evidence from numerous observational studies, along with recently completed randomized clinical trials.
2. Predictive models can be produced which contain multiple patient risk factors. These models can provide accurate pre-treatment estimates of prognosis from sepsis. This is a grade "B" conclusion. It is supported by observational studies and evidence from one recently completed clinical trial.
3. Categorical definitions such as sepsis syndrome, sepsis syndrome with shock, and various definitions of organ system failure identify sepsis patients with a wide variation in individual patient risks. This is a grade "A" conclusion, based both on recently published observational studies and randomized clinical trials.
4. Clinical trials relying on categorical descriptors of sepsis patients, such as sepsis syndrome or organ system failure, have failed to establish efficacy for new adjunctive therapy. This is a grade "B" conclusion, based on randomized trials with relatively low power.

Recommendations

1. Individual predicted risk of mortality based on a comprehensive set of risk factors modelled from an independent database should be measured at study entry in all trials of patients with sepsis. Grade A−/B+.
2. Relationship of individual predicted risk of mortality and outcome should be confirmed in placebo group. Risk distribution in placebo and treatment groups can be used to confirm randomization of risks and to test for interaction between risk and efficacy of new therapy. Grade B.
3. The relationship of individual predicted risk of mortality and mediator and soluble receptor levels should be investigated by measuring them at study entry and then daily during period of drug administration. Grade C.

Acknowledgements: Supported by the Agency for Health Care Policy and Research (HSO 7137).

References

1. Bone RC (1991) The pathogenesis of sepsis. Ann Intern Med 115:457–469
2. Bone RC, Fisher C, Clemmer TP, et al (1989) Sepsis syndrome: A valid clinical entity. Crit Care Med 17:389–394
3. Bone RC, Balk RA, Cerra FB, et al (1992) Definitions of sepsis and organ failure and guidelines for the use of innovative therapies in sepsis. Chest 101:1644–1655
4. Knaus WA, Sun X, Nystrom PO, Wagner DP (1992) Evaluation of definitions for sepsis. Chest 101:1656–1662

5. Fisher CJ Jr, Dhainaut JF, Pribble JP, Knaus WA, and the IL-1 Receptor Antagonist Study Group (1993) A study evaluating the safety and efficacy of human recombinant interleukin-1 receptor antagonist in the treatment of patients with sepsis syndrome. Clin Intensive Care 4:8 (Abst)
6. Cross AS, Sadoff JC, Kelly N, Bernton E, Gemski P (1989) Pretreatment with recombinant murine tumor necrosis factor α/cachectin and murine interleukin-1α protects mice from lethal bacterial infection. J Exp Med 169:2021–2027
7. Fisher CJ, Opal SM, Dhainaut JF, et al (1993) Influence of an anti-tumor necrosis factor monoclonal antibody on cytokine levels in patients with sepsis. Crit Care Med 21:318–327
8. Dinarello CA, Gelfand JA, Wolff SM (1993) Anticytokine strategies in the treatment of the systemic inflammatory response syndrome. JAMA 269:1829–1835
9. Dinarello CA (1992) Role of interleukin-1 in infectious diseases. Immunol Rev 127:119–146
10. Wortel CH, von der Mohlen MAM, van Deventer SJH, et al (1992) Effectiveness of a human monoclonal antiendotoxin antibody (HA-1A) in gram-negative sepsis:Relationship to endotoxin and cytokine levels. J Infect Dis 166:1367–1374
11. Tracey KJ (1992) Tumor necrosis factor in the biology of septic shock syndrome. Circ Shock 35:123–128
12. Waage A, Halstensen A, Espevik T (1987) Association between tumour necrosis factor in serum and fatal outcome in patients with meningococcal disease. Lancet 1:355–357
13. Calandra T, Gerain J, Heumann D, Baumgartner JD, Glauser MP (1991) High circulating levels in interleukin-6 in patients with septic shock: Evolution during sepsis, prognostic value, and interplay with other cytokines. Am J Med 91:23–29
14. Debets JMH, Kampmeijer R, van der Linden MPMH, Buurman WA (1989) Plasma tumor necrosis factor and mortality in critically ill septic patients. Crit Care Med 17:489–494
15. Girardin E, Grau GE, Dayer JM, Roux-Lombard P, and the J5 Study Group (1988) Tumor necrosis factor and interleukin-1 in the serum of children with severe infectious purpura. N Engl J Med 319:397–400
16. Lowry SF (1993) Anticytokine therapies in sepsis. New Horizons 1:120–126
17. Hack CE, DeGroot ER, Felt-Bersma RJF, et al (1989) Increased plasma levels of interleukin-6 in sepsis. Blood 74:1704–1710
18. Waage A, Brandtzaeg P, Halstensen A, Kierulf P, Espevik T (1989) The complex pattern of cytokines in serum from patients with meningococcal septic shock. J Exp Med 169:333–338
19. Hamilton G, Hofbauer S, Hamilton B (1992) Endotoxin, TNF-alpha, interleukin-6 and parameters of the cellular immune system in patients with intra-abdominal sepsis. Scand J Infect Dis 24:362–368
20. Dinarello CA, Wolff SM (1993) The role of interleukin-1 in disease. N Engl J Med 328:106–113
21. Calandra T, Baumgartner JD, Grau GE, et al (1990) Prognostic values of tumor necrosis factor, interleukin-1, interferon-α, snf interferon-γ in the serum of patients with septic shock. J Infect Dis 161:982–987
22. Uaun O, Akalin HE, Hayran M, Unal S (1992) Factors influencing prognosis in bacteremia due to gram-negative organisms: Evaluation of 448 episodes in a Turkish university hospital. Clin Infect Dis 15:866–873
23. Gracia de la Torre M, Romero-Vivas T, Martinez-Beltran J, Guerrero J, Meseguer M, Bouza E (1985) Klebsiella bacteremia: An analysis of 100 episodes. Rev Infect Dis 7:143–150
24. Bouza E, Garcia de la Torre M, Erice A, Losa E, Diaz-Borrego JM, Buzon L (1985) Enterobacter bacteremia: An analysis of 50 episodes. Arch Intern Med 145:1024–1027
25. Bisbe J, Gatell JM, Puig J, et al (1988) Pseudomonas aeruginosa bacteremia: Univariate and multivariate analyses of factors influencing the prognosis in 133 episodes. Rev Infect Dis 10:629–635

26. Gallager PG, Watanakunakorn C (1989) Pseudomonas bacteremia in a community teaching hospital, 1980–84. Rev Infect Dis 11:846–852
27. Hilf M, Yu VL, Sharp J, Zuravleff JJ, Korvick JA, Muder RR (1989) Antibiotic therapy for pseudomonas aeruginosa bacteremia: Outcome correlations in a prospective study of 200 patients. Am J Med 87:540–546
28. Gatell JM, Trilla A, LaTorre X, et al (1988) Nosocomial bacteremia in a large Spanish teaching hospital: Analysis of factors influencing prognosis. Rev Infect Dis 10:203–210
29. Ashkenazi S, Leibovici L, Samra Z, Konisberger H, Drucker M (1992) Risk factors for mortality due to bacteremia and fungemia in childhood. Clin Infect Dis 14:949–951
30. Cooper GS, Havlir DS, Shlaes DM, Salata RA (1991) Polymicrobial bacteremia in the late 1980's: Predictors of outcome and review of the literature. Medicine 69:114–123
31. Knaus WA, Wagner DP, Lynn J (1991) Short-term mortality predictions for critically ill hospitalized adults: Science and ethics. Science 254:389–394
32. Knaus WA, Harrell FE, Fisher CJ, Wagner DP, Opal SM, Sadoff JC (1993) The clinical evaluation of new drugs for sepsis: A prospective study design based on survival analysis. JAMA 270:1233–1241
33. Graninger W, Ragette R (1992) Nosocomial bacteremia due to enterococcus fecalis without endocarditis. Clin Infect Dis 15:49–57
34. Hoge CW, Adams J, Buchanan B, Sears SD (1991) Enterococcal bacteremia, to treat or not to treat, a reappraisal. Rev Infect Dis 13:600–605
35. Malone DA, Wagner RA, Myers JP, Watanakunakorn C (1986) Enterococcal bacteremia in two large community teaching hospitals. Am J Med 81:601–606
36. Fidalgo S, Vazquez F, Mendoza MC, Perez F, Mendez FJ (1990) Bacteremia due to staphylococcus epidermidis: Microbiologic, epidemiologic, clinical, and prognostic features. Rev Infect Dis 12:520–528
37. Elebute EA, Stoner HB (1983) The grading of sepsis. Brit J Surg 70:29–31
38. Stevens LE (1983) Grading the severity of surgical sepsis. Arch Surg 118:1190–1192
39. Knaus WA, Zimmerman JE, Wagner DP, Draper EA, Lawrence DE (1981) APACHE-acute physiology and chronic health evaluation: A physiologically based classification system. Crit Care Med 9:591–597
40. Dellinger EP, Wertz MJ, Meakins JL, et al (1985) Surgical infection stratification system for intra-abdominal infection. Arch Surg 120:21–29
41. Knaus WA, Draper EA, Wagner DP, Zimmerman JE (1985) APACHE II: A severity of disease classification system. Crit Care Med 13:818–829
42. Goris RJA, te BoeDherst TPA, Nuytinek JKS, et al (1985) Multiple organ failure: Generalized autodestructive inflammation. Arch Surg 120:1109–1115
43. Knaus WA, Draper EA, Wagner DP, Zimmerman JE (1985) Prognosis of organ-system failure. Ann Surg 202:685–693
44. Knaus WA, Wagner DP, Wagner DP, et al (1991) The APACHE III prognostic system: Risk prediction of hospital mortality for critically ill hospitalized adults. Chest 100:1619–1636
45. Meck M, Munster AM, Winchurch RA, Dickerson C (1991) The Baltimore sepsis scale: Measurement of sepsis in patients with burns using a new scoring system. J Burn Care Rehabil 12:564–568
46. Baumgartner JD, Bula C, Vaney C, Wu M, Eggiman P, Perret C (1992) A novel score for predicting the mortality of septic shock patients. Crit Care Med 20:953–960
47. Ziegler EJ, Fisher CJ, Sprung CL, et al (1991) Treatment of gram-negative bacteremia and septic shock with HA-1A human monoclonal antibody against endotoxin. N Engl J Med 324:429–436
48. Greenman RL, Schein RMH, Martin MA, Wenzel RP, MacIntyre NR, Emmanuel G (1991) A controlled clinical trial of E5 murine monoclonal IgM antibody to endotoxin in the treatment of gram-negative sepsis. JAMA 266:1097–1102

SAPS II and MPM II Models for Early Severe Sepsis

J. R. Le Gall and S. Lemeshow

Introduction

The "Sepsis syndrome" refers to the clinical and biological manifestations of infection, no matter the intensity of the symptoms or the type and timing of infection.

What are the Problems?

Two main problems exist about definition and grading of sepsis.

Firstly, the sepsis syndrome is not a diagnosis. It includes urinary infection, pneumonia, septicemia of all origins, bacteriological, fungal, viral infections. Is it possible to use a unique model for all these pathologies? Besides, the definitions used in compiling the database may be different from the target population. Since the appearance of the anti-endotoxin or anti-cytokine antibodies, therapeutic trials among septic patients have been more frequently conducted. The results, however, are often controversial, which may be due at least in part to the inclusion of all septic patients in the studies, without taking in account the many different types of sepsis. Is it reasonable to include in the same study patients who are septic from urinary sources and patients who have pneumonia, peritonitis, or catheter-related infection? An obviously limiting factor has been the necessity to obtain information on a sufficiently large number of patients to perform the desired statistical comparisons.

Secondly, until recently, there was no proposed grading of sepsis. It is why the reports of mortality rates from sepsis have differed widely: 30% in the steroid trials [1], 20% in the Veterans Administration Cooperative Study [2], 35% in the HA-1A [3].

Subjective Grading of Sepsis

In 1991, the American College of Chest Physicians (ACCP) proposed a grading of severity of sepsis based on clinical and biological symptoms available at the bedside [4]. According to the definitions, four stages of increasing severity were defined: sepsis, severe sepsis, septic shock, and multiple organ dysfunction syndrome. One of the primary criticisms of the proposed grading system is that, in order to be useful for the selection of patients, the severity of illness as reflected in a probability of mortality should be accurately assessed, in addition to the grading of sepsis. For instance, in the European-North American database, the repartition of risk of death varies in the group of severe sepsis from 0.01 to 0.99, showing the necessity to add a probability model to analyse the results.

Model Development Strategy

Since the multipurpose models do not calibrate correctly, the development of a specific probability model for sepsis patients is necessary. There are 3 ways to develop a specific model: from a specific database, from an existing database using an expanded model, and from an existing database using the customization technique.

Ideally, models could be developed on samples of sepsis patients on whom data were collected for the express purpose of model development. A large number of specifically defined patients could be enrolled and the data would be used to generate an entirely new model with a unique set of variables. This would be, of course, a time-consuming and expensive developmental effort.

Another way is to use an existing database, from which the patients of interest are selected and a new model is generated using a unique set of important variables. For instance, a model for sepsis, using physiology, primary disease, previous intensive care, age, clinical history of cirrhosis and other data, has been recently developed [5]. The model was based on a scoring system into which additional risk factors have been incorporated.

The third way is to use the customization technique. This was our method, using the European-North American Study Data Base. Although this study was not specifically designed to build models for septic patients, we could isolate the group of patients with severe sepsis. We collected data for the first ICU day, so the proposed models are only for the early ICU sepsis. The definition of confirmed infection at the 24th hour was as follows: Enter "yes" only if cultures, gram-stains, or X-rays confirm a suspected admission infection or new infection that developed in the first 24 h, or if there is evidence of gross purulence. Laboratory confirmation (including versal or "FAX-type" confirmation) must be obtained by the 24-hour mark for "Confirmed" to be entered. A confirmed diagnosis from another source was acceptable if cultures are negative because patient has been on antibiotics.

Patient were classified as having severe sepsis if they manifested the systemic inflammatory response syndrome (SIRS) and infection, plus evidence of hypotension, hypoperfusion or multiple organ dysfunction. These criteria for identifying patients with severe sepsis correspond to the ACCP/SCCM guidelines for severe sepsis or worse, including septic shock and sepsis in conjunction with hypotension or multiple organ dysfunction.

For each patient, vital status at hospital discharge was determined, and 28-day survival curve were constructed to examine the differential survival between severe sepsis patients and all others. The risk of death as estimated by the probability of hospital mortality was assessed based on two statistical models: SAPS II (Table 1) [6] and MPM II24 [7], the 24-hour model of the MPM II system (Table 2).

It was determined that the standard SAPS II and MPM II24 did not fit the data well. We decided to modify the models to adapt them for use specifically among severe sepsis patients by using multiple logistic regression techniques to generate a customized SAPS II and a customized MPM II24 models for this subgroup of patients. For SAPS II, the score has been used as a term in a new logistic regression equation, and the logic of the MPM II24 has been used as a term in a different logistic regression equation.

This technique does not necessitate additional data collection by users of the standard SAPS II and MPM II24 models in order for the new models to be implemented in studies of severe sepsis patients. The success of the customization has been evaluated by examining both the calibration and discrimination of the new models.

Validation of a Probability Model

In order to answer the questions about the ability of models to provide accurate estimates of hospital mortality, two important statistical criteria must be defined: discrimination and calibration. Discrimination uses the area under the receiver-operator-characteristics (ROC) curve to evaluate the ability of a model to distinguish patients who die from patients who live, based on the estimated probabilities of mortality [8]. Calibration evaluates the degree of correspondence between a model estimated probabilities of mortality and the actual mortality experience of patients within severity strata using formal goodness of-fit tests [9].

Both discrimination and calibration criteria should be used to evaluate and compare the predictive efficacy of competing models. The area under the ROC curve provides an assessment of a model's ability to discriminate between patients who live and patients who die. Goodness-of-fit testing indicates whether the model is well calibrated. Calibration and discrimination provide different and useful information about a model's performance. Both techniques should be used routinely to evaluate models prior to their dissemination for general use. Whether a model fits well or not tells us nothing about the discrimination ability of the model, and the reverse is also true. Once it has been determined that a model does fit well, ROC analysis should be used to assess a model's performance with regard to discrimination, so that both parameters of model performance are applied to models in development.

Table 1. SAPS II Score

Variable	26	13	12	11	9	7	6	5	4	3	2
Age (years)											
Heart Rate (beat/min)				<40							40.69
Syst Blood Press (mm Hg)		<70						70.99			
Body temperature (°C)											
PaO_2/FiO_2 (mm Hg) Only if VENT or CPAP				<100	100.199	≥200					
Urinary Output (L/day)				<0.500					0.500.0.999		
Blood Urea (mMol/L) (g/L)											
WBC Count (10E3/mL)			<1.0								
Serum K (mEq/L)										<3.0	
Serum Na (mEq/L)								<125			
Serum HCO_3 (mEq/L)						<15				15.19	
Bilirubin (μMol/L)											
Glasgow Coma Score (Points)	<6	6.8					9.10	11.13			
Chronic diseases											
Type of admission											
Sum of Points											

In order to adequately compare observed to expected number of deaths based on a logistic regression model, it is necessary to construct a confidence interval for the ratio of observed to expected number of deaths [10]. Without taking into account these confidence intervals, it is not possible to state with a specific level of confidence that the observed mortality rate in the treatment group is statistically different from that predicted by the model in a similar group of untreated patients.

Validation of a probability model requires that calibration and discrimination be assessed in the new group of patients. Our sepsis models calibrate and discriminate well, but the limited sample size did not permit independent validation of the models. Therefore, validation efforts among other groups of sepsis patients must be undertaken. The area under the ROC curve is important, since it measures the discrimination power of the model. Nevertheless, they do not indicate whether calibration is also good. The success of the customization technique using information already easily collected for the standard SAPS II or MPM II24 calculations means that the data for these models can easily be collected for validation from precisely defined sepsis patients. One could argue that some factors generally considered important on the prognosis of sepsis, such as cirrhosis, hypothermia, anemia, lead-time bias, or origin of sepsis are not adequately addressed by

0	1	2	3	4	6	7	8	9	10	12	15	16	17	18
<40						40.59				60.69	70.74	75.79		>80
70.119				120.159		≥160								
100.199		≥200												
<39°			≥39°											
≥1000														
<10.0 <0.60					10.0.29.9 0.60.1.79				≥30.0 ≥1.80					
1.0.19.9			≥20.0											
3.0.4.9			≥5.0											
125.144	≥145													
≥20														
<68.4 <40.0				68.4.102.4 40.0.59.9				≥102.5 ≥60.0						
14.15														
								Met. Can.	Hem. Mal.				AIDS	
Elec.					Med.		S.Em.							

Total SAPS II = [ ] Pts

Risk of Hospital Death = [ ] %

customizing our standard models for severe sepsis patients. It can be demonstrated that more complex models with additional variables, the number of which could be very large depending on the technique used to decide whether variables should be included, also provide accurate estimates of the probability of mortality of severe sepsis patients. On the other hand, the customization technique resulted in high performance models without them having to be made more complicated.

Use of the SAPS II and MPM II Models for Trials in Early Severe Sepsis

Once developed and validated, how are the probability models useful for a therapeutic trial? When a therapeutic trial is designed to compare outcome in experimental and placebo groups, a model that provides an estimate of the groups at the start of the trial and to evaluate the efficacy of the therapy

Table 2. Variables for the MPM II 24

Admission variables
– Age (10-year odds ratio)
– Metastatic neoplasm
– Cirrhosis
– Intracranial mass effect
– Admission not for elective surgery
24-h variables
– Coma or deep stupor at 24 h
– Urine output <150 ml in 8-h period
– Mechanical ventilation
– Creatine >2.0 mg/dL
– IV vasoactive drug therapy
– Prothrombin time >3 sec above standard
– Confirmed infection
– $PO_2 < 60$ mm Hg

by comparing observed and expected outcome in the two groups within several strata of probability. This method is more accurate and precise than the classical method of comparing global mortality rates. It is possible, for example, to observe a therapeutic effect only in groups of patients at risk of death above a stated probability threshold [5].

All the proposed models are derived from large databases. In these databases, diseases are recorded with definitions spectrum and inclusion criteria which may not be the same than those used in a trial. Inclusion or exclusion criteria in a trial may concern particularities which could hardly be prospectively registered in the original database. It is not conceivable that a large database could contain all the informations which could answer to all the requirements of actual and future trials. This must lead to reject comparisons between an expected mortality rate, given by a model derived from a large database, and an observed mortality rate in a treatment group. In a recent critique of scoring systems, P. Loirat [11] favors the opposite way, by using a more simple tool without any weight for acute disease. For a trial, a specific model could be derived from the score and patients or disease characteristics in one half of the control group. This model could be used to assess comparability between the second control-half and the treatment group, which would be less expensive than repetitive trials because of lack of evidence.

In a recent editorial, HP Selker [12] states that the specific characteristics of the risk adjusted mortality predictors are: time intensive predictive instruments; they must be based on the first minutes of hospital presentation; not affected by whether a patient is hospitalized; use data collected in the usual care of the patients; must have excellent calibration; be computer system integrated, be open for inspection and testing. These criteria are probably utopian. How could a scoring system in the same time be perfectly calibrated, based on the first minutes of hospital presentation, not affected by whether the patient is hospitalized? Other characteristics are reached by the SAPS II and MPM II systems: use of data collected in the usual care of patients, open publication for inspection and testing, time insensitive predictive instruments.

Conclusions

Probability models for well-defined categories of patients, such as early ICU sepsis, have great potential for refining clinical trials among sepsis patients. The models for severe sepsis patients can be easily implemented based on easily collected data for either SAPS II or MPM II24. Model evaluation of these and other models proposed for sepsis patients should be conducted among independent groups of sepsis patients. The methodology used to develop these models must be precisely presented, and the models openly published for validation and use. It would also be desirable to develop models for use among patients whose sepsis develops later in the ICU stay. For SAPS II, this could involve using the score at later days in the ICU stay, with customized models developed to reflect the changing mortality patterns as the ICU increases. For MPM II, the later models in the system, the MPM II48 and MPM II72, could be customized for later developing severe sepsis. Observed and expected probabilities of mortality rise over the course of the ICU stay must be taken into account in efforts to characterize severe sepsis patients.

Recommendations

The SAPS II and MPM II models for early severe sepsis (within the first 24 h) in the ICU are well calibrated, discriminate well and are open to inspection and testing.

Practically speaking, the probability models cannot be used as inclusion criteria for a therapeutic trial on sepsis. The inclusion criteria must be clinical, easy to collect at the bedside. It is why the proposed ACCP/SCCM classification could be useful, to define severe sepsis as we did in this study. The less severe patients, such as those with only SIRS and infection must probably be excluded from the future therapeutic trials, since the mortality rate is relatively low and one study has shown that the effect of IL-1ra was nihil when the risk of death was below 25.

The inclusion criteria of course could be different from ours: it could be for instance the septic shock, defined not only by hypotension but other variables: oliguria, metabolic acidosis. In all cases, the model we propose for early severe sepsis must be checked on the placebo group, and if necessary, customized.

If they are to be used in a specific trial on early ICU sepsis, then they must be verified on the placebo group before comparisons are made with the treatment group.

This chapter did not include the precise coefficients for the SAPS II and MPM II models for sepsis. This is because they are included in a paper being submitted to a journal with copyright laws. They can be communicated upon request.

References

1. Bone RC, Fisher CJ Jr, Clemmer TP, Slotman GJ, Metz CA, Balk RA (1987) A controlled clinical trial of high dose methylprednisolone in the treatment of severe sepsis and septic shock. N Engl J Med 317:653–658
2. The Veterans Administration Systemic Sepsis Comparative Study Groups (1987) Effects of high dose glucocorticoid therapy on mortality in patients with clinical signs of sepsis. N Engl J Med 317:659–665
3. Ziegler EJ, Fisher CJ Jr, Sprung CL, et al (1991) Treatment of gram-negative bacteremia and septic shock with HA-1A human monoclonal antibody against endotoxin. N Engl J Med 324:429–436
4. American College of Chest Physicians/Society of Critical Care Medicine Consensus Conference (1992) Definitions for sepsis and organ failure and guidelines for the use of innovative therapies in sepsis. Crit Care Med 20:864–874
5. Knaus WA, Harrel FE, Fisher CJ, et al (1993) The clinical evaluation of new drugs for sepsis. A prospective study design based on survival analysis. JAMA 270:1233–1241
6. Le Gall JR, Lemeshow S, Saulnier F (1993) A new simplified acute physiology score (SAPS II) based on a European-North American multicenter study. JAMA 270:2957–2963
7. Lemeshow S, Teres D, Klar J, Avrunin JS, Gehlbach SH, Rapoport J (1993) Mortality probability model (MPM II) based on an international cohort of intensive care patients. JAMA 270:2478–2486
8. Hanley JA, McNeil BJ (1982) The meaning and use of the area under a receiver-operator-characteristics (ROC) curve. Radiology 143:29–36
9. Hosmer DW, Lemeshow S (1989) Applied Logistic Regression. John Wiley & Sons, New York
10. Hosmer DW, Lemeshow S (1994) Confidence internal estimates of an index of quality performance based on logistic regression models (in press)
11. Loirat P (1994) Critique of existing scoring systems: Admission scores. Intensive Care Med (in press)
12. Selker HP (1993) Systems for comparing actual and predicted mortality rates: Characteristics to promote cooperation in improving hospital care. Annals Intern Med 118:820–822

Clinical Management of Sepsis

Fluid Therapy in Septic Shock

L. G. Thijs

Introduction

In patients with septic shock, hypovolemia is a major factor contributing to circulatory instability. In the early phase, cardiac filling pressures are often lowered, due to a decrease in venous return, compromising cardiac output and tissue perfusion [1, 2]. A decline in effective circulating volume can be induced by a variety of sepsis-related mechanisms. First, generalized vasodilation increases total vascular capacitance with subsequent *relative* hypovolemia. A decline in systemic vascular resistance, mainly due to arteriolar vasodilation, is a constant feature in human septic shock [3]. Alterations in the venous capacitance system, by far the largest part of the intravascular compartment, are however difficult to assess. The concept of venous pooling as a major factor limiting effective venous return stems from animal experiments [4, 5]. Experimental studies in endotoxin and sepsis models have indicated that in several body areas venous capacitance increases. Although significant increases in venous capacitance in the forearm could not be demonstrated in the clinical study [6], it is likely that also in human septic shock venous pooling in vascular beds other than skeletal muscle (e.g. the splanchnic area) is an important mechanism. The evidence for this is, however, only circumstantial. The observation that large amounts of fluids are usually required for initial resuscitation supports such a concept. Secondly, *absolute* hypovolemia may contribute to a defect in effective circulating volume. This could be due to fever with perspiration and increased insensible loss, vomiting, diarrhea, volume loss by drains or sequestration (e.g. in the gut), and inadequate oral intake. In addition, a generalized increase in microvascular permeability for macromolecules, both in the pulmonary and systemic vascular beds, can contribute substantially to loss of intravascular volume. In particular in areas of localized infection (such as the abdominal cavity in case of peritonitis) large amounts of protein-rich fluids can extravasate.

The often observed hypoalbuminemia (especially in the later stages) due to decreased hepatic production and/or extravasation of albumin, lowers serum colloid osmotic pressure, which further compromises the ability to preserve intravascular volume. In a few patients with septic shock, inappropriate polyuria is observed [7]. Its mechanism is unclear but it is manifested by an increased urine volume despite hypotension and decreased intravascular volume. The volume deficit in septic shock may be extremely large, and failure to appreciate the significance of hypovolemia results in a low cardiac output state and increased mortality rates [8]. Recently, the importance of rapid and liberal fluid resuscitation for outcome also in pediatric septic shock has been demonstrated [9]. Therefore, there is general agreement that vigorous fluid therapy to improve venous return, cardiac output and tissue perfusion and oxygenation is the mainstay of initial resuscitation in septic shock.

In this review, mainly two questions will be addressed:

1. What are the physiologic endpoints of fluid resuscitation?
2. What is the optimal type of resuscitation fluid?

Goals and Endpoints of Fluid Resuscitation

Septic shock is hemodynamically characterized by a hyperdynamic circulation with low systemic vascular resistance, a narrowed a-v oxygen difference and a high cardiac output which sometimes becomes only manifest after restoration of circulating blood volume. This is usually associated with elevated arterial lactate levels, assumed to reflect, at least in part, tissue hypoxia related to a defective capacity to regulate peripheral oxygen extraction and impaired oxygen utilization. Tissue hypoxia, reflecting an imbalance between oxygen demand and uptake of the tissues, is considered an important contributing factor to morbidity and mortality in septic and critically ill patients [10]. Severe sepsis is a hypermetabolic syndrome with marked increases in oxygen requirements related to host defense processes [11]. The primary goal of fluid therapy as part of general supportive treatment in septic shock is to restore adequate circulating blood volume to improve tissue oxygenation in order to sustain organ function.

Oxygen Transport

Optimal levels of oxygen delivery (DO_2) are, *a priori*, significantly higher than under normal physiological circumstances because of increased metabolic needs and diminished effective oxygen extraction. Several clinical studies using indirect methods to calculate systemic oxygen consumption have demonstrated an abnormal dependency of oxygen uptake (VO_2) on oxygen supply, indicating that also at normal or even high levels of DO_2, VO_2 increases following a further increase in DO_2 [12–17]. In some studies, elevated plasma lactate levels predicted this oxygen uptake/supply dependency, supporting the concept of that increased lactate levels indicate covert tissue hypoxia [13, 14, 17]. This view has, however, recently been challenged, as in septic patients directly measured systemic oxygen uptake did not increase upon a marked increase in DO_2, both in patients with and without elevated lactate levels [18, 19].

On the basis of hemodynamic profiles in survivors, Shoemaker et al. [10] developed therapeutic goals to titrate treatment of high risk surgical patients. These include supranormal values for cardiac output and DO_2. Survival improved, also in a subgroup of septic patients, when treatment adhered to these therapeutic goals [10].

In a prospective randomized study (level 2) in septic shock, evaluating the effect of augmenting cardiac output to supranormal values during 72 h, no statistically significant difference in survival was found between treatment aimed at supranormal or at normal levels of cardiac output and DO_2 [20]. This appeared to be related to the (in)ability to reach the preset goals. A significant correlation was, however, demonstrated between DO_2 and survival, and subset analysis showed that patients who were able to increase cardiac index to >4.5 L/min/m^2 had a statistically significant higher VO_2 and lower lactate levels as well as mortality rates than those who were not. Similar observations were presented in a prospective, randomized controlled study (level 2) in critically ill patients with a majority of septic patients [21]. Maintaining $DO_2 \geq 600$ mL/min/m^2 during 24 h resulted in a higher VO_2 and statistically significant lower mortality rate, although the development of organ failure was not affected. A recent study showed two distinct patterns of response to treatment aimed at achieving supranormal DO_2 and VO_2 [22]. In those who achieved target CI, DO_2 and VO_2 simultaneously in the first 24 h, lactate levels fell and all survived. By contrast, almost all who failed to attain these goals died. Failure to increase VO_2 was related predominantly to an inability of tissues to extract or utilize oxygen rather than a failure to increase DO_2 [22]. These studies support the hypothesis that a high level of VO_2 is important for survival but also indicate that in some patients even maximal therapeutic effort may fail in reaching such a level.

Cardiac Filling Pressures

Fluid resuscitation aims at optimizing left (and right) ventricular preload in order to increase cardiac output and at minimizing complications of pulmonary (and systemic) edema which are associated with increased morbidity and mortality. In about 30–40% of the patients, rapid fluid administration alone can be sufficient to restore hemodynamic stability, but in only a few cases volume loading is sufficient to obtain optimal oxygen transport variables, and usually additional inotropic support is necessary [22].

Left ventricular (LV) filling pressure (pulmonary artery occluded pressure, wedge pressure) is usually measured to assess volume status and LV preload. An optimal filling pressure is often defined as the wedge pressure above which LV stroke work does not further increase. This level of filling pressure appears to be in the range of 12–15 mm Hg, but there are marked individual differences [23]. This issue is complicated by intrinsic myocardial abnormalities in addition to the often observed pulmonary hypertension with increased afterload to the right heart in septic shock. LV and RV dilatation associated with diminished ejection fraction, and altered Frank-Starling and pressure-volume relationships characterize myocardial performance in septic shock. RV and LV filling pressures do not correlate with RV and LV end-diastolic volume, respectively [24, 25]. Although volume loading generally results in increases in filling pressures, this response does not adequately reflect concurrent changes in end-diastolic volume [24, 26]. LV end-diastolic volume (LVEDV) may in fact increase or remains unaltered, or even declines in the presence of an increasing wedge pressure [24, 26, 27]. RVEDV usually increases upon volume loading but may also remain unchanged whereas central venous pressure increases [25, 27, 28]. In a not insignificant number of patients, a fluid challenge fails to increase stroke volume, a response which is difficult to predict and related to the complex abnormalities of cardiac performance [24, 25, 27]. In particular, patients with markedly enlarged right ventricles seem to be less likely to benefit from fluid therapy [25, 28]. Enlargement of the right heart may affect LV preload, compliance and function through septal bulging, pericardial constraint and encroachment of the left ventricle. Left ventricular performance may therefore be influenced by the loading conditions and function of the right heart. This is corroborated by the observation that patients not responding to a fluid challenge do not increase LVEDV while wedge pressure is markedly increased [24, 27], and at the same time have the most pronounced enlargement of the right ventricle [25, 27, 28]. Most of these studies included a limited number of patients and often in a heterogeneous population, and their results need to be expanded in larger and more homogeneous groups of patients, it is clear that the hemodynamic response to fluid therapy is inhomogeneous. This is dependent on the various loading conditions of the heart, and changes in myocardial competence.

It is clear that wedge pressure is of limited value in assessing (optimal) LV preload and may in fact be misleading. On the other hand, it is at present the only measurement feasible in clinical practice and wedge pressure still remains an important determinant of microvascular filtration in the lung and, therefore, clinically useful.

Optimal Hematocrit

Since enhanced tissue DO_2 is the desired endpoint of fluid resuscitation, not only the effect on total blood flow but also on arterial oxygen content must be considered. Infusion of asanguinous fluids can actually lower DO_2 while increasing cardiac output by a dilutional effect on hemoglobin concentration [13]. Low hemoglobin levels decrease the oxygen carrying capacity of the blood but also lower total blood viscosity, which may have rheological advantages and may lower vascular resistance. Increasing hemoglobin levels above 10 g/dL has been reported to increase VO_2 only in a subset of septic patients with high lactate levels [14]. In another study, VO_2 increased only in patients with normal lactate levels [29]. In contrast, other studies designed to increase hemoglobin concentration to similar levels in fully resuscitated septic patients failed to demonstrate a significant increase in systemic VO_2, even in patients with lactic acidosis [30, 31]. In one study, improvement was only observed in patients with a very limited oxygen extraction [30]. Red blood cell transfusions failed to improve gastric intramucosal acidosis while increasing systemic DO_2 [31]. These findings may reflect the effects of enhanced viscosity or vasomotor changes, or both, that occur with increases in hematocrit level, which may affect microcirculatory flow [32]. These viscosity effects may be even more pronounced due to increased red cell deformability and enhanced red cell aggregation [33, 34]. In addition, microvascular hematocrit may further increase by augmented microvascular fluid loss and loss of vasomotor control. These findings also suggest that in some cases the benefits of increased oxygen content of the blood can be offset by rheological changes associated with increased blood viscosity.

The optimal hematocrit level, therefore, is a complex issue, also because central hematocrit is not the same as capillary hematocrit. Retrospective studies in critically ill surgical patients suggested that oxygen transport and VO_2 are optimal at hematocrit values ranging from 27–33% [35]. However, the optimal hemoglobin concentration and hematocrit for adequate DO_2 and optimal VO_2 in severe sepsis have not been defined. They may likely be variable for individual patients and may also differ for the various organ systems. No controlled clinical trials have been performed addressing the issue of an optimal hematocrit and one may argue whether they are really possible given the complex pathophysiology of tissue DO_2 and VO_2 in which hemoglobin concentration is just one factor. Therefore, at present, specific recommendations cannot be made but, a hematocrit of 30–35% is usually found acceptable.

Resuscitation Fluids

Crystalloid Solutions

The two most common solutions are normal saline (0.9% NaCl) and lactated Ringer's solution. A 5% solution of glucose does not contain electrolytes and is therefore distributed throughout total body space, including the intracellular space. Only about 8% of infused 5% glucose is retained in the intravascular compartment after one hour and this solution should therefore not be utilized for fluid resuscitation. Normal saline and Ringer's lactate are freely permeable to the vascular membrane and are therefore distributed in the intravascular and interstitial compartment. There is virtually no difference between saline and Ringer's lactate as expanders of plasma volume although their electrolyte composition is different. Usually, less than 25% of the infused volumes of these solutions is retained in the intravascular space after one hour [36, 37]. By nature these solutions lower plasma colloid osmotic pressure (COP).

Small volume resuscitation with hypertonic salt solutions has been advocated for immediate treatment of hemorrhagic/traumatic shock. These solutions decrease intracellular fluid volume which is translocated to the extracellular space. They have potentially advantageous effects including improvement of cardiac contractility and precapillary vasodilation.

Colloid Solutions

Albumin is a naturally occurring plasma protein which provides approximately 80% of the plasma COP. Less than 10% of injected albumin leaves the vascular compartment within 2 h. Normal human serum albumin is available as 5% or 20–25% solution. The oncotic pressure of a 5% solution is about 20 mm Hg, whereas the higher concentrations are definitely hyperoncotic with a COP of 80–100 mm Hg. Even infusion of 5% albumin usually raises plasma COP significantly, especially in patients with low COP.

Adverse reactions to infusion occur in approximately 0.5% of patients, are generally mild and include fever, chills and urticaria. In hypovolemic patients, the 5% solutions rather than the hyperoncotic solutions are used for initial resuscitation. The hyperoncotic albumin solution may expand total plasma volume by translocation of fluid from the interstitial to the intravascular space, particularly in edematous patients. The effect of 5% albumin on expansion of plasma volume is variable, depending on the severity of the volume deficit and initial plasma COP. No selective effects on coagulation variables have been demonstrated.

Dextrans are linear polysaccharide molecules of high molecular weight which behave as colloids when dissolved in normal saline. Two dextran products are available for clinical use: dextran 40 and dextran 70. Dextran 70 is hyperoncotic and one liter of a 6% solution increases intravascular volume by 700–1200 mL [36, 37], but less than 30% of the infused volume remains intravascularly after 24 h. Dextran 40 as a 10% solution is also definitely hyperoncotic but is rapidly removed from the intravascular compartment by renal excretion and diffusion into the interstitial space, and less than 60% is present in the intravascular compartment after 4 h. Dextran 40 reduces red cell sludging and may improve tissue oxygenation. Anaphylactic reactions to dextran include abdominal discomfort, vomiting, diarrhea, urticaria, angioneurotic edema and anaphylactic shock, and occur in less than 5%. Dextrans interfere with plasmatic coagulation and increase the risk of bleeding. They impair platelet function by coating platelets. In patients with severe dehydration, there is an increased risk of acute renal failure when infusing dextran 40.

Hydroxyethyl starch (HES) is a synthetic colloid derived from amylopectin. After infusion as a 6% solution, which has a COP of around 30 mm Hg, it is slowly metabolized intravascularly by amylase. The route of elimination of small weight particles is primarily through the kidneys, and larger weight particles are phagocytized in the reticuloendothelial system. Infusion of one liter of a 6% solution expands the plasma volume by approximately 700 mL to 1 L and as much as 40% of the maximum plasma expansion persists for 24 h. Two major classes of HES are available: a high molecular weight solution (*hetastarch*), which has a prolonged intravascular effect, and a low molecular weight solution (*pentastarch*) with a more transient effect. HES has limited toxicity, anaphylactic reactions occur in approximately 0.8%. Recently, it has been suggested on the basis of experimental observations that pentastarch may have a direct "occlusive" effect on damaged capillaries and may limit extravasation of fluids in sepsis [39].

Gelatins are derivatives of collagen with a relatively low molecular weight, and several preparations are available for clinical use as 3.5–5.5% solutions with a COP slightly higher than plasma. They have been demonstrated to be effective plasma expanders in critically ill patients [39]. Gelatin solutions are rather rapidly eliminated, mainly by the kidneys, and their half life is shorter than of other colloid solutions, necessitating more frequent infusion to maintain an adequate intravascular volume. Neither specific effects on blood clotting mechanisms nor antithrombotic properties have been demonstrated. The most significant toxicity is an anaphylactoid reaction associated in most cases with histamine release. Its incidence varies with the preparation but is usually not higher than 0.8%.

Choice of Resuscitation Fluids: The Colloid-Crystalloid Controversy

For many years, a debate is ongoing on what the best asanguineous resuscitation fluid is for patients in shock. A major issue has been since the 1960's whether to choose cheap crystalloid solutions or expensive colloid solutions. Their major difference is the presence or absence of oncotically active compounds. Notwithstanding a number of clinical trials, this problem has not been solved and the colloid-crystalloid controversy still exists. This disagreement centers on the safest and most effective method to achieve the proper plasma volume to maintain adequate total body perfusion. A wide variety of patients has been studied in comparative trials ranging from young traumatized to older critically ill patients with variable underlying diseases and conditions. Many of these studies in critically ill patients have presented considerable bias. Most studies are characterized by an inhomogeneity of the patient population with a variety of study designs, endpoints and measured variables. Some trials have used a preset amount of fluid to study the effects on clinical or various physiological variables, others have defined a physiological endpoint of resuscitation and studied the amount of fluid necessary to reach such an endpoint as well as effects on various physiological variables. In some studies, whole blood and/or fresh frozen plasma was given in addition in the crystalloid group. Also, the amount of colloids added to the fluids as well as the constituents of the fluids were not the same. In most studies, the number of patients included was relatively small. There is a striking paucity of studies in septic shock or severe sepsis. Although some studies included septic patients, studies with only septic patients or a majority of this type of patients are very limited.

A recent (level 2) meta-analysis of 8 randomized clinical trials comparing the effects of colloid versus crystalloid solutions on survival showed a 5.7% relative difference in mortality rate in favor of crystalloid therapy [40]. However, a 12.3% difference in mortality rate was found in trauma patients in favor of crystalloids, and a 7.8% difference in mortality rate in non-trauma patients in favor of colloids. The confidence intervals were however large, and one may question whether the studies were appropriately assigned to trauma or non-trauma groups. In a more recent analysis of these trials of which one was not included because it was not considered properly randomized [41], the pooled data demonstrated a 13.4% mortality rate for crystalloid-treated patients and a 21.25% mortality rate for colloid-treated patients (not statistically significant at a $p=0.01$ level) [42]. When arbitrarily subdividing the trials according to the severity of the underlying processes, again no statistically significant difference was observed between the two treatment groups, although there was a tendency to a higher mortality in colloid-treated patients with more severe illness [42].

Although mortality is an obvious vital endpoint, this is a complex issue, and fluid therapy is only one factor among many others which may influence outcome. Therefore, to evaluate the relative merits of various resuscitation fluids, the hemodynamic efficacy of crystalloids or colloids and their effects on various organ systems should be reviewed.

Prospective Randomized Clinical Trials

Several clinical studies have attempted to assess whether either type of fluid (colloids or crystalloids) is superior in terms of efficacy and effects on various physiological variables. Theses studies have occurred mainly in three areas: in patients with trauma, during and following abdominal vascular surgery, and in critically ill patients of various origin. Generally, they have a level 2 of evidence (Table 1).

Trauma: One of the earliest studies was performed in patients with abdominal trauma in whom fluid administration was guided by vital signs and urine output [43]. This comparative study was started during operation and in particular the effects on pulmonary function were studied. Patients received lactated Ringer's solution together with washed red blood cells with or without the addition of 50 g of human serum albumin to each liter of Ringer's lactate. No difference was observed between the two groups. The majority of patients were, however, not in shock and mortality rate was extremely low (4.3%).

The same group reported on a comparative trial in trauma patients (including chest injury) who were in shock [44]. Randomization took place on admission and patients received Ringer's lactate with or without albumin ti-

Table 1. Prospective randomized clinical trials

Authors (year)	Reference	Patient group	Crystalloids n (mortality %)	Colloids n (mortality %)	Endpoint of resuscitation
Skillman et al. (1975)	[49]	abdominal vascular surgery	9	7	by formula
Lowe et al. (1977)	[43]	abdominal trauma	84 (4)	57 (5)	vital signs urinary output
Weaver et al. (1978) Lucas et al. (1978)	[45]	trauma with shock	25 (0)	27 (26)	by formula
Virgilio et al. (1979)	[46]	abdominal aortic surgery	14 (7)	15 (7)	wedge pressure cardiac index urinary output
Boutros et al. (1979)	[51]	abdominal aortic surgery	17 (12)	7 (0)	wedge pressure
Dahn et al. (1981)	[47]	trauma	48	46	by formula
Hauser et al. (1980)	[54]	critically ill surgical patients ARDS	11*	11*	by formula
Moss et al. (1981)	[44]	trauma with shock	20 (5)	16 (0)	clinical signs urinary output
Shires et al. (1983)	[52]	aortic surgery	9	9	wedge pressure cardiac output urinary output
Rackow et al. (1983)	[55]	septic and hypovolemic shock	8 (75)	18 (61)	wedge pressure
Modig (1983)	[48]	trauma with shock	11	12	blood pressure central venous pressure
Metildi et al. (1984)	[56]	severe respiratory insufficiency	26 (50)	20 (60)	wedge pressure cardiac output
Hankeln et al. (1989)	[57]	critically il patients	15*	15*	wedge pressure
Dawidson et al. (1991)	[53]	abdominal aortic surgery	10	10	wedge pressure urinary output

* = cross-over study

trated by clinical signs. Hematocrit was maintained by infusion of washed red cells. Although serum protein concentrations were significantly lower on the first day after admission in the crystalloid group, no differences in variables related to pulmonary function or clinical outcome were observed. None of the patients developed pulmonary edema. Weaver et al. [45] prospectively randomized severely traumatized patients in shock after resuscitation with whole blood and fresh frozen plasma to an intra- and postoperative infusion protocol with or without additional albumin (150 g/day). Patients receiving additional albumin demonstrated more signs of pulmonary failure. Mortality in this group was higher than in the crystalloid group [46]. However, the total volume of fluids was uncontrolled and cardiac filling pressures increased substantially more in the albumin group raising serious concern whether the issue of the relative merits of the two infusion regimens was really addressed. The same group reported on a larger group of patients with a similar protocol and suggested that in the group receiving additional albumin, a negative inotropic effect could be observed [47]. However, the same criticism applies also in this study, as evidence provided by their study points to fluid overload as the cause of increased ventricular filling pressure, rather than any selective effect of albumin on the myocardium.

In patients in a serious state of shock following major pelvic and femoral fractures sustained in traffic accidents, Modig [48] compared dextran 70 together with Ringer's acetate versus Ringer's acetate solution alone for initial resuscitation in addition to infusion of whole blood. The interval from the start of fluid therapy until a stable circulating condition was achieved was significantly shorter in the colloid group. In the following 6 days, colloids were infused in the colloid group but not in the crystalloid group. The incidence of ARDS was significantly higher in the crystalloid group. Wedge pressures were, however, not measured.

Abdominal Aortic Surgery: Skillman et al. [49] studied the effects of crystalloids versus colloids in patients undergoing abdominal vascular surgery. In addition to the infusion of whole blood to replace blood loss, the patients received electrolyte solutions with or without albumin. Randomization of treatment was limited to the interval of surgical operation and fluids were given by predetermined formulas rather than titrating to hemodynamic endpoints. However, postoperatively also, the crystalloid group received albumin and three patients in this group were infused with amounts of lactated Ringer's solution in excess of the protocol and developed pulmonary edema. The alveolar-arterial (A-a) oxygen gradient increased significantly more in the crystalloid group but cardiac output and wedge pressure were not measured. The study indicated a more favorable postoperative course in those patients who received colloids intraoperatively but mortality was not reported. In patients undergoing major abdominal aortic surgery, Virgilio et al. [50] compared the effects of a 5% albumin solution versus Ringer's lactate in addition to packed red cells titrated to hemodynamic endpoints. The study was started during operation and the protocol was maintained until the morning after surgery. Mortality was not different and although COP significantly declined by 40%, no clinical or radiographic signs of pulmonary edema were observed in the crystalloid group. Two patients in the colloid group developed pulmonary edema which, however, occurred at wedge pressures higher than 25 mm Hg.

In a study in a similar group of patients, all patients received intraoperatively whole blood and electrolyte solutions and were postoperatively randomized into 3 groups, 2 receiving different types of electrolyte solutions and

1 receiving additional albumin for 48 h [51]. Infusions were titrated to maintain wedge pressure at baseline values. Signs of increased pulmonary venous admixture were only observed in patients receiving crystalloids with high sodium content. The only 2 deaths occurred in the crystalloid groups. This study seems to favor colloid solutions.

Shires and colleagues [52] compared solutions of plasma protein and Ringer's lactate given in addition to packed red blood cells titrated to maintain cardiac output and wedge pressure. The protocol started during operation and was maintained until the next morning. Although twice as much lactated Ringer's solution was required to maintain hemodynamic stability and wedge pressure, cardiac output was higher in the colloid group postoperatively. Although COP decreased by 50% and COP-wedge gradient by 60% in the crystalloid group, while these variables were essentially unchanged in the colloid group, no clinical or radiographic signs of pulmonary edema occurred. Mortality rates were not reported.

Dawidson et al. [53] prospectively randomized 20 consecutive patients to either Ringer's lactate or 3% dextran 60 in Ringer's lactate for infusion during and 24 h postoperative. Fluids were titrated to maintain a wedge pressure of at least 10 mm Hg together with adequate urine output. Three times more volume of crystalloids than of colloids was necessary to reach these endpoints. Plasma volume was significantly higher in the colloid group even though some patients in the crystalloid group received fresh frozen plasma postoperatively.

Critically Ill Patients of Various Type: In a prospective randomized crossover study in critically ill hypovolemic surgical patients with ARDS, Hauser et al. [54] compared the effects of 100 mL 25% albumin and lactate Ringer's solution. The hyperoncotic albumin solution increased plasma volume significantly more than the crystalloid solution, and this was associated with a significant increase in wedge pressure, cardiac index, oxygen availability and uptake which was not observed in the crystalloid group. A-a oxygen gradient and pulmonary venous admixture did not increase upon colloid infusion, but A-a oxygen gradient increased following crystalloid infusion. This study indicated that hyperoncotic albumin effectively expands plasma volume without interfering with pulmonary gas exchange. Rackow et al. [55] studied 26 patients in *septic* (n = 18) or hypovolemic (n = 8) shock. Patients were randomized to treatment with either 5% albumin, 6% hetastarch or 0.9% NaCl solutions infused as a fluid challenge which ended when wedge pressure equalled 15 mm Hg. The protocol was maintained for 24 h. For equivalent hemodynamic effects, between two- and fourfold greater volumes of saline were required, but the quantities for the 2 colloid solutions were not different. The COP decreased by 34% after initial resuscitation with saline and increased with the colloid solutions; the COP-wedge gradient was reduced by 125% in the crystalloid group and by 62 and 43% in the colloid groups, and remained significantly lower in the crystalloid than in the colloid groups. A significantly higher incidence of pulmonary edema, as evidenced on the chest

X-ray, was observed in the saline-treated group (88%) than in the colloid-treated groups (22%) by 24 h. Mortality rate was not different between the groups.

In 46 patients with severe pulmonary insufficiency (intrapulmonary shunt >20%, pulmonary edema on chest X-ray) after acute lung injury, in 24 cases associated with *sepsis,* Metildi et al. [56] compared lactated Ringer's solution with 5% albumin. The infusions were titrated to maintain wedge pressure. Total amount of fluid administered in the crystalloid group was higher than in the colloid group, but this difference was not statistically significant due to large individual variations. Also COP and COP-wedge gradient were not different between the groups nor did they significantly change during the 48 h of the study. In both groups, intrapulmonary shunt fraction improved but was significantly higher in the crystalloid-treated group only at 48 h, also for the sepsis patients. Mortality was high but not different in both groups. So, in this study, there seemed to be no clinical advantage of either solution.

In 15 critically ill patients, a prospective cross-over study was performed by Hankeln et al. [57] to compare the effects of 10% hetastarch and lactated Ringer's solution. Infusions were titrated to a wedge pressure of 15–18 mm Hg and in particular oxygen transport variables were evaluated. The colloid solutions significantly increased both DO_2 and VO_2 whereas the crystalloid solution did not significantly improve oxygen transport variables.

Summarizing the results of these relatively properly although differently designed trials, it is obvious that the results are not conclusive. Some studies have shown no essential differences between the two types of fluids [43, 44, 50, 52, 56], some are an advantage for crystalloids [45–47] others an advantage for colloids [48, 49, 51, 53–55].

Hemodynamic Efficacy

There is no doubt that both with crystalloids and colloids adequate resuscitation can be obtained. However, the amount of fluid necessary to reach the same hemodynamic endpoint is usually 2–4 times higher with crystalloids than with colloids [48, 50, 52, 53, 55]. This results in a higher weight gain and induces the risk of systemic edema [50, 53].

There is convincing evidence that colloid-containing fluids act more promptly than crystalloid solutions to restore hemodynamic stability. In a study in 600 hypotensive patients, it was demonstrated that the mean resuscitation time was shorter with colloids than with crystalloids, also in septic patients [41]. A similar observation was made by Modig [48] in severely traumatized patients. For a given volume of fluids infused, colloid solutions expand the plasma volume to a greater extent than crystalloid solutions. Shoemaker [36] measured plasma volumes in critically ill patients before and after infusion of either 1 L of Ringer's lactate or 500 mL of various colloid solutions. Five hundred mL of 5% albumin or dextran 70 expanded plasma volume by roughly 600–700 mL whereas the same volume of dextran 40 expanded plasma volume by more than 1 L. In contrast, 1 L of Ringer's lactate increased plasma volume by less than 150 mL. The hemodynamic effects as well as the favorable effects on oxygen transport variables of colloids were much more pronounced than those of crystalloid fluids, closely related to the measured expansion of plasma volume. In postoperative patients, Lamke et al. [37] compared plasma volumes before and after infusion of 1 L of either 6% hetastarch, 5% albumin, dextran 70 or saline. They observed the greatest expansion after dextran 70 (790 mL) followed by hetastarch (710 mL), and albumin (490 mL) whereas this increase was smallest following saline infusion (180 mL). In a cross-over study in critically ill patients, it was observed that 100 mL 25% albumin progressively increased plasma volume with an average increase of 465 mL at 45 min post-infusion when 1 L of lactated Ringer's solution produced a maximal increase of 194 ml at the end of infusion after which the plasma volume decreased exponentially [54]. In this study, significant improvements in hemodynamic and oxygen transport variables were only observed following colloid infusion. These studies indicate that colloids are more effective plasma expanders than crystalloids.

A number of studies have been performed to assess the cardiorespiratory effects of albumin and various plasma substitutes, which are considerably less expensive which is an obvious advantage [36, 37, 55, 58–60]. In a prospectively randomized cross-over study, Lazrove et al. [60] compared the cardiorespiratory effects of 500 mL of either 5% albumin or 6% hetastarch infused over a 60 min period in 10 postoperative hypovolemic patients. Both solutions expanded plasma volume to a similar extent but this persisted for a larger period after hetastarch. Also, infusion of either colloid fluid produced comparable increases in COP, cardiac filling pressures, cardiac index and oxygen transport. A more sustained increase in cardiac index was noted following hetastarch infusion. Similar observations have been reported by Puri et al. [58] and Moggio et al. [59] in 50 critically ill and 47 postoperative cardiac surgery patients, respectively.

Rackow et al. [61] randomized 20 patients with severe sepsis to fluid challenge with either 5% albumin or 10% pentastarch. The volume required to achieve a wedge pressure of 15 mm Hg was comparable between the groups and both solutions produced similar increases in cardiac output and decreases in the COP-wedge gradient without an effect on intrapulmonary shunt fraction. From these studies it may be concluded that these various colloid solutions are equivalent in their resuscitative potency.

Pulmonary Function

One of the core issues in the colloid-crystalloid controversy is the potential difference in capability of inducing pulmonary edema of these fluids. Infusion of crystalloids results in a significant and prolonged decline in serum albumin concentration and COP, while infusion with colloids maintains or even increases COP. From experimental studies its is known that a low COP can promote the development of pulmonary edema when microvascular hydrostatic pressures increase above normal [62]. However, increases in hydrostatic pressure can promote the formation of pulmonary edema to a much larger extent than comparable decreases in plasma oncotic pressure [63, 64]. Therefore, hydrostatic pressure plays a much more important role in the fluid exchange in the lung than plasma oncotic pressure. The concept of colloid osmotic pressure-pulmonary artery wedge pressure (COP-wedge) gradient has been introduced as a clinical tool for assessing the risk of pulmonary edema [65]. In critically ill patients, a low COP-PAW gradient was associated with a high incidence of pulmonary edema and a higher mortality rate [66]. This was true both for cardiogenic and (also sepsis-induced) non-cardiogenic edema. Such a relationship was, however, not found in other studies [50, 52, 67]. It should be appreciated that those variables at best represent only 2 factors of the complex starling forces that rule fluid exchange over the capillary-alveolar membrane.

Proponents of colloid solutions for resuscitation have argued that crystalloids alone dilute the plasma proteins, thereby reducing plasma COP, setting the stage for the development of pulmonary edema [49, 55]. Colloids by maintaining plasma oncotic pressure, on the other hand, could aid in the retention of fluid in the intravascular compartment and limit the magnitude of edema formation even in the presence of a permeability defect as this is not an all-or-none phenomenon and the alveolo-capillary membrane is still capable of sieving proteins. A spectrum of membrane permeability-defects has been documented in pulmonary edema [68]. Proponents of crystalloid solutions point out that a significant permeability defect in the pulmonary vasculature favors protein escape into the interstitium. Colloid infusion then could promote a transmicrovascular fluid of colloids resulting in an almost parallel increase in intra- and extravascular COP, thereby worsening the severity of edema.

Experimental studies in models with increased pulmonary permeability have yielded conflicting results. In studies in septic baboons, it was demonstrated that a markedly lowered COP did not further increase the sepsis-induced increases in the intrapulmonary shunt when wedge pressure was kept normal [69]. Extravascular lung water (EVLW), as estimated with a double indicator technique, did not increase upon endotoxin administration in dogs at a low wedge pressure, but markedly increased following resuscitation with low weight molecular dextran resulting in an adequate wedge but high effective pulmonary capillary pressure [70]. In rats subjected to rattle snake venom, 6 times more volume of crystalloids than of colloids was necessary to reverse hemoconcentration [71]. Infusion of crystalloids lowered PaO_2 and increased $PaCO_2$, whereas no changes were found in the colloid group, and resulted in a significantly higher wet-to-dry lung ratio. In sheep in septic shock, resuscitation with crystalloids or a plasma solution aimed at a similar left atrial pressure resulted in a decline in plasma and pulmonary lymph albumin concentration in the crystalloid group, which were significantly lower than in the colloid group. Pulmonary interstitial albumin lymph flux as well as EVLW were significantly higher in the colloid group but total (increased) lymph flow was not different [72]. In a similar model, same amounts of saline or homologous plasma infusion increased lymph flow as well as pulmonary bloodless wet-to-dry ratio to the same extent [64]. In a hemorrhagic shock model in sheep, saline infusion induced a triple increase of lung lymph flow, whereas autologous plasma increased this flow by only 50%, and only saline resuscitated animals developed increases in wet-to-dry lung ratios [73]. In contrast, EVLW as measured with a double indicator dilution technique increased more following resuscitation with a plasma solution than with crystalloids in hemorrhagic shock in baboons [74]. However, in both groups the shed blood was infused as well.

In a study comparing the effects of preoperative isovolemic hemodilution in patients undergoing extensive surgical procedures by either lactated Ringer's solution or a plasma solution, Laks et al. [75] showed an increase in extravascular lung water of 34% in the crystalloid group and a decrease of 18% in the colloid group. Analysis of the above discussed prospective, randomized clinical trials reveals the following. In a series of trauma patients observed for 5 days, no differences were observed in several clinical pulmonary function tests (including A-a oxygen gradient, DV/TV, Qs/Qt) between colloid and crystalloid-treated patients although serum albumin concentration declined significantly in the latter [43]. There was no significant difference in the incidence of pulmonary failure. Extending these observations in trauma patients who were in shock also, Moss et al. [44] could not find differences in the same pulmonary function tests between patients infused with crystalloids or colloids. Pulmonary edema was not seen in any patient in this study. In severely traumatized patients resuscitated from shock by either crystalloids or colloids, Modig [48] noted a significantly higher incidence of ARDS in the crystalloid group during a 6-day observation. In contrast, Weaver et al. [45] reported in seriously injured patients a substantial decrease in PaO_2/FiO_2 as well as a greater dependence on respiratory support in patients receiving additional albumin. However, the administration of excessive quantities of colloidal fluids in this study resulted in hypervolemia and high wedge pressures which has seriously clouded the issue. In patients undergoing abdominal vascular surgery, Skillman et al. [49] found a significantly greater increase in A-a oxygen difference in patients treated with crystalloids than with colloids which was positively correlated with total sodium intake. Also Boutros et al. [51] found an increase in A-a oxygen gradient as well as in Qs/Qt following infusion with high sodium containing crystalloids during a 2-day observation. This did not occur in patients treated with colloids or low sodium containing crystalloids. In contrast, in a similar group of patients, Virgilio et al. [50] observed an increase of Qs/Qt following resuscitation but this was not different between colloid- or crystalloid-treated patients during a 3-day follow-up. Similarly, Shires et al. [52] found an increase in Qs/Qt following infusion of either colloids or crystalloids after abdominal vascular surgery observed for 2 days, but there was no difference between the groups. Extravascular lung water as measured with the double indicator dilution technique did not increase with either fluid and clinical or radiographic signs of pulmonary edema did not occur. In septic and hypovolemic shock patients, Rackow et al. [55] noted that the incidence of pulmonary edema as indicated on a chest X-ray was significantly higher after crystalloid resuscitation than after colloid resuscitation at a similar wedge pressure. No pulmonary function tests were performed. In established pulmonary failure, in majority related to sepsis, Metildi et al. [56] observed no difference in COP-wedge gradients between patients receiving crystalloids or colloids, but intrapulmonary shunt fraction was significantly higher in the crystalloid group at 48 h at comparable wedge pressure. It is obvious that these studies differ in many respects. Trauma patients are usually young and in these cases the amount rather than the type of fluid seems to be important, and it is questionable whether findings in such patients have a bearing on the management of septic patients who usually are older and have a high chance of developing non-cardiogenic pulmonary edema [55]. The same is probably true for the observations in patients undergoing abdominal vascular surgery.

More important with respect to the topic of this review are studies related to patient groups with severe sepsis or with a majority of sepsis patients [55, 56]. Unfortunately, they are scarce. Appel et al. [76] evaluated retrospectively the effects of fluid challenge with various colloids, packed red blood cells, whole blood and lactated Ringer's solution in patients with ARDS. They found no evidence that the administration of colloids altered intrapulmonary shunt fraction or lung function in early ARDS, including ARDS related to sepsis. No significant change in extravascular lung water was observed after albumin infusion in experimentally induced pulmonary edema or patients with ARDS [77]. Using a radiotracer technique with two radioactive tracers (^{111}In-DPTA and ^{125}I-albumin) to detect pulmonary microvascular flux of these high and low molecular tracers, Sibbald et al. [78] studied patients with ARDS among whom many with sepsis. Following infusion with a hyperoncotic albumin solution with furosemide when necessary to prevent increases in wedge pressure, no changes in the clearance of both radiotracers were observed, both in patients with a modest and with a large increase in microvascular permeability. The authors concluded that albumin infusion will not augment the pulmonary transmicrovascular flux of low or high molecular weight solutions.

A major issue is how to assess both the presence and severity of pulmonary edema at the bedside. The most commonly used method is the chest X-ray which, however, may show a time lag between clinical signs and radiographic development or resolution of edema. In many of the clinical trials discussed earlier, various pulmonary function tests have been used to quantitate the effects of fluid resuscitation on the lungs. Although obviously of clinical importance, these variables correlate poorly with double-indicator measurements of extravascular lung water. In patients with pulmonary edema, Sibbald et al. [79] found no correlation between extravascular lung water and intrapulmonary shunt fraction, whereas Brigham et al. [80] could not document a correlation between increases in EVLW and the A-a oxygen gradient in patients with ARDS. Considerable increases in EVLW may occur before overt pulmonary edema is recognized clinically. No controlled trials have been reported comparing the effects of crystalloids or colloids on extravascular lung water in patients with sepsis.

Hypertonic (-hyperoncotic) Solutions

A relatively new approach in resuscitation of hypovolemic and traumatic shock is the use of hypertonic saline solutions (1.7%, 3%, 5%, 7.5%) with or without the addition of (hyper)oncotic substances which substantially prolong their short lasting effects (see review [81, 82]). These solutions are effective and rapid vascular expanders with significantly less volume than necessary with conventional crystalloids. Several studies have demonstrated that effective resuscitation from shock can be achieved with rapid improvement of hemodynamics without significant adverse effects [83, 84]. Also, a decrease in intracranial pressure has been observed which may be advantageous in trauma patients [85]. Experimental studies suggest that these solutions improve microcirculatory flow possibly due to reduction of shock-induced endothelial swelling [81, 82, 86]. Also in endotoxin animal models hypertonic saline has been shown to be more effective than isotonic crystalloids in improving cardiac output and oxygen transport [87], but only very transiently in another study with no overall benefit [88]. To date, no clinical controlled trials on the use of hypertonic-(hyperoncotic) solutions in human septic shock have been published.

Distribution of Flow

In animal models of septic or endotoxic shock, at significant redistribution of blood flow has been documented. No information is available in the distribution of cardiac output in human septic shock because adequate measurement techniques are lacking, but there is clinical evidence that the distribution of total blood flow is altered. In a canine endotoxin shock model it was found that saline infusion restored blood flow to the heart, brain, resting muscle, kidneys and gut to control levels [89]. In a septic shock model in rats, Ottoson et al. [90] compared the effects of lactated Ringer's solution with or without 3% albumin on hemodynamics and organ blood flow. Infusions were titrated to maintain preshock hematocrit values which necessitated the infusion of 4 times more volume in the crystalloid than in the colloid group. Infusion with 3% albumin yielded a higher cardiac output and increased colonic, renal, pancreatic and hepatic blood flow whereas infusion with crystalloids alone did not significantly improve any organ blood flow. In porcine hyperdynamic endotoxemia with isovolemic predilution, Kreimeier et al. [91] compared lactated Ringer's solution and 6% dextran 60 infused to maintain wedge pressure, which needed more than three times the volume of crystalloids than of colloids, while the latter resulted in a higher cardiac output. Blood flow to kidneys, stomach as well as intestines was significantly higher in the colloid-treated animals, whereas no statistically significant differences in blood flow to other organ systems was observed. COP was maintained in the colloid group and significantly fell in the crystalloid group. This group of investigators reported also on the effects of small-volume resuscitation with a bolus (4 mL/kg) of either 7.2% NaCl, 10% dextran 60, or 10% dextran 60 dissolved in 7.2% sodium chloride followed by 6% dextran 60 titrated to maintain wedge pressure in the same model [92]. In a control group only 6% dextran 60 was infused. On small-volume resuscitation cardiac index significantly increased within 5 min in all groups, while mean arterial pressure remained unchanged and fluid requirements were significantly reduced. Lowest requirements in the first hours were observed in the animals receiving the hypertonic-hyperoncotic solutions. Oxygen delivery remained high as well as blood flow to heart, kidneys and splanchnic organs (not different between the 4 groups). This study suggests that addition of 10% dextran to a hypertonic solution could be favorable as cardiac output and regional blood flow were sustained by significantly lower volume requirements. No controlled trials comparing different resuscitation fluids in their effects on organ blood flow or function in patients with sepsis have appeared.

Conclusions

Fluid therapy aimed at reversing hypovolemic and at restoring adequate venous return and cardiac output is the most important initial therapeutic approach in septic shock. Clinical trials have failed to demonstrate beyond any doubt, the superiority of either crystalloids or colloids as resuscitation fluid in hypovolemia and shock. However, the overall number of patients with sepsis or septic shock in these trials is small. Colloid solutions act more promptly than crystalloids in restoring hemodynamic stability and substantially less volume is necessary to achieve this, but successful resuscitation is possible with either type of fluid. In particular in septic patients, the type of fluid is important as they have a high incidence of increased pulmonary microvascular permeability and usually need rather high filling pressures to maintain oxygen transport, reflecting the usually older age of these patients. The major complication of fluid therapy is the development of edema, in particular pulmonary edema. The primary determinant of lung water accumulation in sepsis appears to be pulmonary microvascular hydrostatic pressure rather than oncotic pressure. The clinical importance of low colloid oncotic pressure, as well as the effects of transmicrovascular escape of colloids in the pulmonary circulation, in the formation and maintenance of pulmonary edema in sepsis is still a matter of debate. The COP-wedge gradient has emerged as a practical clinical tool to guide fluid repletion to minimize the risk of pulmonary edema, but its value is not completely beyond doubt.

However, no definite adverse effects on pulmonary function have been demonstrated in patients with sepsis receiving colloids, provided that adequate wedge pressures are maintained. There is some indication that at similar wedge pressures the incidence of pulmonary edema is higher in crystalloid-treated patients than in colloid-treated patients. There is no proof that the use of either fluid has a significant impact on outcome.

Recommendations

With the present state of knowledge, the following recommendations can be made for patients with severe sepsis.

- Prompt and adequate fluid therapy is the mainstay of treatment of septic shock and aims at an optimal filling pressure of the heart, defined as a wedge pressure associated with the highest cardiac output. This wedge pressure should be as low as possible and at least not exceed 16–18 mm Hg (Grade C recommendation).
- Asanguinous fluid therapy lowers hemoglobin concentration, oxygen carrying capacity and whole blood viscosity. The optimal hematocrit in septic shock has not been defined. No specific recommendation can be made, but a hematocrit of 30–35% seems acceptable.
- The choice of fluid should take into account its effect on plasma oncotic pressure. Severe decreases in COP should be avoided and a balance between COP and wedge pressure should be aimed at (Grade B recommendation). The lowest acceptable level of the COP-wedge gradient has not been defined.
- The various plasma substitutes are as effective as albumin in their resuscitative potency and their use is preferred because of their lower costs (Grade C recommendation). Some, however, have (minor) effects on hemostasis which may be undesirable in some particular patients.

These general recommendations leave alone that also volume treatment should be individualized and titrated to individual needs.

References

1. Rackow EC, Kaufmann BS, Falk JL, Astiz ME, Weil MH (1987) Hemodynamic response to fluid repletion in patients with septic shock: Evidence for early depression of cardiac performance. Circ Shock 22:11–22
2. D'Orio V, Mendes P, Saad G, Marcelle R (1990) Accuracy in early prediction of prognosis of patients with septic shock by analysis of simple indices: Prospective study. Crit Care Med 18:1339–1345
3. Groeneveld ABJ, Bronsveld W, Thijs LG (1986) Hemodynamic determinants of mortality in human septic shock. Surgery 99:140–152
4. Teule GJJ, Lingen A van, Verweij-van Vught MAJ, et al (1984) Role of peripheral pooling in porcine Escherichia coli sepsis. Circ Shock 12:115–123

5. D'Orio V, Wahlen C, Naldi M, Fossion A, Juchmes J, Marcelle R (1989) Contribution of peripheral blood pooling to central hemodynamic disturbances during endotoxin insult in intact dogs. Crit Care Med 17:1314–1319
6. Astiz ME, Tilly E, Rackow EC (1991) Peripheral vascular tone in sepsis. Chest 99:1072–1075
7. Lucas CE (1976) The renal response to acute injury and sepsis. Surg Clin North Am 56:953–975
8. Weil MH, Nishijima H (1978) Cardiac output in bacterial shock. Am J Med 64:920–922
9. Carcillo JA, Davis AL, Zaritsky A (1991) Role of early fluid resuscitation in pediatric septic shock. JAMA 266:1242–1245
10. Shoemaker WC, Appel PL, Kram HB, Waxman K, Lee TS (1988) Prospective trial of supranormal values of survivors as therapeutic goals in high-risk surgical patients. Chest 94:1176–1186
11. Kreymann G, Grosser S, Buggisch P, Gottschall C, Matthaei S, Greten H (1993) Oxygen consumption and resting metabolic rate in sepsis, sepsis syndrome, and septic shock. Crit Care Med 21:1012–1019
12. Kaufman BS, Rackow EC, Falk JL (1984) The relationship between oxygen delivery and consumption during fluid resuscitation of hypovolemic and septic shock. Chest 85:336–341
13. Haupt MT, Gilbert EM, Carlson RW (1985) Fluid loading increases oxygen consumption in septic patients with lactic acidosis. Am Rev Respir Dis 131:912–916
14. Gilbert EM, Haupt MT, Mandanas RY, Huaringa AJ, Carlson RW (1986) The effect of fluid loading, blood transfusion, and catecholamine infusion on oxygen delivery and consumption in patients with sepsis. Am Rev Respir Dis 134:873–878
15. Wolf YG, Cotev S, Perel A, Manny J (1987) Dependency of oxygen consumption on cardiac output in sepsis. Crit Care Med 15:198–203
16. Astiz ME, Rackow EC, Falk JL, Kaufman BS, Weil MH (1987) Oxygen delivery and consumption in patients with hyperdynamic septic shock. Crit Care Med 15:26–28
17. Vincent JL, Roman A, De Backer D, Kahn RJ (1990) Oxygen uptake/supply dependency. Effects of short-term dobutamine infusion. Am Rev Respir Dis 142:2–7
18. Ronco JJ, Fenwick JC, Wiggs BR, Phang PT, Russell JA, Tweeddale MG (1993) Oxygen consumption is independent of increases in oxygen delivery by dobutamine in septic patients who have normal or increased plasma lactate. Am Rev Respir Dis 147:25–31
19. Hanique G, Dugernier T, Laterre PF, Dougnac A, Roescher J, Reynart MS (1994) Significance of pathologic oxygen supply dependency in critically ill patients: Comparison between measured and calculated methods. Intensive Care Med 20:12–18
20. Tuchschmidt J, Fried J, Astiz M, Rackow E (1992) Elevation of cardiac output and oxygen delivery improves outcome in septic shock. Chest 102:216–220
21. Yu M, Levy MM, Smith P, Takiguchi SA, Miyasaki A, Myers SA (1993) Effect of maximizing oxygen delivery on morbidity and mortality rates in critically ill patients: A prospective, randomized, controlled study. Crit Care Med 21:830–838
22. Hayes MA, Yau EHS, Timmins AC, Hinds CJ, Watson D (1993) Response of critically ill patients to treatment aimed at achieving supranormal oxygen delivery and consumption. Relationship to outcome. Chest 103:886–895
23. Packman MI, Rackow EC (1983) Optimum left heart filling pressure during fluid resuscitation of patients with hypovolemic and septic shock. Crit Care Med 11:165–169
24. Calvin JE, Driedger AA, Sibbald WJ (1981) The hemodynamic effect of rapid fluid infusion in critically ill patients. Surgery 90:61–76
25. Reuse C, Vincent JL, Pinsky MR (1990) Measurements of right ventricular volumes during fluid challenge. Chest 98:450–454
26. Ognibene FP, Parker MM, Natanson C, Shelhamer JH, Parrillo JE (1988) Depressed left ventricular performance. Response to volume infusion in patients with sepsis and septic shock. Chest 93:903–910
27. Schneider AJ, Teule GJJ, Groeneveld ABJ, Nauta JJP, Heidendal GAK, Thijs LG (1988) Biventricular performance during volume loading in patients with early septic

shock, with emphasis on the right ventricle: A combined hemodynamic and radionuclide study. Am Heart J 116:103–110
28. Redl G, Germann P, Plattner H, Hammerle A (1993) Right ventricular function in early septic shock states. Intensive Care Med 19:3–7
29. Steffes CP, Bender JS, Levison MA (1991) Blood transfusion and oxygen consumption in surgical sepsis. Crit Care Med 19:512–516
30. Conrad SA, Dietrich KA, Hebert CA, Romero MD (1990) Effect of red cell transfusion on oxygen consumption following fluid resuscitation in septic shock. Circ Shock 31:419–429
31. Silverman HJ, Tuma P (1992) Gastric tonometry in patients with sepsis. Effects of dobutamine infusions and packed red blood cell transfusions. Chest 102:184–188
32. Fan FC, Chen RYZ, Schuessler GB, Chien S (1980) Effects of hematocrit variations on regional hemodynamics and oxygen transport in the dog. Am J Physiol 238:H545–H552
33. Voerman HJ, Fonk T, Thijs LG (1989) Changes in hemorheology in patients with sepsis or septic shock. Circ Shock 29:219–227
34. Hurd T, Dasmahapatra K, Rush BF, Mahiedo GW (1988) Red cell deformability in human and experimental sepsis. Arch Surg 123:217–220
35. Czer LSC, Shoemaker WC (1978) Optimal hematocrit values in critically ill postoperative patients. Surg Gynecol Obstet 147:363–368
36. Shoemaker WC (1976) Comparison of the relative effectiveness of whole blood transfusions and various types of fluid therapy in resuscitation. Crit Care Med 4:71–78
37. Lamke LO, Liljedahl SO (1976) Plasma volume changes after infusion of various plasma expanders. Resuscitation 5:85–92
38. Webb AR, Tighe D, Moss RF, Al-Saady N, Hynd JW, Bennett ED (1991) Advantages of a narrow-range, medium molecular weight hydroxyethyl starch for volume maintenance in a porcine model of fecal peritonitis. Crit Care Med 19:409–416
39. Edwards JD, Nightingale P, Wilkins RG, Faragher EB (1989) Hemodynamic and oxygen transport response to modified fluid gelatin in critically ill patients. Crit Care Med 17:996–998
40. Velanovich V (1989) Crystalloid versus colloid fluid resuscitation: A meta-analysis of mortality. Surgery 105:65–71
41. Shoemaker WC, Schluchter M, Hopkins JA, Appel PL, Schwartz S, Chang PC (1981) Comparison of the relative effectiveness of colloids and crystalloids in emergency resuscitation. Am J Surg 142:73–84
42. Bissoni RS, Holtgrave DR, Lawler F, Marley DS (1991) Colloids versus crystalloids in fluid resuscitation: An analysis of randomized controlled trials. J Fam Pract 32:387–390
43. Lowe RJ, Moss GS, Jilek J, Levine HD (1977) Crystalloid vs colloid in the etiology of pulmonary failure after trauma: A randomized trial in man. Surgery 81:676–683
44. Moss GS, Lowe RJ, Jilek J, Levine HD (1981) Colloid or crystalloid in the resuscitation of hemorrhagic shock: A controlled clinical trial. Surgery 89:434–438
45. Weaver DW, Ledgerwood AM, Lucas CE, Higgins R, Bouwman DL, Johnson SD (1978) Pulmonary effects of albumin resuscitation for severe hypovolemic shock. Arch Surg 113:387–392
46. Lucas CE, Weaver D, Higgins RF, Ledgerwood AM, Johnson SD, Bouwman DL (1978) Effects of albumin versus non-albumin resuscitation on plasma volume and renal excretory function. J Trauma 18:564–570
47. Dahn MS, Lucas CE, Ledgerwood AM, Higgins RF (1979) Negative inotropic effect of albumin resuscitation for shock. Surgery 86:235–241
48. Modig J (1983) Advantages of dextran 70 over Ringer's acetate solution in shock treatment and in prevention of adult respiratory distress syndrome. A randomized study in man after traumatic-haemorrhagic shock. Resuscitation 10:219–226
49. Skillman JJ, Restall DS, Salzman EW (1975) Randomized trial of albumin vs. electrolyte solutions during abdominal aortic operations. Surgery 78:291–303

50. Virgilio RW, Rice CL, Smith DE, et al (1979) Crystalloid vs. colloid resuscitation: Is one better? A randomized clinical study. Surgery 85:129–139
51. Boutros AR, Ruess R, Olson L, Hoyt JL, Baker WH (1979) Comparison of hemodynamic, pulmonary, and renal effects of use of three types of fluids after major surgical procedures on the abdominal aorta. Crit Care Med 7:9–13
52. Shires GT, Peitzman AB, Albert SA, et al (1983) Response of extravascular lung water to intraoperative fluids. Ann Surg 197:515–519
53. Dawidson IJA, Willms CD, Sandor ZF, Coorpender LL, Reisch JS, Fry WJ (1991) Ringer's lactate with or without 3% dextran 60 as volume expanders during abdominal aortic surgery. Crit Care Med 19:36–42
54. Hauser CJ, Shoemaker WC, Turpin I, Goldberg SJ (1980) Oxygen transport responses to colloids and crystalloids in critically ill surgical patients. Surg Gynecol Obstet 150:811–816
55. Rackow EC, Falk JL, Fein IA, et al (1983) Fluid resuscitation in circulatory shock: A comparison of the cardiorespiratory effects of albumin, hetastarch, and saline solutions in patients with hypovolemic and septic shock. Crit Care Med 11:839–850
56. Metildi LA, Shackford SR, Virgilio RW, Peters RM (1984) Crystalloid versus colloid in fluid resuscitation of patients with severe pulmonary insufficiency. Surg Gynecol Obstet 158:207–212
57. Hankeln K, Rädel C, Beez M, Laniewski P, Bohmert F (1989) Comparison of hydroxyethyl starch and lactated Ringer's solution on hemodynamics and oxygen transport of critically ill patients in prospective crossover studies. Crit Care Med 17:133–135
58. Puri VK, Howard M, Paidipaty B, et al (1983) Resuscitation in hypovolemia and shock: A prospective study of hydroxyethyl starch and albumin. Crit Care Med 11:518–523
59. Moggio RA, Rha CC, Somberg ED, Praeger PI, Pooley RW, Reed GE (1983) Hemodynamic comparison of albumin and hydroxyethyl starch in postoperative cardiac surgery patients. Crit Care Med 11:943–945
60. Lazrove S, Waxman K, Shippy C, Shoemaker WC (1980) Hemodynamic, blood volume, and oxygen transport responses to albumin and hydroxyethyl starch infusions in critically ill postoperative patients. Crit Care Med 8:302–306
61. Rackow EC, Mecher C, Astiz ME, Griffel M, Falk JL, Weil MH (1989) Effects of pentastarch and albumin infusion on cardiorespiratory function and coagulation in patients with severe sepsis and systemic hypoperfusion. Crit Care Med 17:394–398
62. Guyton AC, Lindsey AW (1959) Effect of the elevated left arterial pressure and decreased plasma protein concentration on the development of pulmonary edema. Circ Res 7:649–657
63. Prewitt RM, McCarthy J, Wood LDH (1981) Treatment of acute low pressure pulmonary edema in dogs: Relative effects of hydrostatic and oncotic pressure, nitroprusside and positive end-expiratory pressure. J Clin Invest 67:409–418
64. Nylander WA, Hammon Jr JW, Roselli RJ, Tribble JB, Brigham KL, Bender Jr HW (1981) Comparison of the effects of saline and homologous plasma infusion on lung fluid balance during endotoxemia in the unanesthetized sheep. Surgery 90:221–226
65. Da Luz DA, Shubin H, Weil MH, Jacobson E, Stein L (1975) Pulmonary edema related to changes in colloid osmotic and pulmonary artery wedge pressure in patients with acute myocardial infarction. Circulation 51:330–357
66. Rackow EC, Fein IA, Siegel J (1982) The relationship of the colloid osmotic-pulmonary artery wedge pressure gradient to pulmonary edema and mortality in critically ill patients. Chest 82:433–437
67. Rafferty TD, Ljungquist R, Firestone L, et al (1983) Plasma colloid oncotic pressure pulmonary artery occlusion pressure gradient: A poor predictor of pulmonary edema in surgical intensive care unit patients. Arch Surg 118:841–843
68. Sprung CL, Rackow ED, Fein A, Jacob AI, Isikoff SK (1981) The spectrum of pulmonary edema: Differentiation of cardiogenic, intermediate and non-cardiogenic forms of pulmonary edema. Am Rev Resp Dis 124:178–222

69. Kohler JP, Rice CL, Zarins CK, Cammack III BF, Moss GS (1981) Does reduced colloid oncotic pressure increase pulmonary dysfunction in sepsis? Crit Car Med 9:90–93
70. D'Orio V, Mendes P, Carlier P, Fatemi M, Marcelle R (1991) Lung fluid dynamics and supply dependency of oxygen uptake during experimental endotoxic shock and volume resuscitation. Crit Care Med 19:955–962
71. Haupt MT, Teerapong P, Green D, Schaeffer Jr RC, Carlson RW (1984) Increased pulmonary edema with crystalloid compared to colloid resuscitation of shock associated with increased vascular permeability. Circ Shock 12:213–224
72. Sturm JA, Carpenter MA, Lewis Jr FR, Graziano C, Trunkey DD (1979) Water and protein movement in the sheep lung after septic shock: Effect of colloid versus crystalloid resuscitation. J Surg Res 26:233–248
73. Mckeen CR, Bowers RE, Harris TR, Hobson JE, Brigham KL (1986) Saline compared to plasma volume replacement after volume depletion in sheep: Lung fluid balance. J Crit Care 1:133–141
74. Holcroft JW, Trunkey DD (1974) Extravascular lung water following hemorrhagic shock in the baboon: Comparison between resuscitation with Ringer's lactate and plasmanate. Ann Surg 180:408–415
75. Laks H, O'Connor NE, Anderson W, Pilon RN (1976) Crystalloid versus colloid hemodilution in man. Surg Gynecol Obstet 142:506–512
76. Appel PL, Shoemaker WC (1981) Evaluation of fluid therapy in adult respiratory failure. Crit Care Med 9:862–869
77. Baudendistel L, Dahms JE, Kaminski DL (1982) The effect of albumin on extravascular lung water in animals and patients with low-pressure pulmonary edema. J Surg Res 33:285–293
78. Sibbald WJ, Driedger AA, Wells GA, Myers ML, Lefcoe M (1983) The short-term effects of increasing plasma colloid osmotic pressure in patients with non-cardiac pulmonary edema. Surgery 93:620–633
79. Sibbald WJ, Warshawski FJ, Short AK, et al (1983) Clinical studies of measuring extravascular lung water by thermal dye technique in critically ill patients. Chest 85:725–732
80. Brigham KL, Kariman K, Harris TR, Snapper JR, Bernard GR, Young SL (1983) Correlation of oxygenation with vascular permeability-surface area but not with lung water in humans with acute respiratory failure and pulmonary edema. J Clin Invest 72:339–349
81. Kramer GC, Wallfisch HK (1992) Recent trends in fluid therapy. Cur Opinion Anaesth 5:272–277
82. Kreimeier U, Frey L, Messmer K (1993) Small-volume resuscitation. Cur Opinion Anaesth 6:400–408
83. Holcroft JW, Vassar MJ, Turner JE, Derlet RW, Kramer GC (1987) 3% NaCl and 7.5% NaCl/dextran 70 in the resuscitation of severely injured patients. Ann Surg 206:279–288
84. Mattox KL, Maningas PA, Moore EE, et al (1991) Prehospital hypertonic saline/dextran infusion for post-traumatic hypotension. Ann Surg 213:482–491
85. Prough DS, Whitley JM, Taylor CL, Deal DD, DeWitt DS (1991) Regional cerebral blood flow following resuscitation from hemorrhagic shock with hypertonic saline. Anesthesiology 75:319–327
86. Mazzoni MC, Borgström P, Intaglietta M, Arfors KE (1990) Capillary narrowing in hemorrhagic shock is rectified by hyperosmotic saline-dextran reinfusion. Circ Shock 31:407–418
87. Luypaert P, Vincent JL, Domb M, et al (1986) Fluid resuscitation with hypertonic saline in endotoxic shock. Circ Shock 20:311–320
88. Kristensen J, Modig J (1990) Ringer's acetate and dextran 70 with or without hypertonic saline in endotoxin-induced shock in pigs. Crit Care Med 18:1261–1268
89. Hussain SNA, Rutledge F, Roussos C, Magder S (1988) Effects of norepinephrine and fluid administration on the selective blood flow distribution in endotoxic shock. J Crit Care 3:32–42

90. Ottosson J, Dawidson I, Brandberg Å, Idvall J, Sandor Z (1991) Cardiac output and organ blood flow in experimental septic shock: Effect of treatment with antibiotics, corticosteroids, and fluid infusion. Circ Shock 35:14–24
91. Kreimeier U, Ruiz-Morales M, Messmer K (1993) Comparison of the effects of volume resuscitation with dextran 60 vs. Ringer's lactate on central hemodynamics, regional blood flow, pulmonary function, and blood composition during hyperdynamic endotoxemia. Circ Shock 39:89–99
92. Kreimeier U, Frey L, Dentz J, Herbel T, Messmer K (1991) Hypertonic saline dextran resuscitation during the initial phase of acute endotoxemia: Effect on regional blood flow. Crit Care Med 19:801–809

Role of RBC Transfusion Therapy in Sepsis

W. J. Sibbald, G. S. Doig, and H. Morisaki

Introduction

Sepsis is a clinical syndrome that arises because of an inappropriate and excessive host inflammatory response. Recent work has demonstrated that this syndrome is also characterized by the development of quantifiable injury in both the lungs and extra-pulmonary organs. This process is clinically expressed as Multiple Organ Dysfunction Syndrome (MODS). Sepsis is also a hypermetabolic state, where tissue O_2 needs may be markedly increased. In this context, research has linked the widespread tissue injury typical of this syndrome with an inability to match tissue O_2 delivery (DO_2) with these elevated tissue O_2 needs. Thus, the emergence of *metabolic dysregulation* of tissue O_2 availability in sepsis may contribute to the genesis of MODS [1]. For example, mortality in septic patients has been positively correlated with elevated arterial lactates [2] and "pathologic" VO_2/DO_2 dependency has been demonstrated both in animal [3] and clinical [4] studies of sepsis. As short term increases in arterial lactate and evidence of "pathologic" VO_2/DO_2 dependency are regarded as evidence for underlying tissue ischemia [1, 5], it seems probable that MODS complicating sepsis reflects, in whole or in part, the summative effects of tissue injury on a hypoxic-ischemic basis.

With research suggesting that a tissue O_2 debt likely contributes to the evolution and/or progression of MODS in sepsis, other work has coincidentally claimed that maintaining a "supranormal" systemic DO_2 reduces the incidence of both MODS and mortality in this syndrome [6, 7]. Hence, metabolic O_2 dysregulation in sepsis is generally countered by treatment strategies that attempt to maintain "supranormal" convective-DO_2's. Increasing systemic DO_2 is achieved by applying either or both of two clinical strategies: 1) increase the cardiac output, by intravascular volume expansion or inotropic therapy, and 2) increase arterial O_2 content, by transfusing packed red blood cells (RBC) and adopting measures to improve arterial oxygenation, i.e. positive end-expiratory pressure and supplemental O_2.

It is not uncommon to find modest anemia in critically ill septic patients, probably the consequence of both occult blood loss and depressed erythropoiesis. The "appropriateness" of transfusing RBCs to increase tissue O_2 availability (sometimes to "supranormal" levels) is therefore frequently discussed in the critical care literature [8-12]. These debates have been frustrated in efforts to gain agreement regarding the transfusion trigger (the lowest hemoglobin level where transfusion would be recommended) by the lack of explicit evidence demonstrating clinical benefit from approaches that maintain different hemoglobin levels in septic patients (*vide infra*). Thus, while the effect of increasing the cardiac output on systemic DO_2 and tissue VO_2 is frequently reported, this chapter will demonstrate that the clinical benefit of increasing systemic DO_2 by RBC transfusion therapy has not been carefully examined in sepsis.

Existing Clinical Guidelines

There are two existing statements which constitute guidelines for decisions regarding RBC transfusions. In 1988, the National Institutes of Health reviewed that the main objective of a RBC transfusion should be to improve the O_2 carrying capacity of blood [11]. In this consensus document, it was noted that the decision to transfuse a specific patient should take into consideration the duration of anemia, the intravascular volume, the extent of the operation, the probability for massive blood loss, and the presence of coexisting conditions such as impaired pulmonary function, inadequate cardiac output, myocardial ischemia, or cerebral vascular or peripheral circulatory disease. Without providing specific guidelines, it was concluded "these factors are representative of the universe of considerations that comprise judgement". Finally, it was concluded that available evidence did not support the "100/0.30 rule", that is the application of arbitrary decisions to transfuse patients when the hemoglobin was less than 100 g/L (or the hematocrit was less than 0.30). However, it was acknowledged that patients with acute anemia, where hemoglobin values were less than 70 g/L, frequently required RBC transfusions.

In 1992, the American College of Physicians published more explicit recommendations concerning RBC transfusion therapy, the theoretic basis for which was derived from an extensive literature review [12]. This statement noted that normovolemic anemia (hemoglobin, 70–100 g/L) is well tolerated in asymptomatic patients. Categorization of patients into one of two groups was proposed to guide decisions regarding the need for RBC transfusion: 1) patient groups at risk from intravascular volume depletion, and 2) patients with signs and symptoms requiring blood transfusion (Table 1). Transfusion therapy was not proposed in asymptomatic, normovolemic patients with anemia who are a risk (Table 1, panel a) unless a deterioration in vital signs is observed or unless the patient develops symptoms (Table 1, panel b). In symptomatic patients (Table 1, panel b), it was proposed that crystalloid should initially be used to replace intravascular volume. If symptoms persist after volume repletion, the patient should receive a RBC transfusion with autologous blood. When transfusion therapy is initiated, a unit-by-unit basis approach should be used, with patient evaluation after each unit.

Table 1. Patient groups "at risk" from intravascular volume depletion and anemia (Adapted from [13])

Panel A: Patients "at risk" for myocardial ischemia
1. Coronary artery disease
2. Valvular heart disease (for example, hemodynamically significant aortic stenosis)
3. Congestive heart failure
4. Patients at risk for cerebral ischemia
5. History of transient ischemic attacks
6. Previous thrombotic stroke
Panel B: Signs and symptoms requiring blood transfusion in normovolemia
1. Syncope
2. Dyspnea
3. Postural hypotension
4. Tachycardia
5. Angina
6. Transient ischemic attack

Although existing recommendations in either of the two previous statements have not made explicit reference to the treatment of septic patients, we assume there will be no debate about recommending that a *minimal* transfusion trigger in sepsis approximates 70 to 80 g/L (i.e. the minimal hemoglobin level considered acceptable in perioperative patients) and those clinical trials investigating new treatments of sepsis might therefore require that the hemoglobin concentration be maintained above this level.

Where existing recommendations regarding the acceptable hemoglobin level in clinical sepsis appear in conflict is whether transfusion therapy is necessary between hemoglobin levels of 70 to 80 g/L and normal values of 130 to 150 g/L. Arguments used to support suggestions that septic patients be transfused to normal or near-normal hemoglobin levels [9] have generally concentrated on evidence demonstrating that the circulatory compensation required to maintain tissue O_2 availability during modest anemia is significantly perturbed in this syndrome (reviewed in [1]). In an editioral summarizing treatment principles for sepsis, Weg [9] recognized that circulatory dysfunction in sepsis might interfere with the normal process of metabolically regulating tissue O_2 availability and therefore recommended: "the most assured means of increasing DO_2 is to increase arterial O_2 content by increasing hemoglobin. Hemoglobin or hematocrits should be maintained at normal values in patients with potential DO_2 problems, such as sepsis and ARDS". In contrast, others have not concluded that transfusion therapy is required when the hemoglobin exceeds 100 g/L [8, 10].

In summary, areas in which there is evidence for disparate view in the treatment of sepsis include: 1) should systemic DO_2 be therapeutically increased to supranormal levels, and 2) should RBC transfusions to greater than 70–80 g/L be used to support either normal or supra-normal systemic DO_2? Our review of this issue will therefore be limited to asking whether the adoption of a treatment strategy that includes maintaining a *normal* or *near-normal* hemoglobin level can be considered effective therapy?

Determining the Efficacy of RBC Transfusion

The NIH consensus stated that the main objective of a RBC transfusion should be to improve the O_2 carrying capacity of blood. We suggest that modification of this statement is necessary to acknowledge that the explicit objective of a RBC transfusion is to *increase tissue O_2 availability.* Thus, it cannot be concluded that therapy that elevates the O_2 carrying capacity of blood necessarily results in improved tissue O_2 availability.

In the majority, previous work has concluded that transfusing RBC is efficacious when the following is demonstrated: 1) acceptable levels of 2, 3-DPG and p50 in preserved cells, and 2) greater than 80% *in vivo* survival 24 h post-transfusion. This approach assumes (perhaps incorrectly) that tissue DO_2 acutely increases post-transfusion if storage preservation techniques have resulted in RBC with acceptable function and viability.

Another surrogate measure commonly used to determine the efficacy of RBC transfusions is the systemic DO_2. This approach assumes that increasingly systemic DO_2 by RBC transfusions is followed by a reasonably immediate and parallel increase in tissue DO_2. In the presence of circulatory dysfunction, however, this assumption may be invalidated.

It is probably more appropriate that questions regarding the efficacy of RBC transfusions be discussed using direct, not inferential, data. Thus, when RBC transfusions are prescribed to counteract a tissue O_2 debt, efficacy could be concluded by demonstrating a temporally related increase in systemic (or specified organ) VO_2. For example, when the tissues are in a state of O_2 need (when the systemic VO_2 is supply-dependent), the gold standard evidence for efficacy would be an increase in systemic VO_2 post-transfusion (Figure 1). Demonstrating a temporally related fall in elevated arterial lactate levels may be another way to demonstrate RBC transfusion efficacy since changes in arterial lactates have been used to represent parallel changes in the balance between tissue O_2 need and availability.

Relevant Physiology

Although transfusing RBC elevates convective DO_2 by increasing both cardiac preload and arterial O_2 content, there is no consensus on the role of transfusion therapy to support the typically elevated tissue O_2 needs found in sepsis. In contrast, expert panels have recommended that hemoglobin concentrations of 70–80 g/L in hospitalized patients may not require transfusion therapy if the intravascular volume has been normalized [11, 12]. Such recommendations, which have lowered the transfusion trigger for hospital-

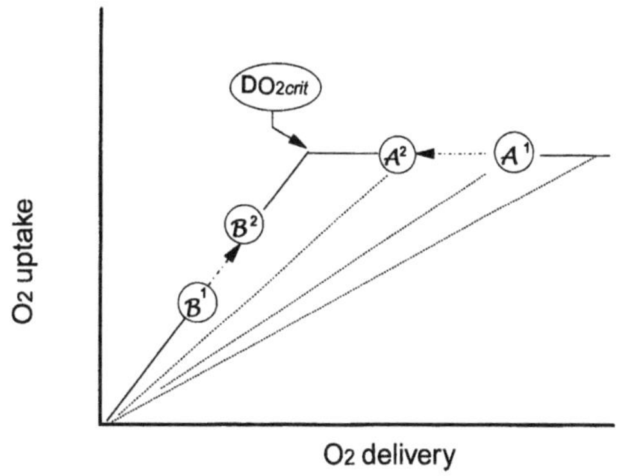

Fig. 1. When DO_2 falls, increasing VO_2 maintains O_2 uptake (A_1 to A_2). When this compensation is exceeded, O_2 uptake becomes supply-dependent, that is, ischemia occurs because O_2 uptake falls as DO_2 is further reduced (B_2 to B_1).
As the objective of RBC transfusion is to increase tissue O_2 availability, the 'gold standard' test of efficacy could be post-transfusion demonstration of increases O_2 uptake from a position of initial supply-dependence.

ized patients over the last decade, are supported by data establishing that both the circulatory and hematopoietic systems autoregulate with respect to tissue DO_2 (reviewed in [13]).

Under normal conditions, blood flow, and therefore DO_2, is distributed to ensure that tissue O_2 availability is matched to the tissue's metabolic O_2 need [14–16]. This is a finely regulated control system involving all levels of the circulation, including the heart and the regional and microregional circulations. For example, an increase in cardiac output maximizes systemic DO_2 at a peak of 110% of pre-anemic control variables when the hematocrit is 30% [13, 16]. An elevated cardiac output during anemia is a function of the degree of hemodilution, with the majority of the increase due to an elevated stroke volume. This increase in stroke volume is explained by: 1) a depressed ventricular afterload since viscosity is depressed in anemia; 2) augmented inotropic and chronotropic cardiac stimulation due to increased circulating catecholamines; and 3) an increased venous return that augments ventricular preload.

Regional control of overall systemic DO_2 is also important in the normal circulatory adaptation to anemia. Below a hematocrit of 30%, the matching of O_2 supply to demand requires a redistribution of blood flow between organs. In health, isovolemic hemodilution is therefore accompanied by: 1) an increase in blood flow to the heart and brain to maintain DO_2 to these vital organs; and 2) no change in the pattern of blood flow to all of the kidneys, intestine and liver [13–16]. Therefore, relative DO_2 to these non-vital organs falls during modest anemia (and it is redistributed to the heart and brain), although tissue O_2 availability is maintained by an increase in O_2 extraction (*vide infra*).

Adaptation to anemia also occurs in the microcirculation, where adjustments combine to elevate O_2 extraction when hematocrits are depressed to as low as 20% [17]. Increasing the number of capillaries with RBC flow when the hematocrit is depressed permits tissues to extract more of the available O_2 for the following reasons: 1) increasing capillary density reduces the diffusion distance for O_2; and 2) reducing the velocity of RBC in each capillary is accompanied by a reduction in the time for O_2 diffusion.

Finally, changes in the molecular dynamics of the hemoglobin molecule result in more efficient DO_2 in anemia. Thus, a rightward shift of the oxyhemoglobin dissociation curve enhances O_2 release at constant O_2 tensions. In anemia, this rightward shift begins at hemoglobin levels of 90 g/L and is prominent when levels are less than 65 g/L. This rightward shift of the oxyhemoglobin dissociation curve in anemia is the result of increased synthesis of 2, 3-DPG, which is seen with declining hemoglobins by 12–36 h.

What is the overall effectiveness of this circulatory compensation to anemia? In a comprehensive review of the human tolerance of anemia, Welch et al. [12] listed a number of studies, both animal and clinical, which support the argument that anemia can be tolerated to a hemoglobin level as low as 50–70 g/L, provided that intravascular volume replacement has been adequate to support the increase in cardiac output that accompanies acute anemia. The evidence reviewed included examples where patients with hemoglobin levels was less than 50–70 g/L (and presumably without major associated risk factors), underwent surgery, yet had no subsequent evidence for mortality or cardiac failure.

Is There any Theoretical Basis for Increasing the Currently Recommended Transfusion Trigger in Sepsis?

As previously reviewed, recent guidelines for RBC transfusion practice have incorporated transfusion triggers into appropriateness criteria. Thus, a lower hemoglobin threshold of 70 g/L was suggested by the NIH consensus conference on perioperative blood transfusion [11]. Increasing the transfusion trigger, that is, providing RBC transfusions to maintain the hemoglobin level greater than 70 g/L, may be acceptable in patients with an underlying disease which would limit the acute circulatory compensation to an anemia.

The best clinical example of this exception to existing clinical guidelines is the patient with coronary artery disease (CAD). In this situation, underlying CAD limits the extent to which the cardiac output can be increased to maintain tissue DO_2 in circumstances where the arterial O_2 content is depressed by anemia. In these patients, the need to augment tissue O_2 availability when the hemoglobin is less than 70 g/L, for example, during the hypermetabolic postoperative period, might well exceed the circulation's ability to maintain adequate tissue O_2 availability. Therefore, transfusion to a hemoglobin level approximating 100 g/L may well be considered acceptable in this circumstance. A more appropriate practice, however, would include close monitoring of these patients for size and symptoms of organ dysfunction due to an

O_2 deficit. At this time, that is with explicit evidence of tissue O_2 need (Table 1), RBC transfusion therapy would be prescribed on a unit-by-unit basis.

There are a number of reasons why sepsis might be another clinical situation where the transfusion trigger should be elevated, for example:

1. Sepsis is a hypermetabolic process and increasing the metabolic rate in healthy animal models elevates the optimal hematocrit both in the intestine [18] and skeletal muscle [19]. The optimal hematocrit is considered to be that level where the ability to compensate for depressed tissue O_2 availability during the stress of either increased O_2 needs or depressed DO_2's is maximized;
2. Sepsis is characterized by significant circulatory abnormalities, all of which likely impact on the ability to maintain tissue O_2 availability when systemic DO_2 is depressed by modest anemia. For example, sepsis limits the cardiac output reserve, the extent to which the cardiac output can be augmented in response to increased tissue O_2 needs [20]. Redistributing DO_2 from the splanchnic organs to the heart and brain normally accompanies anemia, but the ability to shunt delivery between the regional circulations (to maintain DO_2 to the vital organs) is also limited in sepsis [21]. Although the precise cause of this lesion is unknown, it is likely related to the demonstration that arterial hyporesponsiveness is common in this syndrome [22]. In addition, microcirculatory adjustments during anemia normally subserve an increase in O_2 extraction, but the ability to extract O_2 is depressed in sepsis [23].
   Recent animal data confirm that sepsis alters the normal circulatory compensation to modest anemia. In a retrospective analysis of a database of septic sheep, we found that the hemoglobin concentration exerted independent and negative effects on DO_2, at both the central and regional levels of the circulation [24]. Subsequently, a prospective study in a murine model of normotensive sepsis demonstrated that normal to modestly elevated hemoglobin concentrations supported DO_2 to the heart more effectively that was noted when hemoglobin levels were reduced to only 80–100 g/L [25]. Table 2 summarizes where sepsis might adversely affect normal physiologic adaptations to anemia.
3. There is also evidence that sepsis alters the ability of the oxyhemoglobin dissociation curve to rightward shift. In a large animal model of hyperdynamic sepsis, we found that the oxyhemoglobin dissociation curve was left-shifted, compared to when the animal model was non-septic [26]. This would further reduce the ability to maintain tissue O_2 availability and anemia complicates sepsis.

Both circulatory and hematopoetic systems autoregulate to maintain tissue O_2 availability during anemia. The efficiency of these systems is sufficient to support guidelines indicating that the transfusion trigger may be lowered to as low as 70 g/L in perioperative patients.

Table 2. "Septic effects" on physiologic adaptations to anemia

1. On O_2 release
– depressed O_2 extraction "reserve"
– left shift of oxyhemoglobin dissociation curve
2. Depressed O_2 "reserve"
– tachycardia
– depressed contractility
– impaired regional distribution of blood flow

In patients with sepsis, however, abnormalities in the normal compensation found within anemia in the hematopoetic and circulatory system may be significantly constrained. The remainder of this review will examine whether there is clinical data to support the notion that the transfusion trigger should be greater in sepsis than has been proposed for non-septic, perioperative patients.

Levels of Evidence and Grades of Recommendation

The objectives of this section are: 1) to assess the clinical evidence which could be used to justify elevating the transfusion trigger in sepsis above levels currently recommended for other hospitalized patients; and 2) to assess the impact of current transfusion practices on the septic patient.

To identify the relevant papers on RBC transfusion therapy in sepsis, a computerized search of the National Library of Medicine's Medline and the Institute for Scientific Information's Current Contents: Clinical Medicine was performed using BRS On-line search services. Searching from 1966 to December 1993, using the key descriptors (MESH headings) "sepsis" or "septic" and cross-referenced with the descriptor "transfusion", more than 250 abstracts were downloaded and reviewed.

A search of these abstracts revealed 120 papers using random allocation and 75 dealing with human subjects. Of these 75 papers, 7 were based on results from large multicenter randomized control trials, which could qualify as Level I evidence. A much smaller subset of these papers actually dealt with RBC transfusion in sepsis. It is this subset that will be reviewed in this section.

The most compelling grades of recommendation on which to base clinical decisions are supported by Level I and Level II studies on human subjects (see chapter by Cook). A summary of the grades of recommendations relevant to this chapter can be found in Table 3. *We found no randomized trials which compared different transfusion strategies in clinical sepsis.*

Therefore, we will now discuss our second objective, to investigate the impact of current transfusion practices on the septic patient.

Table 3. Grades of recommendation and supporting levels of evidence

Grade A
– supported by Level I evidence (large well designed RCT)
– proven beneficial effect
Grade B
– supported by a least one Level II study (smaller well designed RCT)
– adverse effects no rules out
Grade C
– no support from level I or level II evidence
– level III trials suggest further research is required
– no proven benefit/adverse effects not ruled out

Relevant Outcomes

Survival: The categorical outcome in any clinical treatment study in septic patients is evidence for a survival advantage conferred by the treatment under study. Survival to discharge from hospital, survival to discharge from ICU and 28-day survival have all been employed to examine efficacy of treatment strategies in critically ill patients. If a new therapy proves itself to be equally efficacious as a currently accepted therapy with respect to survival, then quality-of-life measures, surrogate measures of severity of illness, or overall cost of therapy can be evaluated to support clinical recommendations. *We found no study that has evaluated the impact of RBC transfusion on survival, severity of illness, quality-of-life or overall cost of therapy.*

Transfusion and the Systemic VO_2/DO_2 Relationships (Table 4): Since the primary goal of RBC transfusion therapy is to increase tissue oxygenation, changes in systemic DO_2 and systemic VO_2 are two most commonly outcome measures in clinical experiments. This approach assumes that increasing systemic DO_2 by RBC transfusions will be followed by a reasonably immediate and parallel increase in tissue DO_2. In the preceding section, we argued that circulatory dysregulation in sepsis may contravene this assumption.

It is probably more appropriate, therefore, that questions regarding the efficacy of RBC transfusions be discussed using direct, not inferential, data. Thus, when RBC transfusions are prescribed to counteract a tissue O_2 debt in sepsis, efficacy could be concluded by demonstrating a temporally related increase in systemic (or specified organ) VO_2. For example, when tissues are in a state of O_2 need (when the systemic VO_2 is 'supply dependent' see Fig. 1), the gold standard evidence for efficacy would be an increase in systemic VO_2 post-transfusion (Fig. 2). Demonstrating a temporally related fall in elevated arterial lactate levels may be another way to demonstrate efficacy of RBC transfusion, as acute changes in arterial lactate have been used to rep-

Table 4. Brief overview of trials investigating RBC transfusion in septic patients

Authors	Ref.	Level	Methodology	Population (n)	Intervention	Outcomes
Lorente et al. (1993)	[27]	II	randomized, cross over	septic patients (16)	Dobutamine and RBC transfusion	DO_2? VO_2
Marik et al. (1993)	[28]	III	case series	septic patients (23)	RBC transfusion	?VO_2
Dietrich et al. (1990)	[29]	III	case series	septic patients (19)	RBC transfusion	?VO_2, ?lactate
Fenwick et al. (1990)	[31]	III	case series	ARDS patients (24)	RBC transfusion	VO_2 lactate
Steffes et al. (1991)	[32]	III	case series	septic patients (21)	RBC transfusion	DO_2,
Lucking et al. (1990)	[33]	III	case series	septic patients (pediatrics, 8)	RBC transfusion	DO_2, VO_2
Mink et al. (1990)	[34]	III	case series	septic patients (pediatrics, 8)	RBC transfusion	DO_2, ?VO_2

resent changes in the balance between tissue O_2 need and availability [2, 3].

Although it has been proposed that achieving supranormal levels of systemic DO_2 is important for survival in sepsis [6, 7, 9], we found surprisingly few studies that had explicitly examined the hypothesis that increasing systemic DO_2 with RBC transfusion in sepsis would elevate systemic VO_2.

In an interesting cross-over design which investigated the impact of dobutamine and transfusion with 800 mL packed red blood cells on both systemic DO_2 and VO_2, Lorente et al. [27] found that dobutamine significantly increased both DO_2 and VO_2 whereas RBC transfusion increased only DO_2. This trial randomized 16 consecutive septic patients with hemoglobin levels less than 10 g/dL to receive either RBC transfusions or dobutamine followed by RBC transfusion.

In a series of 23 critically ill septic patients undergoing mechanical ventilation, Marik and Sibbald [28] failed to find a statistically significant increase in systemic VO_2 in response to transfusion with up to 3 units of packed red blood cells. These patients were followed for up to 6 h post-transfusion and systemic VO_2 was measured by indirect calorimetry.

In a series of 19 patients with sepsis and a mean pre-transfusion Hgb of 8.3 g/dL, Dietrich et al. [29] failed to show a significant increase in systemic VO_2 or a significant decrease in lactate levels as a result of RBC transfusion.

In 30 euvolemic, hemodynamically stable surgical ICU patients with hemoglobins below 10 g/dL, Babineau et al. [30] demonstrated that 58% of all patients failed to show an improvement in systemic VO_2 with RBC transfusion.

Fenwick [31] transfused 24 consecutive adult patients with ARDS with two units of packed RBC. In 11 patients with a normal plasma lactate preceding transfusion, VO_2 did not change from baseline, although O_2 extraction decreased significantly. In 13 patients with an elevated plasma lactate preceding transfusion, systemic VO_2 increased and O_2 extraction was unchanged. The authors concluded that increasingly systemic DO_2 by RBC transfusion identified pathologic dependence of systemic VO_2 on DO_2 patients with ARDS and increased plasma lactates.

In 1991, Steffes et al. [32] showed that 21 patients defined to be septic either post-surgery or post-trauma responded to RBC transfusion with a statistically significant increase in systemic VO_2 (from 145 ± 39 to 160 ± 56 mL/min/m). The pre-transfusion average hemoglobin was 9.3 ± 1.1 g/L and the post-transfusion hemoglobin concentration was 10.7 ± 1.5 g/L. In this study, stratification of the patients into two groups based on pre-transfusion lactate levels resulted in the demonstration of a statistically significant increase in systemic VO_2 in response to RBC transfusion in patients with normal lactate levels (less than 1.6 mmol/dL, $n=10$). In contrast, patients with an elevated pre-transfusion lactate ($n=17$) demonstrated no significant increase in systemic VO_2 in response to RBC transfusion, despite a significant increase in systemic DO_2.

In 8 children with hyperdynamic septic shock, Lucking et al. [33] reported that after resuscitation with volume loading and pharmacologic support, transfusion with packed RBC resulted in an increase in systemic VO_2 and DO_2 without increasing cardiac output. Patients were only considered for entry into this study if they already demonstrated significant derangements in systemic DO_2, which was defined as a systemic VO_2 less than 180 mL/min/m and O_2 extraction less than 24%.

In a study of 8 hemodynamically stable septic shock pediatric patients, Mink and Pollack [34] failed to find a statistically significant increase in systemic VO_2 after patients were transfused with 8–10 mL/kg of packed RBC over a 1–2 h period. These transfusion resulted in a significant increase in the hemoglobin concentration from an average of 10.2 to 13.2, in the hematocrit from 0.30 to 0.39, and in the systemic DO_2 from 599 to 818 mL/min/m [34].

Review of the available clinical literature therefore demonstrates that studies are inconsistent in their ability to demonstrate that transfused RBC augment systemic VO_2. This could be explained by consideration of the following. First, there may have been no explicit need, therefore, no O_2 deficit to correct by transfusing RBC to increase O_2 availability. For example, if RBC were transfused when systemic VO_2 was supplied-independent (Figure 1 point A_1), it would not have been possible to demonstrate efficacy. In contrast, were RBC to be transfused when systemic VO_2 was supply-dependent (Fig. 1, point B_1), efficacy could easily have been demonstrated by an increase in systemic VO_2.

Second, the inability to demonstrate efficacy might occur if the transfused RBC could not gain access to the microcirculation to unload their O_2 during the time that post-intervention measures were made. For example, we found that a paradoxic depression in gastric pHi despite an increase in systemic DO_2 when septic patients were administered RBC which had been stored for greater than 12 to 15 days [27]. We hypothesized that the normal loss in deformability of stored RBC renders them inaccessible to the damaged septic microcirculation until *in vivo* rejuvenation occurs (and deformability is thereby restored) approximately 6 h post-transfusion.

Finally, if RBC are transfused after storage has resulted in depletion of 2, 3 DPG, again efficacy would not be demonstrable.

Risks of Transfusion

Since there is a lack of evidence in the literature with which to guide transfusion therapy in the septic patient, it is relevant to investigate the risks more closely. Complications associated with blood transfusion are rare, but well-documented (Table 5) [35]. Rigorous attention to details of collection, storage, reissuing of infusion of blood products along with aggressive screening for contaminated blood products [36] reduces this risk of complications. It is interesting to note, especially in the context of the septic patient, that

Table 5. Complications associated with blood transfusion

Immunological
1. Red cell antigens
– hemolytic reactions (delayed or immediate)
– alloimmunization
2. White cell antigens
– febrile reactions
– transfusion related lung injury
– alloimmunization
3. Platelet antigens
– post-transfusion purpura
– alloimmunization
4. Plasma proteins
– hypersensitivity
Infectious
1. Hepatitis A, B, non-A non-B (C), others
2. HIV-1, HIV-2, HTLV
3. CVM, Epstein-Barr
4. Syphilis, malaria, babesiosis, trypanosomiasis
5. Bacterial contamination
Complications related to massive transfusion
1. Fluid overload
2. Thrombocytopenia
3. Hyperkalemia
4. Hypothermia
5. Hypocalcemia

some work questions whether RBC transfusion could be implicated in the amplification of the inflammatory process and subsequent onset of ARDS [37].

Future Directions

Although meta-analysis can be used to increase the strength of a recommendation, there is insufficient evidence to support such an approach to the question of the effectiveness of transfusion therapy to normal or near-normal levels in sepsis. There are, however, at least 7 well conducted multicenter randomized control trials (Level I) which could support a hypothesis-generating process.

The Methylprednisolone Severe Sepsis Study Group [38] enrolled 382 patients at 19 study centers based on a rigid definition of sepsis and septic shock and accounts for 4 of the 7 multicentered, randomized clinical trials regarding the treatment of sepsis that we reviewed. In this trial, patients were randomized to receive either high-dose (30 mg/kg) methylprednisolone or placebo and the data failed to demonstrate any clinical benefit of methylprednisolone treatment in sepsis. Three additional articles using data from the Methylprednisolone Severe Sepsis Study Group have been published. The first described the progression of clinical signs and outcomes in the sepsis syndrome, and used only patients in the control arm of the study [42]. The second report [43] described the clinical outcomes of patients with hypothermia and the sepsis syndrome and recently, Slotman et al. [44] reported the detrimental effects of the high-dose methylprednisolone treatment on markers of hepatic and renal function.

In 1988, Calandra et al. [39] reported a rather small 100 patient multicenter trial which compared the efficacy of administering human IgG antibody to *E. coli* J5 with the standard IgG preparation. The HA-1A Sepsis Study Group [40] enrolled 543 patients with presumed gram-negative sepsis from multiple study centers and in a similar study, the XOMA Sepsis Study Group enrolled 486 patients from 33 university affiliated study centers [41]. None of these three studies failed to show a significant impact of these new approaches to treating septic patients on mortality.

Although none of these major Level I studies directly investigated the effects of RBC transfusion or reported the hematocrit or hemoglobin levels, data from these clinical trials could provide intriguing information. Combined, these studies enrolled approximately 1500 patients into treatment and control arms. If the data could be combined into a single database, and depending on the quality and quantity of the information available in each study, a meta-analysis could provide valuable insights into the optimal trigger for RBC transfusion in a septic patient. They could also provide insight into potential complications of transfusions in the septic patient, such as multiorgan system failure or ARDS. Any hypothesis generated as a result of such a project would require confirmation with a randomized control trial.

Conclusion

1. Current clinical guidelines [11, 12] emphasize:
   - adequate intervascular volume resuscitation is the first objective in the anemic patient.
   - RBC transfusion with a deterioration in vital signs or when the patient develops symptoms of O_2 need.
2. In the absence of patient risks, RBC transfusion above hemoglobins levels of 70 g/L is likely not indicated.
3. In "at risk" patients, clinical judgement should be used to justify transfusing to hemoglobin levels greater than 70 g/L, and this should be done on a unit-by-unit basis in a goal-orientated approach.
4. There is no current evidence to support explicit recommendations for an optimal hematocrit or hemoglobin level at which to transfuse in septic patients.

However, we believe that septic patients are "at risk" by virtue of: 1) their usually elevated tissue O_2 needs, and 2) the explicit evidence for a depression in the circulatory "reserve" required to maintain tissue O_2 availability with modest anemia. Furthermore, there is some support from Level II trials to suggest that transfusion does increase systemic DO_2 and VO_2 in the septic patient. If increases in systemic DO_2 which can be shown to elevate systemic VO_2 are accepted as valid surrogate outcome measures of RBC transfusion therapy in septic patients, then a Grade B recommendation for the statement that hemoglobin level be maintained greater than 100 g/L is appropriate.

Recommendations

1. Hemoglobin levels should be maintained above 100 g/L in septic patients (Grade B/C+).
2. A clinical trial is needed to determine the effectiveness of a clinical strategy which maintains hemoglobin levels >100 g/L in sepsis.

References

1. Bersten AD, Sibbald WJ (1989) Circulatory disturbances in multiple systems organ failure. Crit Care Clinics 5:233–254
2. Rashkin MC, Bosken C, Baughman RP (1985) Oxygen delivery in critically ill patients. Relationship to blood lactate and survival. Chest 87:580–584
3. Nelson DP, Samsel RW, Wood LDH, Schumacker PT (1988) Pathological supply dependence of systemic and intestinal O_2 uptake during endotoxemia. J Appl Physiol 64:2410–2419
4. Haupt MT, Gilbert EM, Carlson RW (1985) Fluid loading increases oxygen consumption in septic patients with lactic acidosis. Am Rev Respir Dis 131:912–916

5. Hersch M, Gnidec AD, Bersten AD, Troster M, Rutledge FS, Sibbald WJ (1990) Histologic and ultrastructural changes in non-pulmonary organs during early hyperdynamic sepsis. Surgery 107:397–410
6. Tuchschmidt J, Fried J, Astiz M, Rackow E (1992) Elevation of cardiac output and oxygen delivery improves outcome in septic shock. Chest 102:216–220
7. Shoemaker WC, Appel PL, Kram HB, Waxman K, Lee TS (1988) Prospective trial of supranormal values of survivors as therapeutic goals in high-risk surgical patients. Chest 94:1176–1186
8. Cane RD (1990) Hemoglobin: How much is enough? Crit Care Med 18:1046–1047
9. Weg JG (1991) Oxygen transport in adult respiratory distress syndrome and other acute circulatory problems: Relationship of oxygen delivery and oxygen consumption. Crit Care Med 19:650–657
10. Greenberg AG (1990) To transfuse or not to transfuse – That is the question? Crit Care Med 18:1045
11. Office of Medical Applications for Research, NIH (1988) Perioperative cell transfusion. JAMA 260:1700
12. Welch GH, Meehan KR, Goodnough LT (1992) Prudent strategies for elective red blood cell transfusion. Ann Intern Med 117:441–442
13. American College of Physicians (1992) Practice strategies for elective red blood cell transfusion. Ann Intern Med 116:403–406
14. Fan FC, Chen RYZ, Schuessler GB, Chien S (1980) Effects of hematocrit variations on regional hemodynamics and oxygen transport in the dog. Am J Physiol 238:H545–622
15. Jan KM, Chien S (1977) Effect of hematocrit variations on coronary hemodynamics and oxygen utilization. Am J Physiol 233:H106–113
16. Berstein D, Teitel DF (1990) Myocardial and systemic oxygen ultilization during severe hypoxia in ventilated lambs. Am J Physiol 258:H1856–1864
17. Lipowsky HH, Firrell JC (1986) Microvascular hemodynamics during systemic hemodilution and hemoconcentration. Am J Physiol 250 (Heart Circ Physiol 19):H908–H922
18. Kiel JW, Shepherd AP (1989) Optimal hematocrit for canine gastric oxygenation. Am J Physiol 256:H472–H477
19. King SE, Cain SM (1987) Regional O_2 uptake during hypoxia and recovery in hypermetabolic dogs. J Appl Physiol 63:381–386
20. Ognibene FF, Parker MM, Natanson CN, Parrillo JE (1988) Depressed left ventricular performance. Response to volume infusion in patients with sepsis and septic shock. Chest 93:903–910
21. Bersten A, Gnidec A, Rutledge FS, Sibbiald WJ (1990) Hyperdynamic sepsis modifies a PEEP-mediated redistribution in organ blood flows. Am Rev Respir Dis 141:1198–1208
22. Martin CM, Yaghi A, Sibbald WJ, McCormack D, Paterson NAM (1993) Differential impairment of vascular reactivity of small pulmonary and systemic arteries in a rat model of hyperdynamic sepsis. Am Rev Respir Dis 148:164–172
23. Shumaker PT, Samsel RW (1989) Oxygen delivery and uptake by peripheral tissues: Physiology and pathophysiology. Crit Care Clinics 5:255–269
24. Fox GA, Bersten A, Lam C, Neal A, Rutledge F, Imman K, Sibbald WJ (1994) The hematocrit modifies the circulatory control of systemic and myocardial oxygen utilization in septic sheep. Crit Care Med (in press)
25. Morisaki H, Bloos F, Cross L, et al (1992) Colloid infusion preserves microvascular integrity better than crystalloid in hyperdynamic sepsis. Crit Care Med 20:4 (Suppl); S 101
26. Bloos MF, Neal A, Pitt A, Martiin CM, Ellis CG, Sibbald WJ (1993) The O_2 dissociation curve in hyperdynamic septic sheep. Clin Invest Med 16 (Suppl):157
27. Lorente JA, Landin L, De Pablo R, Renes E, Rodriguez-Diaz R, Liste D (1993) Effects of blood transfusion on oxygen transport variables in severe sepsis. Crit Care Med 21:1312–1318

28. Marik PE, Sibbald WJ (1993) Effect of stored-blood transfusion on oxygen delivery in patients with sepsis. JAMA 269:3024–3029
29. Dietrick KA, Conrad SA, Hebert CA, Levy GL, Romero MD (1990) Cardiovascular and metabolic response to red blood cell transfusion in critically ill volume-resuscitated non-surgical patients. Crit Care Med 18:940–944
30. Babineau TJ, Dzik WH, Borlase BC, Baxter JK, Bistrian BR, Benotti PN (1992) Reevaluation of current transfusion practices in patients in surgical intensive care units. Am J Surg 164:22–25
31. Fenwick JC, Dodeck PM, Ronco JJ, Phang PT, Wiggs B, Russell JA (1990) Increased concentrations of plasma lactate predict pathologic dependence of oxygen consumption on oxygen delivery in patients with adult respiratory distress syndrome. J Crit Care 5:81–86
32. Steffes CP, Bender JS, Levison MA (1991) Blood transfusion and oxygen consumption in surgical sepsis. Crit Care Med 19:512–517
33. Lucking SE, Williams TM, Chaten FC, Metz RI, Mickell JJ (1990) Dependence of oxygen consumption on oxygen delivery in children with hyperdynamic septic shock and low oxygen extraction. Crit Care Med 18:1316–1319
34. Mink RB, Pollack MM (1990) Effect of blood transfusion on oxygen consumption in pediatric septic shock. Crit Care Med 18:1087–1091
35. Nacht A (1992) The use of blood products in shock. Crit Care Clinics 8:255–291
36. Gottlieb T (1993) Hazards of bacterial contamination of blood products. Anaesth Intensive Care 21:20–23
37. Malouf M, Glanville AR (1993) Blood transfusion related adult respiratory distress syndrome. Anaesth Intensive Care 21:44–49
38. Bone RC, Fisher CJ Jr, Clemmer TP, Slotman GJ, Metz CA, Balk RA (1987) A controlled clinical trial of high-dose methylprednisolone in the treatment of severe sepsis and septic shock. N Engl J Med 317:653–658
39. Calandra T, Glauser MP, Schellekens J, Verhoef J (1988) Treatment of gram-negative septic shock with human IgG antibody to Escherichia coli J5: A prospective, double-blind, randomized trial. J Infect Dis 158:312–319
40. Ziegler EJ, Fisher CJ Jr, Sprung CL, et al (1991) Treatment of gram-negative bacteremia and septic shock with HA-1A human monoclonal antibody against endotoxin. A randomized, double-blind, placebo-controlled trial. The HA-1A Sepsis Study Group. N Engl J Med 324:429–436
41. Greenman RL, Schein RM, Martin MA, et al and The XOMA Sepsis Study Group, (1991) A controlled clinical trial of E5 murine monoclonal IgM antibody to endotoxin in the treatment of gram-negative sepsis. JAMA 266:1097–1102
42. Bone RC, Fisher CJ Jr, Clemmer TP, et al and the Methylprednisolone Severe Sepsis Study Group (1989) Sepsis syndrome: A valid clinical entity. Crit Care Med 17:389–393
43. Clemmer TP, Fisher CJ Jr, Bone RC, et al and The Methylprednisolone Severe Sepsis Study Group (1992) Hypothermia in the sepsis syndrome and clinical outcome. Crit Care Med 20:1395–1401
44. Slotman GJ, Fisher CJ Jr, Bone RC, et al and The Methylprednisolone Severe Sepsis Study Group (1993) Detrimental effects of high-dose methylprednisolone sodium succinate on serum concentrations of hepatic and renal function indicators in severe sepsis and septic shock. Crit Care Med 21:191–195

Vasoactive Drug Therapy in Sepsis

K. Reinhart, F. Bloos, and C. Spies

Introduction

The hemodynamic alterations of septic shock may impair the determinants of cellular O_2 supply on all levels. First, myocardial depression and peripheral vasodilation may result in inadequate perfusion pressure and global O_2 transport. Second, the distribution of regional blood flow may be mismatched in the face of changes in the regional metabolic demands (i.e. the hepato-splanchnic region). Third, microvascular blood flow and the tissue's O_2 extraction capability may be disturbed for various reasons. The aim of vasoactive drug therapy in septic shock is therefore to correct the cardiocirculatory alterations as far as possible in order to achieve adequate tissue oxygenation. It has to be stressed however that the basic concept for therapy of septic shock is an adequate fluid resuscitation which never can be replaced by any vasoactive drug therapy.

Only when proper volume expansion fails to restore cardiocirculatory function and cellular O_2 supply, vasoactive drugs such as inotropes, vasopressors, prostacyclins etc. are used to re-establish blood pressure, cardiac output, and possibly nutritive blood flow.

The development of guidelines on the proper use of vasoactive drugs in sepsis and septic shock is hampered because catecholamines, which are still the basis in the treatment of sepsis, have been primarily developed and investigated for cardiac patients. However, it is evident that the hemodynamic effects of the various catecholamines are different under septic and non-septic conditions. Little is known about the effect of different catecholamines on regional blood flow and tissue oxygenation in septic shock patients.

Criteria for the Evaluation of Vasoactive Drugs

In contrast to the current studies on new therapeutic strategies in sepsis (anti-endotoxin and anti-TNF antibodies, IL-1 receptor antagonist, etc.), with the exception of prostaglandin E_1 (PGE_1, see below), catecholamines have never been investigated with respect to their impact on patient morbidity and mortality. There is only indirect evidence that it might be beneficial to increase DO_2 above supranormal levels by using vasoactive drugs [1].

Therefore, the use of catecholamines and other vasoactive drugs in the treatment of septic shock is mainly based on their effects on different vascular beds and the alteration of organ function. In sepsis, the commonly expected effects of catecholamines may be altered. Endogenic plasma catecholamines are elevated in sepsis which is associated with a diminished response to catecholamines [2]. This may lead to the administration of unusually high dosages to achieve the desired hemodynamic effects [1] and induce negative side effects. Beneficial effects of vasopressors on organ perfusion pressure may outweigh the negative effects on the nutritive blood flow on the microcirculatory level. On the other hand, some vasodilators may improve global blood flow to some areas at the expense of a drop in blood pressure followed by no longer adequate perfusion of other organs. An increased intrapulmonary right/left shunting accompanied with a drop in arterial O_2 content may also counterbalance the beneficial effects of catecholamines and vasodilators on cardiac output and DO_2. Catecholamines may deteriorate myocardial O_2 balance by increasing the myocardial O_2 need due to an increase in contractility, heart rate, and O_2 wasting [3]. Vasodilators may be harmful as they lower coronary perfusion pressure beyond the autoregulatory level. Catecholamines increase DO_2 and therefore, improve whole body O_2 balance but at the same time, can increase O_2 demands due to calorigenic effects [4].

For ethical reasons, it is not possible to perform placebo controlled studies on the efficacy of inotropic and vasopressor support in patients with septic shock. However, comparative studies between different catecholamine-treatment models on patient morbidity and mortality should be performed. Before completion of these studies, no definitive recommendations for the use of specific catecholamines can be given. This also holds true for the use of vasoactive drugs that are used to support catecholamine therapy, i.e. prostacyclins and N-acetylcysteine.

Parameters for the Bedside Assessment of the Efficacy of Vasoactive Drugs

It has become evident that blood pressure and heart rate monitoring alone provide only scant information on the adequacy of tissue oxygenation in patients with septic shock. However, the measurement of cardiac output accompanied by the calculation of DO_2 as well as VO_2, aiming for the optimization of these parameters, is not without technical problems either. It may result in under- as well as overresuscitation of individual patients with unpredictable effects on organ function. Global indicators of tissue hypoxia, such as lactate levels and arterial-venous CO_2 content difference, may be used on sequential basis to judge the efficacy of vasoactive drug therapy. Indicators of regional tissue oxygenation, such as measuring gastric mucosal pH by tonometry [5], may prove helpful as a guide to therapy and at least, prove short-term efficacy. However, it must not be forgotten that the goal of treatment in sepsis is to preserve or improve organ function.

Catecholamines

The effects of catecholamines on cardiocirculatory function and regional blood flow is determined and mediated by their specific effects on the different catecholamine receptors (Table 1).

Dopamine

Depending on the dosage, dopamine affects all receptor types. In low doses (<3 μg/kg/min), dopamine dilates the vasculature of the splanchnic and renal region, increasing urinary output by stimulation of the dopaminergic receptors DA1 and DA2. Application of 2–10 μg/kg/min dopamine (medium dosage) results in an increase in cardiac contractility due to β_1-receptor stimulation and general vasoconstriction as a consequence of α_1-receptor stimulation. In higher doses beyond 10 μg/kg/min, vasoconstriction becomes more and more apparent and may override DA1/DA2 induced vasodilation. However, it should be considered that even low-dose dopamine may have unpredictable inotropic or vasoconstricting effects when used in critically ill patients [6].

As septic shock consists of depression in myocardial contractility and severe systemic vasodilation, dopamine in medium or high doses has been propagated as the catecholamine of choice for its management [7]. Due to

Table 1. Effects of catecholamines on the myocardium and the vasculature

Catecholamine	α_1	α_2	β_1	β_2	DA1	DA2	Effects
Dopamine							
0–3 μg/kg/min	∅	+	∅	∅	+++	++	Splanchnic and renal blood flow ↑
2–10 μg/kg/min	+	+	++	+	++	++	Vasoconstriction, +inotrope
>10 μg/kg/min	++	++	++	+	+	+	Vasoconstriction, +inotrope, splanchnic and renal blood flow ↓
Dobutamine	++	∅	+++	++	∅	∅	+Inotrope, vasodilation, coronary blood flow ↑
Epinephrine	+++	+++	++	+++	∅	∅	↑ Cardiac output, ↑ perfusion pressure
Norepinephrine	+++	+++	++	+	∅	∅	+Inotrope, vasoconstriction
Dopexamine	∅	∅	+	+++	++	+	Vasodilation

+, ++, +++ weak to strong receptor agonist, ∅ no effect on this receptor the pharmacological effects mentioned above, dopamine increases cardiac index, maintains systemic vascular resistance and increases arterial blood pressure [8, 9]. Additionally, dopamine increases muscle tissue pO_2 [10] which may point to an improved tissue O_2 availability.

Despite the beneficial properties of dopamine, some doubts have been expressed as to whether dopamine is a reliable drug for the treatment of septic patients. After application of dopamine, an increase in the pulmonary shunt followed by a drop in arterial pO_2 and a rise in the pulmonary capillary wedge pressure were observed [11, 12]. Of more importance however is the question of whether a dopamine-induced increase in whole body DO_2 is accompanied by an increase in regional as well as microregional blood flow and signs of improved tissue oxygenation. Alpha-receptor mediated vasocontriction may actually reduce O_2 supply to some areas despite increased systemic flow [11, 13]. Despite an increase in DO_2, VO_2 did not increase significantly in septic patients treated with dopamine [11] or was significantly less than in septic patients treated with dobutamine [14]. As other catecholamines, dopamine induces a calorigenic effect [4] causing an increase in tissue O_2 demand.

When dopamine was used to reverse hypotension in septic shock patients, both splanchnic DO_2 and VO_2 were increased [15]. We found that low-dose dopamine administered to patients with hyperdynamic septic shock, combined with norepinephrine, increased hepatic splanchnic flow in 8 out of 10 patients. This went along with a significant increase in O_2 uptake in the hepatic-splanchnic region [16]. Whether this increase in regional VO_2 was the result of an improved tissue oxygenation or only due to the calorigenic effect of dopamine has to remain uncertain as gastric mucosal pH and lactate levels remained unchanged. Increasing dosage of dopamine increases hepatic-splanchnic VO_2 more than DO_2, which might be interpreted as a deleterious side effect on the splanchnic oxygenation [17, 18].

Low-dose dopamine is often added in combination with other vasoactive drugs to increase renal blood flow and urinary output. In patients with congestive heart failure, low-dose dopamine significantly increased renal blood flow. This was accompanied by an increase in inulin clearance, and sodium excretion [8, 19]. Furthermore, the addition of low-dose dopamine to norepinephrine in anesthetized dogs preserved renal blood flow better than norepinephrine alone [20]. This has been taken as evidence that low-dose dopamine could counteract renal dysfunction observed during norepinephrine administration [21]. Whether these findings obtained under non-septic conditions can be transferred to patients with septic shock or whether low-dose dopamine affects the incidence of renal failure in septic patients remains to be investigated.

Dobutamine

Dobutamine increases myocardial contractility by β_1-adrenergic action and causes vasodilation by β_2-stimulation. Since coronary vasodilation is mediated via β_2-receptors, the rise in dobutamine-induced myocardial O_2 need is accompanied by an increase in coronary blood flow. In contrast to dopamine and norepinephrine, dobutamine is known not to induce significant O_2 wasting in the heart [3]. Determinants of myocardial O_2 need, i.e. peak wall stress, were significantly lower in dobutamine-treated cardiac surgery patients than in a dopamine treated group despite a greater increase in cardiac contractility in the former group [22]. These studies indicate that myocardial O_2 need is well maintained despite the increase in heart work. Whether this holds true in sepsis has not been investigated.

Dobutamine is the drug of choice to increase myocardial inotropy in cases of ventricular dysfunction accompanied by an impaired tissue perfusion [23]. In septic shock patients with low cardiac output, the positive inotropic effect of dobutamine increased cardiac output and consecutively DO_2 [14, 24–26]. This was accompanied by an increase in VO_2. A rise in VO_2 was observed especially in septic patients who had elevated lactate values [27]. This has been interpreted to mean that dobutamine unmasks tissue ischemia and that the increase of VO_2 after dobutamine infusion is due to an improvement of tissue oxygenation. However, the extent to which the increase in VO_2 may be due to a calorigenic effect is unknown. Dobutamine can have serious cardiac side effects. Hayes and coworkers [1] used dobutamine in doses up to 200 μg/min/kg to achieve a supranormal DO_2. At these doses, severe tachyarrhythmias, that were sometimes unresponsive to treatment, have been observed. Thus, the practice of dosing dobutamine as high as 200 μg/min/kg to achieve a high cardiac output has to be questioned.

As opposed to dopamine, dobutamine does not cause a significant drop in PaO_2 as the pulmonary shunt fraction remains unchanged when patients were ventilated with positive end-expiratory pressure (PEEP) [24]. After proper fluid administration, the dobutamine-induced vasodilation might be beneficial for organ perfusion. In septic patients, infusion of dobutamine improved splanchnic perfusion, seen by a rise in gastric mucosal pH [5]. However, dobutamine did not affect regional blood flows to the splanchnic region in pigs rendered septic by bacteria infusion [28]. In healthy volunteers, there was only a minor increase in renal blood flow after dobutamine infusion [19].

Beta-2 mediated vasodilation can cause hypotension in septic shock patients but sufficient fluid loading prior to dobutamine application prevents the drop in blood pressure [26]. Thus, the development of hypotension after the onset of dobutamine infusion is a sign of hypovolemia. Animal experiments have shown that dobutamine increases the fluid tolerance of septic dogs allowing for additional fluid resuscitation achieving an additional increase in DO_2 and VO_2 [13].

Norepinephrine

Norepinephrine (NE) increases myocardial contractility via β_1-and α-receptor stimulation. Due to its strong α_1-adrenergic effects, norepinephrine is also a powerful vasopressor. Thus, there are similar considerations for the use of norepinephrine in septic patients as with high-dose dopamine. The strong vasopressor properties of NE increase blood pressure even in severe shock. However, the increase in blood pressure is due to a rise in peripheral vascular resistance while nutritive blood flow may actually be decreased. Renal and hepatic dysfunction during NE treatment has been reported as a consequence of NE administration [29]. Since vasoconstriction can induce a high perfusion pressure, NE application in septic patients may mask a fluid underresucitation. In septic shock patients, NE administration resulted in a lower splanchnic perfusion than in a catecholamine regimen with dobutamine and NE [16]. Dasta reviewed several studies in regard of the effects of NE on O_2 transport [30], and it was concluded that NE has unpredictable effects on systemic O_2 availability and that it actually may increase O_2 debt in septic shock patients [30]. Whether combining dobutamine with NE is superior in terms of tissue oxygenation and preserving of organ function remains open. We found no differences in whole body VO_2 between NE versus NE combined with dobutamine despite a significant drop in DO_2 with norepinephrine as a monotherapy [31].

However, it is not always possible to maintain blood pressure with one catecholamine alone. A sufficient perfusion pressure is important, especially in sepsis where there is evidence that autoregulation of organ blood flow is impaired. NE application can increase urinary output and creatinine clearance in septic patients when perfusion pressure is severely depressed [32]. It has to be pointed out that patients in these studies were severely hypotensive and fluid resuscitation might not have been completely adequate.

Because of its side effects, NE is considered to be better as a secondary additional catecholamine when other drugs, i. e. dobutamine or dopamine, have failed to restore blood pressure. In this setting, NE increased mean arterial pressure by elevation of vascular resistance, cardiac output, creatinine clearance and urinary output while heart rate remained unchanged [33]. This combination may also be beneficial in terms of myocardial O_2 needs. Despite NE dosages up to 10 times of what is recommended for non-septic patients, systemic vascular resistance still remains below normal in adequately fluid resuscitated patients with septic shock.

Epinephrine

Epinephrine is a strong α-agonist with vasopressor properties while low-dose epinephrine has primarily β_2-mimetic effects causing vasodilation. Additionally, epinephrine stimulates the release of norepinephrine within 10 min after application [34]. Epinephrine is mainly used in the resuscitation of cardiac failure but during the last few years, studies have been undertaken to investigate epinephrine as a primary as well as an additional catecholamine in the treatment of septic shock.

When epinephrine is used as only sympathomimetic in fluid resuscitated septic patients, application started with 0.1 μg/kg/min and was titrated to a normal blood pressure or systemic vascular resistance as endpoint. Cardiac index, systolic blood pressure, and peripheral vascular resistance increased in a dose-dependent manner [35, 36]. This was accompanied by an increase in DO_2 and VO_2 [36, 37]. These results were interpreted to be beneficial in septic shock. However, Wilson and coworkers [38] found no increase in VO_2 but a rise in arterial lactate levels when epinephrine was added after fluid resuscitation.

Little is known about whether the reported changes are translated into an improved tissue oxygenation. An increased VO_2 after catecholamine application might be due to metabolic stimulation rather than a relief of tissue hypoxia. Especially epinephrine has been reported to increase metabolic activity to up to 25% [39]. This may be the reason for the controversy in the results from the studies cited above. Furthermore, we found that epinephrine reduced splanchnic DO_2 and splanchnic VO_2 representing a deterioration of splanchnic oxygenation in septic patients [40]. This confirms results that epinephrine reduces mucosal blood flow and intestinal O_2 extraction combined with intestinal lactate production in a bowel preparation of the dog [21].

Epinephrine has also been investigated as a possible replacement for NE as an additional catecholamine to dopamine or dobutamine. The disadvantage of NE is that cardiac output may be depressed due to increased afterload. In fact, several studies with NE found inconsistent effects on cardiac output [32, 33] which was taken as evidence that the action of NE on cardiac output is unpredictable [41]. Epinephrine in doses of about 0.5–0.9 μg/kg/min in addition to dopamine increased mean arterial blood pressure and cardiac output in a consistent manner [41]. In a similar study, the addition of epinephrine to the standard catecholamine and fluid regimen increased VO_2, urinary output, and decreased lactate levels in patients with severe hypotension [42]. Therefore, it was concluded that epinephrine is a possible replacement for NE especially when catecholamine treatment is complicated by tachyarrhythmias [43].

However, the large interindividual differences in the dosage of epinephrine required to achieve a sufficient perfusion pressure makes it difficult to use this drug. Since it cannot be ruled out that epinephrine results in impaired hepatic blood flow and deterioration of tissue oxygenation despite favorable effects on global DO_2 and VO_2, the use of epinephrine in sepsis cannot be recommended at this time.

Dopexamine

Dopexamine is a new catecholamine with β_2- and dopaminergic-receptor activity. Similar to low-dose dopamine, dopexamine can increase blood flow to the renal and slanchnic region [44, 45]. As opposed to dopamine, dopexamine lacks vasoconstrictive properties. Therefore, unlike dopamine, β_2-mediated vasodilation is not counteracted by α_1-mimetic vasoconstriction.

In septic patients, dopexamine increased cardiac index combined with a decrease in systemic vascular resistance [46]. In surgical high-risk patients, dopexamine increased global DO_2 followed by a 75% reduction in mortality compared to the control group [47]. In experimental sepsis, dopexamine increased both DO_2 and VO_2 [48]. These effects were accompanied by less histological alterations in liver tissue [49] and lower gut lactate production [50]. Therefore, it is unlikely that the increase in cellular metabolism accounts for the rise in VO_2. These results would suggest an improvement of nutritive blood flow and tissue oxygenation, at least in the splanchnic region. However, no difference in regional blood flows was observed between dopexamine- and dobutamine-treated endotoxemic rats [51]. The data are promising and suggest that dopexamine might be useful in the treatment of septic patients. However, too few data are currently available to offer guidelines and indications for this new catecholamine.

Nonadrenergic Substances

Vasodilating Prostaglandins

Both animal and human studies provide considerable evidence that the vasodilating prostaglandins prostacyclin PGI_2 and PGE_1 may have beneficial effects on tissue perfusion in ARDS, sepsis and septic shock. These effects include substantial vasodilation, increasing the number of perfused capillaries, maintaining blood flow to the splanchnic region, inhibition of platelet, neutrophil as well as monocyte-macrophage activation, and pulmonary vasodilation with a reduction in pulmonary artery pressure and calculated vascular resistance.

Animal Studies: In different animal models of endotoxic shock, PGI_2 and PGE_1 were able to decrease pulmonary hypertension, elevated pulmonary vascular resistance (PVR) and interstitial edema produced by endotoxin [52]. This was primarily caused by their vasodilating properties. However, PGI_2 did not improve the oxygenation or intrapulmonary shunting [52]. There is evidence from animal studies that PGI_2 infusion attenuates both hypoxia-induced pulmonary hypertension and hypoxic vasoconstriction which allows the flow to be maintained to hypoxic alveoli, resulting in a reduced systemic pO_2 [53].

In a porcine model of severe respiratory failure due to continuous infusion of live *Pseudomonas aeruginosa* [54] and in a model of lethal endotoxic shock [55], PGI_2 increased cardiac output and prevented the depression and disruption of the cardiac mitochondria produced by endotoxemia. Thus, in the latter model, PGI_2 infusion protected myocardial function. The prophylactic use of PGI_2 in a canine model of endotoxic shock as well as the infusion of PGI_2 after the application of endotoxin significantly increased survival rates [56].

Human Studies: In patients suffering from primary and secondary pulmonary hypertension, short-term and long-term PGI_2 infusion can be associated with significant reductions in total PVR and increases in cardiac output [57]. In patients with ARDS, short-term infusion of PGI_2 reduces pulmonary artery pressure (PAP), PVR, and pulmonary capillary wedge pressure (PCWP) without deleterious effects on arterial oxygenation [58]. These effects on PAP and PVR have also been observed in patients with ARDS during PGE_1 infusion [59, 60]. However, the effects of PGE_1 infusion on survival in patients with ARDS remain controversial. Holcroft et al. [60] demonstrated a significant improvement in survival rates in a small group of ARDS patients initially free of severe organ failure. These results could not be confirmed in a randomized double-blind multicenter study of PGE_1 infusion in patients with severe ARDS [61, 62].

In critically ill patients with sepsis, it has been demonstrated that PGI_2 significantly increased VO_2 and microvascular blood flow to the skin [63]. Bihari et al. [64] found substantial increases in DO_2 after PGI_2 infusion in critically ill patients and a higher increase in VO_2 in non-survivors. This suggests that PGI_2 unmasked a tissue O_2 debt. However, DO_2 values were within the normal range, and in another clinical study where PGI_2 was infused in hyperdynamic septic shock patients (submitted for publication), an increase in DO_2 was not matched by an increase in global VO_2. Furthermore, PGI_2 and dobutamine infusion in compensated septic patients resulted in a similar increase in DO_2 in both groups, whereas whole body VO_2 significantly increased only during dobutamine infusion [65]. In this study, dobutamine increased DO_2 more consistently and was better tolerated than PGI_2. On the other hand, in a recent study of patients with septic shock, PGI_2 infusion improved gastric intramucosal pH [66]. Thus, PGI_2 probably improved regional tissue oxygenation in these patients.

In summary, many of these potential benefits of vasodilating prostaglandin infusion, which have been demonstrated in experimental studies, have been confirmed in clinical studies. A definite assessment of the value of these substances especially with respect to the improvement of the outcome in critically ill patients, is not yet clear and requires further investigation.

N-acetylcyteine

Endothelium-derived relaxing factor (EDRF) is considered to be important in maintaining nutritive blood flow, and nitric oxide (NO) has been identified as EDRF [67]. It was demonstrated that sepsis may induce depletion of EDRF due to the increased oxygen radical load but nitric oxide-dependent vasodilator tone is vital for organ perfusion and survival during endotoxin shock [68]. Myers and coworkers [69] showed that endotoxin decreased EDRF activity and NO production. N-acetylcysteine (NAC) has antioxidant properties and as a sulfhydryl donor, may contribute to the regeneration of EDRF and glutathione [70]. Further effects of NAC that might be beneficial in the treatment of sepsis include inhibition of granulocyte aggregation and prevention of progression of microvascular permeability.

There is increasing evidence that NAC has action pertinent to microcirculatory blood flow and tissue oxygenation. NAC has been shown to enhance whole body VO_2 by increasing oxygen extraction in patients 18 h after the onset of fulminant liver failure [70]. NAC is undergoing clinical trials to evaluate its usefulness in sepsis [71] and ARDS [72]. In a previous study [71] in maximum conventionally resuscitated septic shock patients, we infused NAC over 90 min according to the standard regimen for acetaminophen-induced liver failure. A subset of almost half the patients treated with NAC responded with a significant increase in whole body VO_2, DO_2, cardiac index and gastric intramucosal pH, and a decrease in veno-arterial carbon dioxide gradient. Subsequently, these patients who responded to NAC treatment had a much higher survival rate than the non-responding patients. The fact that those parameters changed after optimized conventional therapy suggests an effect on the extraction capability of the tissues [73].

Our results were supported by an experimental study of Zhang et al. [74]. Pretreatments with NAC in a dog model of endotoxic shock maintained a higher cardiac index, DO_2, and left ventricular stroke work index, and lowered systemic and pulmonary vascular resistance. The oxygen uptake levels at critical DO_2 were not different between groups. However, critical DO_2 was significantly lower in the NAC group. Critical oxygen extraction ratio and the slope of the VO_2/DO_2-dependent line were higher in the NAC group. As suggested also in our study, they showed that the oxygen extraction capabilities as well as the myocardial function was improved.

As have previously been observed in patients with fulminant liver failure [70], we found an increase in cardiac output, stroke volume index and left ventricular stroke work index, as well as a decrease in SVR in a subset of almost half the septic shock patients treated with NAC [71]. Brigham and coworkers [75] also found an increase in cardiac output and DO_2 in patients with established ARDS. The reason for the increases in stroke volume and left ventricular stroke work index during NAC infusion is unclear; NAC itself is not known to have a positive inotropic action, and the effect occurred only when the patients were critically ill [70, 71]. Thus it is possible that critically ill patients who responded to the NAC treatment had some combination of increased contractility, decreased afterload and microcirculatory or tissue effects.

In septic animals, NO is reported to promote protection from hepatic, intestinal mucosal, and cardiac damage. Inhibition of NO synthesis resulted in increased hepatic damage during acute murine endotoxemia and NO synthesis was found to play an important role in preserving intestinal mucosal integrity in rats.

The role of NO in sepsis, however, is still controversial. The benefit of NO promoting agents such as NAC in sepsis may be time dependent. NO inhibits mitochondrial respiration and hence VO_2 *in vitro*. It reacts with oxygen free radicals to form for example hydroxyl radicals. However, the effects of NO on VO_2 *in vivo* are not known, and changes in blood flow coupled with a direct effect on respiratory chain enzymes may lead to alterations in oxygen consumption that are only metabolic effects [76].

Clinical and experimental studies directly implicate the overproduction of NO by an inducible NO synthase in the medication of hypotension in septic shock [68, 77]. In patients with life-threatening septic shock and severe refractory hypotension, non-responsive to fluid replacement and catecholamine management, treatment with the NO synthase inhibitor N^G monomethyl-L-arginine has been shown to produce dose-dependent increases in blood pressure [78].

Biochemical evidence for increased production of NO in sepsis is provided by studies showing increased plasma concentrations of nitrite and nitrate, breakdown products of NO, in patients with septic shock [77]. In addition, plasma concentrations of arginine, the substrate for NO synthesis, are reduced in patients with sepsis, particularly in those patients who do not survive [79]. This finding is consistent with the increased activity of the L-arginine/NO pathway.

Induction of the NO synthase in the coronary circulation of the rabbit causes vasodilation and a reduced response to vasoconstrictors. Meyer et al. [80] found that inhibition of NO synthesis reversed the hyperdynamic response to continuous endotoxin administration. As reported by Finkel and coworkers [81] in an isolated hamster papillary muscle model, the negative inotropic effects of cytokines on the heart are also mediated by the overproduction of NO.

The cytotoxic effects of endotoxin, interferon γ, and tumor necrosis factor α (TNF) *in vitro* are mediated in part by NO [82]. In addition to damaging endothelial cells, NO increases vascular permeability [83], although the mechanisms are not fully understood. NO-mediated damage to hepatocytes and pancreatic islet cells has been demonstrated *in vitro*.

In most of the studies where treatment with NAC had no effect, no detrimental effects were observed. The only reproducible finding after NAC treatment was a moderate deterioration in gas exchange, but no alterations in lung mechanics [84]. This might be due to reverse reflex hypoxic pulmonary vasoconstriction as a typical response to pulmonary vasodilators such as prostacyclin in critically ill patients [64]. NAC at high concentrations, however, can have cytotoxic effects upon sheep leukocytes as seen in both aggregation in enzyme release studies [84]. It is unlikely that such concentrations are achieved *in vivo*. Under normal conditions, NAC may be excreted via the kidneys only slowly, while under conditions of oxidant stress, it is readily metabolized by cells via the glutathione reductase pathway and the metabolites are readily excreted via the kidneys [84].

Despite the rapid expansion of studies exploring the nature of the interface between hemodynamic environment on the one hand, and mediators and endothelial structure and function on the other hand, many important unsolved questions remain on the pathogenesis of sepsis. It seems likely that the beneficial or harmful effects of NO synthase promoting or inhibiting agents are dose- and time-dependent. However, there are many unsolved riddles on the exact role of agents like NAC in the management of sepsis.

Phosphodiesterase Inhibitors

Phosphodiesterase III decomposes cyclic phosphate 3′5′ monophosphate (cAMP) in the myocardium. Inhibiting this enzyme, i. e. by enoximone or amrinone, results in elevating cAMP levels in cardiac cells. In cardiogenic shock patients, enoximone increases left ventricular stroke work index and decreases pulmonary capillary wedge pressure [85]. This goes along with a significant increase in DO_2 and VO_2 [86]. A further increase in myocardial contractility can be achieved by combining phosphodiesterase inhibitors with a catecholamine such as dobutamine [87]. This potentially desired boost of cardiac function could also be observed in an endotoxemic shock model where amrinone was combined with norepinephrine [88].

Side effects of phosphodiesterase inhibitors include an increase in pulmonary shunt volume accompanied with a drop in PAO_2 [89] and marked vasodilation. The latter can reduce venous return making it necessary to restore cardiac filling pressures by fluid administration [89]. Furthermore, a long half-life of these substances makes handling of these drugs difficult [15]. Phosphodiesterase inhibitors have not been investigated on septic patients in a controlled manner. Therefore, these substances should only be used in this syndrome if cardiac failure occurs that does not respond to conventional catecholamine treatment.

Conclusions

Due to the lack of large clinical trials with morbidity and mortality as study endpoints, the use of vasoactive drugs for the treatment of patients with septic shock is based only on still limited knowledge about their effects on parameters like blood pressure, cardiac output and other indirect indicators of the adequacy of cellular O_2 supply. Most clinical studies assessed only systemic DO_2/VO_2, but an increase in DO_2 does not always improve regional blood flow. Sepsis-induced low pancreatic blood flow could not be reversed with any catecholamine treatment. Furthermore, even a change in systemic DO_2/VO_2 does not necessarily mean that tissue perfusion is altered in the same manner. There is therefore, a need for clinical studies that address different vasoactive drug treatment models and their effects on patient outcome.

Many authors recommend dopamine as the drug of first choice in the treatment of sepsis since it counteracts the features of septic shock vasodilation and myocardial depression by vasoconstriction and positive inotropism. However, as shown by the potentially beneficial effects of vasodilating substances like dopexamine, protacyclins or N-acetylcysteine, unspecific vasoconstriction might not always achieve the desired improvement of tissue oxygenation. There are also good arguments to use dobutamine as first choice agent if the patient is properly fluid resuscitated and hypotension is not predominant. Only when blood pressure remains inadequate, a vasopressor such as norepinephrine may be added to achieve a mean arterial pressure greater than 70 mmHg. Primarily, the individual hemodynamic pattern of a septic patient should always be considered in choosing a vasoactive agent. A patient with a low cardiac output might be treated with dobutamine while a patient with a high cardiac output but marked hypotension might benefit from a vasopressor such as dopamine in high dosages or norepinephrine. Epinephrine should not be used as a single catecholamine in the treatment of septic shock due to the increase in tissue O_2 demand and its potentially negative effects on hepato-splanchnic perfusion. Organ function has to be closely monitored to assure the efficacy of the chosen catecholamine regimen. It is still to early to give guidelines for the use of dopexamine, prostacyclins or N-acetylcysteine in the treatment of sepsis but it might turn out that these drugs specifically improve nutritive blood flow due to direct effects on the microcirculatory level.

Phosphodiesterase inhibitors are not the drug of first choice in the treatment of septic patients. Indication for phosphodiesterase inhibitors in patients with septic shock may include a low cardiac output that does not respond to fluid and conventional catecholamine treatment, i. e. in patients with pre-existing severe cardiac dysfunction. Vasodilation has to be taken into account and may require additional fluid administration.

Recommendations

1. Before the use of vasoactive drugs, adequate volume therapy is crucial, i. e. give volume as long as further fluid resuscitation increases cardiac output and/or blood pressure without seriously impairing pulmonary gas exchange.
2. Use inotropes before applying pure vasopressors, i. e. dopamine 5–20 μg/kg/min or dobutamine 5–20 μg/kg/min. High vasopressor doses may mask a volume deficit whereas dobutamine may unmask it.

3. In patients without primary hypertension, increase vasopressor support if mean arterial pressure remains below 65–70 mm Hg despite adequate volume loading and inotropic support.
4. There is no scientific evidence that low dose dopamine can prevent renal failure although low dose dopamine may sometimes increase urinary output.
5. Epinephrine is not recommended as a drug of first choice in patients with septic shock.
6. Phosphodiesterase inhibitors should only be taken into consideration when cardiac output remains inadequate with the procedures mentioned above.
7. Dopexamine, prostacyclin, and N-acetylcysteine may find a place in the future as adjuvants to conventional inotropic and vasopressor support if future studies can confirm beneficial effects on some regional circulations.

References

1. Hayes MA, Yau EH, Timmins AC, Hinds CJ, Watson D (1993) Response of critically ill patients to treatment aimed at achieving supranormal oxygen delivery and consumption. Relationship to outcome. Chest 103:886–895
2. Benedict CR, Grahame-Smith DG (1978) Plasma noradrenaline and adrenaline concentrations in dopamine-beta-hydroxilase activity in patients with shock due to septicaemia, trauma and hemorrhage. Q J Med 47:1–20
3. Rooke GA, Feigl EO (1982) Work as a correlate of canine left ventricular oxygen consumption, and the problem of catecholamine oxygen wasting effect. Circ Res 50:273–286
4. Regan CJ, Duckworth R, Fairhurst JA, Maycock PF, Frayn KN, Campbell IT (1990) Metabolic effects of low-dose dopamine infusion in normal volunteers. Clin Sci 79:605–611
5. Silverman HJ, Tuma P (1992) Gastric tonometry in patients with sepsis. Effects of dobutamine infusion and packed red blood cell transfusion. Chest 102:184–188
6. Edwards JD, Tweedle DE (1986) The haemodynamic effects of dopamine in severe human shock. Br J Surg 73:503 (Abst)
7. Vincent JL, Preiser JC (1993) Inotropic agents. New Horizons 1:137–144
8. Goldberg LI (1972) Cardiovascular and renal actions of dopamine. Potential clinical applications. Pharmacol Rev 24:1–29
9. Wilson RF, Sibbald WJ, Jaanimagi JL (1976) Hemodynamic effects of dopamine in critically ill patients. J Surg Res 20:163–172
10. Fleckenstein W, Reinhart K, Kersting T, et al (1984) Dopamine effects on the oxygenation of human skeletal muscle. Adv Exp Med Biol 180:609–613
11. Shoemaker WC, Appell PL, Kram HB, Duarte D, Harrier HD, Ocampo HA (1989) Comparison of hemodynamic and oxygen transport effects of dopamine and dobutamine in critically ill surgical patients. Chest 96:120–126
12. Regnier B, Safan D, Carlot J, et al (1979) Comparative haemodynamic effects of dopamine and dobutamine in septic shock. Intensive Care Med 5:115–119
13. Vincent JL, van der Linden P, Domb M, Blecic S, Azimi G, Bernard A (1987) Dopamine compared with dobutamine in experimental septic shock: Relevance to fluid administration. Anesth Analg 66:565–571
14. Shoemaker WC, Appel PL, Kram HB (1991) Oxygen transport measurements to evaluate tissue perfusion and titrate therapy: Dobutamine and dopamine effects. Crit Care Med 19:672–688

15. Ruokonen E, Takala J, Kari A, Saxen H, Mertsola J, Hansen EJ (1993) Regional blood flow and oxygen transport in septic shock. Crit Care Med 21:296–303
16. Meier-Hellmann A, Reinhart K (1994) Influence of catecholamines on regional perfusion and tissue oxygenation in septic shock patients. In: Reinhart K, Eyrich K, Sprung C (eds) Sepsis: Current perspectives in pathophysiology and therapy. Springer-Verlag, Berlin, Heidelberg, New York, pp 274–291
17. Pawlik W, Shepherd AD, Jacobson ED (1975) Effects of vasoactive agents on intestinal oxygen consumption and blood flow in dogs. J Clin Invest 56:484–490
18. Roytblat L, Gelman S, Bradley EL, Henderson T, Parks D (1990) Dopamine and hepatic oxygen supply-demand relationship. Can J Physiol Pharmacol 68:1165–1169
19. Mousdale S, Clyburn PA, Mackie AM, Groves ND, Rosen M (1988) Comparison of the effects of dopamine, dobutamine, and dopexamine upon renal blood flow: A study in normal healthy volunteers. Br J Clin Pharmacol 25:555–560
20. Schaer GL, Fink MP, Parrillo JE (1985) Norepinephrine alone versus norepinephrine plus low-dose dopamine: Enhanced renal blood flow with combination pressor therapy. Crit Care Med 13:492–496
21. Zaritsky A, Horowitz M, Chernow B (1988) Complications of the pharmacotherapy of septic shock. In: Lumb PD, Bryan-Brown CW (eds) Complications in critical care medicine. Year Book Medical Publishers, Chicago, pp 66–80
22. van Trigt P, Spray TL, Pasque MK, Peyton RB, Pellom GL, Wechsler AS (1984) The comparative effects of dopamine and dobutamine on ventricular mechanics after coronary artery bypass grafting: A pressure-dimension analysis. Circulation 70 (Suppl I):I112–I117
23. Leier CV, Underferth DV (1983) Dobutamine. Ann Int Med 99:490–496
24. Shoemaker WC, Appel PL, Kram HB (1986) Haemodynamic and oxygen transport effects of dobutamine in critically ill general surgical patients. Crit Care Med 14:1032–1037
25. Jardin F, Spomche M, Bazine M (1981) Dobutamine: A haemodynamic evaluation in human septic shock. Crit Care Med 9:329–333
26. Vincent JL, Roman A, Kahn RJ (1990) Dobutamine administration in septic shock: Addition to a standard protocol. Crit Care Med 18:689–693
27. Vincent JL, Roman A, de Backer D, Kahn RJ (1990) Oxygen uptake/supply dependency. Effects of short-term dobutamine infusion. Am Rev Respir Dis 142:2–7
28. Schneider AJ, Groeneveld ABJ, Teule GJJ, Nauta J, Heidendal GAK, Thijs LG (1987) Volume expansion, dobutamine and noradrenaline for treatment of right ventricular dysfunction in porcine septic shock: A combined invasive and radionuclide study. Circ Shock 23:93–106
29. Lam C, Tyml K, Martin C, Sibbald WJ (1991) The skeletal muscle microcirculation in sepsis. Microcirc Res 15:A113 (Abst)
30. Dasta JF (1990) Norepinephrine in septic shock: Renewed interest in an old drug. Ann Pharmacother 24:153–156
31. Sprecht M, Meier-Hellmann A, Hannemann L, et al (1993) Effects of dobutamine vs norepinephrine therapy on oxygen supply and oxygen consumption in septic patients. Crit Care Med 21 (Suppl):S276 (Abst)
32. Desjars P, Pinaud M, Potel G, Tasseau F, Touze MD (1987) A reappraisal of norepinephrine in human septic shock. Crit Care Med 15:134–137
33. Hesselvik JF, Brodin B (1989) Low dose norepinephrine in patients with septic shock and oliguria: Effects on afterload, urine flow, and oxygen transport. Crit Care Med 17:179–180
34. Fellows IW, Bennett T, MacDonald IA (1985) The effect of adrenaline upon cardiovascular and metabolic function in man. Clin Sci 69:215–222
35. Lipman J, Roux J, Kraus P (1991) Vasoconstrictor effects of adrenaline in human septic shock. Anaesth Intens Care 19:61–65
36. Moran JL, O'Fathartaigh MS, Peisach AR, Chapman MJ, Leppard P (1993) Epinephrine as an inotropic agent in septic shock: A dose-profile analysis. Crit Care Med 21:70–77

37. Mackenzie SJ, Kapadia F, Nimmo GR, Armstrong IR, Grant IS (1991) Adrenaline in treatment of septic shock: Effects on haemodynamics and oxygen transport. Intensive Care Med 17:36–39
38. Wilson W, Lipman J, Scribante J, et al (1992) Septic shock: Does adrenaline have a role as a first line inotropic agent? Anaesth Intens Care 20:470–474
39. Giraud GD, MacCannell KL (1984) Decreased nutrient blood flow during dopamine- and epinephrine-induced intestinal vasodilation. J Pharmacol Exp Ther 230:214–220
40. Meier-Hellmann A, Specht M, Spies C, Larscheid P, Bartels K, Reinhart K (1994) Impairment of splanchnic perfusion and tissue oxygenation by epinephrine in patients with septic shock. Clin Int Care 5 (Suppl):23 (Abst)
41. Bollaert PE, Bauer P, Audibert G, Lambert H, Larcan A (1990) Effects of epinephrine on hemodynamics and oxygen metabolism in dopamine-resistant septic shock. Chest 98:949–953
42. Gregory JS, Bonfiglio MF, Dasta JF, Reilley TE, Townsend MC, Flancbaum L (1991) Experience with phenylephrine as a component of the pharmacologic support of septic shock. Crit Care Med 19:1395–1400
43. Bonfiglio MF, Dasta JF, Gregory JS, Townsend MC, Reilly TE, Flancbaum L (1990) High-dose phenylephrine infusion in the hemodynamic support of septic shock. Ann Pharmacother 24:936–939
44. Lokhandwala MF, Jandhyala BS (1992) Effects of dopaminergic agonists on organ blood flow and function. Clin Int Care 3 (Suppl):12–16
45. Leier CV (1988) Regional blood flow responses to vasodilators and inotropes in congestive heart failure. Am J Cardiol 62:86E–93E
46. Colardyn FC, Vandenbogaerde JF, Vogelaers DP, Verbeke JH (1989) Use of dopexamine hydrochloride in patients with septic shock. Crit Care Med 17:999–1003
47. Boyd O, Grounds RM, Bennett ED (1993) A randomized clinical trial of the effect of deliberate perioperative increase of oxygen delivery on mortality in high-risk surgical patients. JAMA 270:2699–2707
48. Bredle DL, Cain SM (1991) Systemic and muscle oxygen uptake/delivery after dopexamine infusion in endotoxic dogs. Crit Care Med 19:198–204
49. Webb AR, Moss RF, Tighe D, al-Saady N, Bennett ED (1991) The effects of dobutamine, dopexamine and fluid on hepatic histological responses to porcine faecal peritonitis. Intensive Care Med 17:487–493
50. Cain SM, Curtis SE (1991) Systemic and regional oxygen uptake and delivery and lactate flux in endotoxic dogs infused with dopexamine. Crit Care Med 19:1552–1560
51. van Lambalgen AA, van Kraats AA, Mulder MF, van den Bos GC, Teerlink T, Thijs LG (1993) Organ blood flow and distribution of cardiac output in dopexamine- or dobutamine-treated endotoxemic rats. J Crit Care 8:117–127
52. Steinberg SM, Dehring D, Gower WR, Vento JM, Lowery BD, Cloustier CT (1983) Prostacyclin in experimental septic acute respiratory failure. J Surg Res 34:298–302
53. Öwall A, Davilén J, Sollevi A (1991) Influence of adenosine and prostacyclin on hypoxia-induced pulmonary hypertension in the anaesthetized pig. Acta Anaesthesiol Scand 35:350–354
54. Slotman G, Machiedo G, Casey K, Lyons M (1982) Histological and haemodynamic effects of prostacyclin and prostaglandin E_1 following oleic acid infusion. Surgery 92:93
55. Utsunomiya T, Krausz MM, Kobayashi M, Shepro D. Hechtman HB (1982) Myocardial protection with prostacyclin after lethal endotoxemia. Surgery 92:101–108
56. Fletcher JR, Raumwell PW (1980) The effects of prostacyclin (PGI_2) on endotoxic shock and endotoxin-induced platelet aggregation in dogs. Circ Shock 7:299–308
57. Rubin LJ, Mendoza J, Hood M, et al. (1990) Treatment of primary pulmonary hypertension with continuous intravenous of prostacyclin (epoprostenol), resulsts of a randomized trial. Ann Int Med 112:485–491
58. Jones K, Higenbottam T, Wallwork MB (1989) Pulmonary vasodilation with prostacyclin in primary and secondary pulmonary hypertension. Chest 96:784–789

59. Shoemaker WC, Appel PL (1985) Effects of prostaglandin E_1 in adult respiratory distress syndrome. Surgery 99:275–283
60. Holcroft JW, Vassar MJ, Weber CJ (1985) Prostaglandin E_1 and survival in patients with the adult respiratory distress syndrome. Ann Surg 203:371–378
61. Bone RC, Slotman G, Maunder R, et al (1989) Randomized double-blind, multicenter study of prostaglandin E_1 in patients with the adult respiratory distress syndrome. Chest 96:114–119
62. Silverman HJ, Slotman G, Bone RC, et al (1990) Effects of prostaglandin E_1 on oxygen delivery and consumption in patients with adult respiratory distress syndrome. Chest 98:405–410
63. Pittet JF, Lacroix JS, Gunning K, Laverriere MC, Morel DR, Suter PM (1990) Prostacyclin but not phentolamine increases oxygen consumption and skin microvascular blood flow in patients with sepsis and respiratory failure. Chest 98:1467–1472
64. Bihari D, Smithies M, Grimson A, Tinker J (1987) The effects of vasodilation with prostacyclin on oxygen delivery and uptake in critically ill patients. N Engl J Med 317:397–403
65. De Backer D, Bérré J, Zhang H, Kahn R, Vincent JL (1993) Relationship between oxygen uptake and oxygen delivery in septic patients: Effects of prostacyclin versus dobutamine. Crit Care Med 21 1659–1664
66. Radermacher P, Buhl R, Kemnitz J, et al (1993) Prostacyclin improves gastric mucosal pH in patients with septic shock. Clin Int Care 4:9
67. Palmer RMJ, Ferrige AG, Moncada S (1987) Nitric oxide release accounts for the biological activity of endothelium-derived relaxing factor. Nature 327:524–526
68. Wright C, Rees D, Moncada S (1992) Protective and pathological roles of nitric oxide in endotoxin shock. Cardiovasc Res 26:48–57
69. Myers PR, Minor RL Jr, Guerra R Jr, et al (1990) Vasorelaxant properties of the endothelium-derived relaxing factor more closely resemble S-nitrosocysteine than nitric oxide. Nature 345:161–163
70. Harrison PM, Wendon JA, Gimson AES, et al (1991) Improvement by acetylcysteine of hemodynamics and oxygen transport in fulminant hepatic failure. N Engl J Med 324:1852–1857
71. Spics C, Reinhart K, et al (1994) Influence of N-Acetylcysteine on O_2 consumption and gastric intramucosal pH in septic patients. Crit Care Med (in press)
72. Bernard GR, Swindell BB, Meredith MJ, et al (1989) Glutathione repletion by N-acetylcysteine (NAC) in patients with the adult respiratory distress syndrome. Am Rev Respir Dis 139:A221 (Abs)
73. Fiddian-Green RG (1993) Associations between intramucosal acidosis in the gut and organ failure. Crit Care Med 21:S103–S107
74. Zhang H, Spapen H, Nguyen DN, Benlabed M, Buurman WA, Vincent JL (1994) Protective effects of N-acetylcysteine in endotoxemia. Am J Physiol (in press) 266:H1746–H1754
75. Brigham KL (1991) Oxygen radicals – an important mediator of sepsis and septic shock. Klin Wochenschr 69:1004–1008
76. Boyd O, Bennett ED (1992) Is oxygen consumption an important clinical target? In: Vincent JL (ed): Yearbook of Intensive Care and Emergency Medicine. Springer, Berlin pp 310–324
77. Ochoa JB, Ukdekwu AO, Billiar TR, et al (1991) Nitrogen oxide levels in patients after trauma and during sepsis. Ann Surg 214:621–626
78. Petros A, Bennett D, Vallance P (1991) Effect of nitric oxide synthase inhibitors on hypotension in patients with septic shock. Lancet 338:1557–1558
79. Freund H, Atamian S, Holroyde J, et al (1979) Plasma amino acids as predictors of the severity and outcome of sepsis. Ann Surg 190:571–576
80. Meyer J, Traber LD, Nelson S, et al (1992) Reversal of hyperdynamic response to continuous endotoxin administration by inhibition of NO synthesis. J Appl Physiol 73:324–328

81. Finkel MS, Oddis CV, Jacob TD, et al (1992) Negative inotropic effects of cytokines on the mediated by nitric oxide. Science 257:387–389
82. Estrada C, Gomez C, Martin C, et al (1992) Nitric oxide mediates tumor necrosis factor-α cytotoxicity in endothelial cells. Biochem Biophys Res Commun 186:475–482
83. Hughes SR, Williams TJ, Brain SD, et al (1990) Evidence that endogenous nitric oxide modulates oedema formation induced by substance P. Eur J Pharmacol 191:481–484
84. Bernard GR, Lucht WD, Niedermeyer ME, et al (1984) Effect of N-acetylcysteine on the pulmonary response to endotoxin in the awake sheep and upon in vitro granulocyte function. J Clin Invest 73:1772–1784
85. Chaterjee K (1988) Enoximone in heart failure: Mechanisms of action. Br J Clin Pract 64:19–25
86. Vincent JL, Carlier E, Berré J, et al (1988) Administration of enoximone in cardiogenic shock. Am J Cardiol 62:419–423
87. Gage J, Rutman H, Lucido D, et al (1986) Additive effects of dobutamine and amrinone on myocardial contractility and ventricular performance in patients with severe heart failure. Circulation 74:367–373
88. De Boelpape C, Vincent JL, Contempré B (1989) Combination of norepinephrine and amrinone in the treatment of endotoxin shock. J Crit Care 4:202–207
89. Vincent JL, Domb M, van der Linden P, et al (1988) Amrinone administration in endotoxic shock. Circ Shock 26:75–83

Evidence-Based Analysis of Nutrition Support in Sepsis

F. B. Cerra

Introduction

Nutrition support has become a standard of care in the management of intensive care unit (ICU) patients with the Systemic Inflammatory Response Syndrome (SIRS) with or without sepsis. Much of critical care therapy has been delivered on a physician preference basis. Worldwide, there is a major effort to shift to evidence-based medical decision-making. This effort requires the evaluation of medical literature that is based on objective methodologies for evaluating the quality of the data as well as the strength of the data in promoting evidence-based medical decision-making. This technology is available today.

This chapter applies an evidence-based approach to the medical literature regarding nutrition support in ICU patients with SIRS-Sepsis [1].

Minimum Improvements in Clinical Benefit

The first step in the evidence-based approach was to define the minimum improvement(s) in clinical benefit (MICB) that would qualify to be used as an outcome that evidence could be gathered for. The second step was to gather the evidence through a review of the medical literature. The third step was to apply the standards of evidence to the data gathered.

The MICB chosen for this analysis were a combination of disease-related and patient-related outcomes. The disease-related outcome was the ability of nutrition support to achieve nitrogen retention. The patient-related outcomes were length of hospital stay and the incidence of acquired infectious complications. The considerations used in selecting the MICB were the type, magnitude and clinical relevance of the medical benefit demonstrated, the risks and benefits of the therapy, and the cost of the therapy. Since little evaluable cost data for nutrition support was available in the literature, the definition of the MICB occurred from the first two criteria.

The literature search was performed on Medline for the years 1970 to 1993. The patient groups that the search was restricted to were: adults, received the therapy at least in part in an ICU, had a reason for ICU admission that included polytrauma, surgical intervention, surgical complication or infection, and had data to support the presence of SIRS-Sepsis during the ICU stay. With these constraints, the search was performed to seek either primary research (individual studies or multicenter trials), or overview studies of nutrition support.

A total of 536 studies were found in the medical literature. Each of these studies was then evaluated for information pertaining to the MICB. This evaluation included: statement of hypothesis and primary and secondary outcome variables, description of patients included in the study and whether or not they were accounted for in the results, a description of the nutrition therapy provided and an analysis of study design and data collection (randomization, blinding, concurrent or prospective enrollment and data collection). Fifty-three suitable studies were found in the pool and subjected to evidence analysis.

Each of the primary research studies (single center and multicenter trials), were evaluated by criteria and a judgement made as to the appropriate level of evidence [1]. Each of the scientific overviews was likewise evaluated. Two key aspects were quality and heterogeneity. The quality evaluation included an analysis of the methodology employed in the analysis and the appropriateness and design of the primary studies. Heterogeneity was assessed from the patient descriptions, presence and analysis of co-morbidities, and descriptions of the treatment employed. The relationship of the 95% confidence interval to the MICB was then assessed. Based on these variables, the level of review quality was assigned. For this review, only studies that were ranked as I or II are reported.

A total of 18 studies qualified for this report. Four areas of efficacy of nutrition support were assessed:

1. The effect of perioperative total parenteral nutrition (TPN) on surgical complications (including infections);
2. The effect of enteral nutrition (EN) on infectious complications;
3. The effect of enhanced EN on length of hospital stay; and
4. The effect of amino acid formula on nitrogen retention in TPN.

The therapeutic impact of nutrition support was estimated by calculating the number of patients that would need to be treated to realize the effect in similar clinical circumstances. The evidence was then used as a basis for recommendations for the use of nutritional support in the ICU in patients with SIRS-Sepsis.

Evidence Analysis

The results of the evidence analysis is presented for each of the defined MICB. This is followed by the therapeutic impact analysis.

Perioperative Total Parental Nutrition Affect on Complications

There were 6 studies that met evidence-level criteria for reporting (Table 1). Of these, one was a meta-analysis [7] and one was prospective, but not ran-

Table 1. Evidence summary for perioperative TPN

Patient Type	Number		Days Pre-operative	Complications			Evidence Level	Reference
	Control	TPN		Major	Infections	Mortality		
UGI cancer	59	66	10	$P<0.05$	—	$P<0.05$	I⁻	[2]
General surgery: Abdominal	145 Patients	50 All Post-Op	>7	$P<0.05$ with PNI > 50%		$P<0.05$ with PNI > 50%	III	[3]
General surgery: Abdominal	51	40	7		$P<0.05$ with mod/severe MTN		II	[4]
General surgery: Abdominal and thoracic multi-center trial	228	231	7–15	$P<0.05$ (decreased) with severe MTN	$P<0.05$ (increased) with mild MTN		II	[5]
General surgery	149	151	Only Post-Op	No difference based on intent-to-treat			II	[6]
Meta-analysis	11 randomized trials 18 controlled trials			$P<0.05$			II⁻	[7]

UGI = upper gastrointestinal; Post-Op = postoperative; MTN = malnutrition; PNI = prognostic nutrition index domized [3]. Of the randomized trials, 2 stratified patients based on the degree of malnutrition present at entrance to the study [4, 5].

Four of 5 primary studies and the meta-analysis observed clinically relevant improvement in patient outcomes. However, in 3 studies, this benefit was only observed in the presence of moderate to severe malnutrition [3–7]. In one study in patients with a moderate level of malnutrition, the complication rate was increased with TPN use [6]. In the meta-analysis, the reduction in major complications associated TPN was 7.1% (95% confidence; 2.1 to 12.4%). However, therapy-related complications (pneumothorax, line infection, vein thrombosis) occurred at 6.7% (95% confidence: 4 to 10%). No significant effect on mortality was observed [7].

Route of Nutrition Administration Affect on Infectious Complications

There were 3 studies that met evidence-level criteria for reporting (Table 2). Two studies were randomized and prospective [8, 9], one was a meta-analysis [10]. There were 8 prospective, randomized trials in the meta-analysis, 6 of which were unpublished data. Of the two published studies used, one is reported here [8], and one was judged to be of low quality and not included in this report.

All of the studies reported in Table 2 use infectious complications as the primary outcome variable. Nutrition was begun within 72 h of surgery; the patients were well-nourished. A reduction in infectious complications (pneumonia, wound, intra-abdominal abscess, central venous line) was observed in all 3 studies. In one study where the data is present [9], the central line sepsis incidence was increased in the patients receiving TPN (1.9% EN vs 13.3%

Table 2. Evidence summary for EN

Patient Type	Number		Initiation of feeding	Infectious Complications	Evidence Level	Reference
	Control	EN				
Abdominal trauma with laparotomy	39	36	within 12 h after surgery	reduced in EN $p<0.05$	I	[18]
Abdominal trauma with laparotomy	51	45	within 24 h after surgery	reduced in EN $p<0.05$	I	[9]
Meta-analysis: abdominal trauma with laparotomy General surgery: 8 trials	118	112	within 72 h after surgery	reduced in EN $p<0.05$	II⁻	[10]

TPN). When the data in the meta-analysis was analyzed without line infections, the incidence of infectious complications was still reduced ($p<0.05$). The study populations are more homogeneous than in most nutrition studies: younger, non-malnourished patients with high injury severity scores and abdominal trauma requiring laparotomy and subsequent ICU care. It is of note that the nutrition support was begun within 72 h of injury and that the MICB was observed in the absence of malnutrition at entrance to the study.

Enhanced Enteral Nutrition Affect on Length of Hospital Stay

There were 2 studies that evaluated the effect of enhanced EN on hospital length of stay (Table 3). The patients did not have moderate to severe malnutrition at entrance into the study. Both studies compared the same diets. The control diet was OsmoliteHN (Ross Laboratories). The experimental diet was Impact (Sandoz Nutrition). This experimental diet was nutritionally complete and fortified with arginine, yeast RNA and menhadin oil, as well as increased amounts of antioxidant vitamins.

The first study was a single center trial in patients undergoing elective surgery for upper gastrointestinal cancer [11]. The second study was a multicenter trial of patients admitted to the ICU with SIRS or sepsis. Polytrauma patients comprised 83% of the study entrants.

In both studies, length of hospital stay was the primary outcome variable. In the single center study, the reduction in the treatment group was 4.4 days on the mean ($p<0.01$) [10]. In the multicenter trial, there was a significant trend for a decreased LOS based on intent-to-treat. Statistical significance

Table 3. Evidence summary for enhanced EN

Patient Type	Number		Initiation of feeding	Reduction in LOS	Evidence Level	Reference
	Control	EN				
UGI cancer surgery	44	41	Full feeds by day 4 postoperative	4.4 days on the mean $p<0.01$	I	[11]
SIRS and sepsis	158	168	Full feeds within day 4 of event precipitating ICU admission	Intent-to-treat 6 days on the median $p<0.27$	II	[12]
	77	74		Fed ≥7 days on the median $p<0.01$		

LOS = length of hospital stay; SIRS = Systemic Inflammatory Response Syndrome was achieved in the subgroup that was fed ≥7 days (50% of the patients in each group). This subgroup was defined pre-hoc. The reduction in length of hospital stay was 7 days on the median ($p<0.01$) [12].

Nitrogen Retention Affect of Amino Acid Formula

Nitrogen retention was judged to meet criteria as a minimum important clinical benefit. It is not a clinical outcome in the same way as infectious complications and length of hospital stay are. Rather, it is an outcome that is directly influenced by the magnitude of the metabolic stress response and the ability of nutrition support to affect that response. In addition, the ability to achieve nitrogen retention is correlated with survival potential [13]. Thus, the ability of nutrition support to influence nitrogen retention is a relevant disease-related outcome.

The question addressed in this section relates to the ability of the amino acid composition in modulating metabolism to promote nitrogen retention without increasing ureagenesis as the principal metabolic effect. The formulations tested for this capacity were those with an increased fractional composition of the branched-chain amino acids, leucine, isoleucine, and valine. The data suitable for analysis reside in studies utilizing TPN.

There were 6 studies that met evidence-level criteria for consideration (Table 4). Five of these were single center studies [14–18], and one was a multicenter trial [19]. The patient groups were surgical ICU patients with significant metabolic stress following polytrauma or infection. The control solutions contained 15–25% BcAA; the modified solutions 45–70% BcAA. The 5 single center studies all demonstrated greater nitrogen retention 3 days post-injury and more cumulative nitrogen retention over the duration of the studies (7–21 days). The multicenter trial [4] also demonstrated that the greatest effect of the modified amino acid solutions occurred during moderate to high level metabolic stress. Unfortunately, no studies have been of a design to adequately evaluate a clinical outcome.

Number Needed to Treat (NNT) Analysis (Therapeutic Impact)

Three studies are of sufficient quality to permit NNT analysis (Table 5). Two of these are multicenter trials [15, 19] and one is a meta-analysis [18]. The relevant clinical outcomes are complications after surgical intervention, infectious complications, and length of hospital stay. In all of the clinical settings, the NNT would indicate significant potential clinical benefit when nutrition support is provided in clinical situations the same or similar to those used in these clinical studies. In addition, it must be clarified that appropriate administration and monitoring techniques must be used. This is particularly so with TPN where complications related to the therapy have the potential of offsetting much of the benefit of the therapy itself.

Table 4. Evidence summary for MICB: nitrogen retention

Patient Type	Number		% BcAA	Effect on Nitrogen Retention	Evidence Level	Reference
	Control	Treatment				
Polytrauma	10	10	21 vs 46%	Improved day 3–21 $p<0.05$	II	[14]
Surgical patients with sepsis	40	40	22.5 vs 45%	7 day cumulative $p<0.005$	I	[15]
Surgical patients with sepsis	14	14	25 vs 45%	Improved day 5–10 $p<0.05$	I	[16]
Trauma and general surgery	8	24	15 vs 30, 50 and 70% (8 each)	Improved day 3–7 in 50 and 70% $p<0.05$ retention proportional to BcAA dose $R^2=0.77$	II	[17]
Trauma and general surgery	7	8	15.5 vs 50%	Improved day 3–6 $p<0.01$	I	[18]
Trauma, general surgery and sepsis multicenter trial	34	53	18 vs 50%	Improved day 3–7 $p<0.05$	I	[19]

MICB = minimum important clinical benefit; BcAA = branched-chain amino acids (leucine, isoleucine, valine)

Table 5. Therapeutic impact analysis based on number needed to treat

Clinical Setting	Complication	Risk of Developing Complication, %	Reduction in Risk from Therapy, %	NNT	Reference
Perioperative TPN in severe malnutrition	Major non-infectious complications	42.9	88	2.0	[15]
EN after abdominal trauma	Major infectious complications	35	54	5.3	[18]
Enhanced EN in SIRS and sepsis	Length of hospital stay of 30 days	50	26.6	8.8	[19]
Enhanced EN in SIRS and sepsis	Length of hospital stay of 27 days after an acquired pneumonia	50	29.6	6.8	[19]

NNT = number needed to heat

Conclusions

1. Perioperative nutrition support as TPN can be associated with a reduction in the incidence of postoperative surgical complications. Two qualifications must be added to this Grade B conclusion:
   - The patient's need to be moderately to severely malnourished; and
   - The complications related to TPN must be kept low, preferably under 4–5%.
2. EN begun within 72 h of injury from trauma requiring surgical intervention and ICU admission is associated with a reduction in the incidence of major septic complications. (Grade A^-/B^+)
3. EN formulas fortified with immune-enhancing nutrients and antioxidants is associated with a reduction in the length of hospital stay when it is initiated within 96 h of an event necessitating ICU care and continued for at least 7 days. (Grade A^-/B^+)
4. TPN formulations, with at least 45% branched-chain amino acids within a balanced amino acid formula, are associated with increased nitrogen retention in ICU patients admitted after polytrauma, surgical complications, and/or sepsis. (Grade is A^-/B^+)

Recommendations

1. Perioperative TPN can be utilized to reduce surgical complications if:
   - The patient is moderately to severely malnourished;
   - Seven days of preoperative therapy are given;
   - The therapy related complications are kept under 4–5%; and
   - The enteral route of nutrition administration is not possible. (Grade B)
2. Branched-chain amino acid enriched amino acid formulas as part of a TPN regimen can improve nitrogen retention:
   - in settings of moderate to high metabolic stress following trauma, surgery or sepsis; and
   - in the absence of pre-existing malnutrition. (Grade A^-/B^+)
3. EN should be initiated whenever possible within 72 h of polytrauma requiring surgical intervention, even in the absence of malnutrition. (Grade A^-/B^+)
4. Enhanced EN should be given strong consideration when EN therapy is provided:
   - in ICU settings of trauma, complications of major surgery and sepsis;
   - within 96 h of an event requiring ICU admission; and
   - in the absence of malnutrition. (Grade A^-/B^+)

References

1. Cook DJ (1994) Clinical trials in the treatment of sepsis: An evidence-based approach. See chapter by Cook in this book
2. Muller JM, Brenner U, Dienst C, Pichlmaier H (1982) Preoperative parenteral feeding in patients with gastrointestinal carcinoma. Lancet 1:68–71
3. Mullen JL, Buzby GP, Matthews DC, Smale BF, Rosato EF (1980) Reduction of operative morbidity and mortality by combined preoperative and postoperative nutritional support. Ann of Surg 192:604–613
4. Bellantone R, Doglietto GB, Bossola M, et al (1990) Preoperative parenteral nutrition in the high risk surgical patient. Am Soc Parent Ent Nutr 12:195–197
5. The Veterans Affairs Total Parenteral Nutrition Cooperative Study Group (1991) Perioperative total parenteral nutrition in surgical patients. N Engl J Med 325:525–532
6. Sandstrom R, Drott C, Aforvidsson B, et al (1993) The effect of postoperative TPN on outcome following major surgery evaluated in a randomized study. Ann Surg 217:185–195
7. Detsky AS, Baker JP, O'Rourke K, Goel V (1987) Perioperative parenteral nutrition: A meta-analysis. Am Col Phys 107:195–203
8. Moore FA, Moore EE, Jones TN, McCroskey BL, Peterson VM (1989) TEN versus TPN following major abdominal trauma – reduced septic morbidity. J Trauma 29:916–923
9. Kudsk KA, Croce MA, Fabian TC, et al (1992) Enteral versus parenteral feeding. Ann Surg 215:503–513
10. Moore FA, Feliciano DV, Andrassy RJ, et al (1992) Early enteral feeding, compared with parenteral, reduces postoperative septic complications. Ann Surg 215:172–183
11. Daly JM, Lieberman MD, Goldfine J, et al (1992) Enteral nutrition with supplemental arginine, RNA and omega-3 fatty acids in patients after operation. Immunologic, metabolic, and clinical outcome. Surg 112:56–67
12. Bower RH, Lavin PT, Cerra FB, et al (1994) Early enteral administration of a formula supplemented with arginine, nucleotides and fish oils reduces length of stay of ICU patients: A randomized, prospective trial (in press)
13. Cerra FB, Cheung NK, Fischer JE, et al (1985) Disease-specific amino acid infusion (F080) in hepatic encephalopathy: A prospective, randomized, double-blind controlled trial. JPEN 9:288–295
14. Kuhl DA, Brown RO, Vehe KL, et al (1990) Use of selected visceral protein measurements in the comparison of branched-chain amino acids with standard amino acids in parenteral nutrition support of injured patients. Surg 107:503–510
15. Jimenez Jimenez FJ, Leyba CO, Mendez SM, Perez MB, Garcia JM (1991) Prospective study on the efficacy of branched-chain amino acids in septic patients. JPEN 15:252–261
16. Bower RH, Muggia-Sullam M, Vallgren S, et al (1986) Branched-chain amino acid-enriched solutions in the septic patient: A randomized, prospective trial. Ann of Surg 203:13–20
17. Cerra FB, Mazuski J, Teasley K, et al (1983) Nitrogen retention in critically ill patients is proportional to the branched-chain amino acid load. Crit Car Med 11:775–778
18. Cerra FB, Upson D, Angelico R, et al (1982) Branched-chains support postoperative protein synthesis. Surg 82:192–199
19. Cerra FB, Blackburn G, Hirsch J, Mullen K, Luther W (1987) The effect of stress level, amino acid formula and nitrogen dose on nitrogen retention in traumatic and septic stress. Ann Surg 205:282–287

Investigational Therapy of Sepsis

Anti-Endotoxin Therapy

T. Calandra and J. D. Baumgartner

Introduction

In a recent national hospital discharge survey, sepsis was the 13th leading cause of death in the United States [1]. Between 1979 and 1987, the rate of septicemia increased 139%, from 73.6 to 176 per 100000 persons. Approximately 400000 cases of sepsis occur annually in the US. Bacteria, mainly gram-negative bacilli (*Enterobacteriaceae* and *Pseudomonadaceae*), gram-negative cocci (*Neisseria meningitidis*) and gram-positive cocci (*Staphylococci,* streptococci, *Enterococcus* species) are the most frequent microbial pathogens isolated from blood or from primary infectious sites of patients with documented sepsis. Half of the documented episodes of sepsis are due to gram-negative bacteria. Today, gram-negative bacteremia accounts for approximately 1% of all hospital admissions [2–4] and is associated with an overall mortality of 20 to 35% [5]. However, fatality ratios may be 50 to 80% in patients who present with septic shock [6–11], which is the most common cause of death in non-coronary ICU [12].

Most of the toxic manifestations induced by gram-negative bacteria are caused by endotoxin (lipopolysaccharide, LPS), which is a component of the outer membrane of these bacteria. Antibiotic therapy does not prevent the toxic manifestations of LPS, and may even promote the release of LPS from bacteria [13]. In eukaryotic cells endotoxin provokes a wide variety of responses. Animals exposed to LPS develop fever and an acute phase response. Responsiveness to LPS is an ancient and well-conserved mechanism for responding to infection and is widely distributed in the animal kingdom. Endotoxin stimulates mononuclear phagocytes and immune cells to secrete cytokines, such as tumor necrosis factor (TNF), the interleukins (IL-1, IL-1 receptor antagonist, IL-6, IL-8 and IL-10) or other mediators, such as platelet activating factor (PAF), which all play an important role in host defense mechanisms against infection. However, exaggerated responses to LPS, as seen in patients with gram-negative septic shock, may trigger a cascade of events leading to hypotension, multiple organ failure and death. So far, no adjunctive therapy has increased the modest survival rate achieved with appropriate anti-infective therapy and supportive care. Therefore, the development of new therapeutic approaches for the treatment of patients with severe sepsis is a major challenge of modern medicine. The purpose of this chapter is to review the background, rationale and clinical experience with anti-endotoxin antibodies.

Background

Endotoxin Structure

The endotoxin (LPS) is composed of three major parts. The innermost part, the lipid A, made of fatty acids linked to a diglucosamine, is the structure responsible for the toxic effects of LPS (for an extensive review of the structure-function relationship of endotoxin see reference [14]). Attached to the lipid A by a saccharide molecule called 3-deoxy-D-manno-2-octulo-sonate (KDO) is the core region, which is composed of a few sugars, phosphate and ethanolamine. The outer part of LPS, the side-chains, consists of repeating units of oligosaccharides, which vary among gram-negative strains. These side-chains (O-polysaccharide or O-antigens) are responsible for antigenic specificity (serotypes). In humans, gram-negative infections are caused by several hundreds of serotypes. In contrast, the core-LPS structure (lipid A and core region) is more conserved. However, analyses of the chemical structure of the core region have revealed that this part of LPS also is subject to inter- and intra-species variability [15–18]. Antibodies can be elicited against any of the three endotoxin parts.

Antibody to O-antigen

Immunization with gram-negative bacilli that possess a complete LPS molecule on their surface induces antibodies directed to the immunodominant species-specific O-antigens (anti-O antibodies). Studies in animals have shown that strain-specific anti-O-antibodies are highly protective against infections caused by the immunizing bacterial strain [19, 20]. However, they do not afford protection against infections caused by bacteria with different O-antigens. The specificity of protection precludes the use of antibodies to O-antigens in patients with gram-negative infections. Two approaches were taken to circumvent this problem.

The first approach was to administer purified polyvalent immunoglobulins. Purified immunoglobulins contain the antibodies present in the pool of plasma from which they were extracted. Since plasma from thousands of donors are pooled to purify immunoglobulins, they contain a large repertoire of antibodies. Intravenous immunoglobulins G (IVIG) have good opsonic activity against many bacteria and have been shown to be protective in various experimental models of infection. The high diversity of bacterial serotypes remains however a major problem. Up to 25 g of IVIG can be administered with one IV infusion. Yet, this amount of IgG represents only 15 to 25% of total human IgG and it may be insufficient to confer protection. Although it is possible to infuse higher doses of IVIG over several days, such treatment would be costly and might be detrimental in patients with infections, insofar as large doses of IgG may block the reticulo-endothelial system. This property has been utilized to reduce the clearance of circulating platelets in idiopathic thrombocytopenia.

The administration of IVIG to prevent infections in ICU patients or neonates has been successful to some extent [21–25]. However, none of these studies showed any reduction of mortality and the cost-effectiveness of prophylaxis was not analyzed. IVIG have also been used as adjunctive therapy for documented infections. Some reports have claimed that the administration of IVIG was beneficial [26–30], but most of these studies had problems related to study design (unblinded evaluations, retrospective analyses), small sample size, or to the quality of the documentation of infections. Moreover, IVIG were shown to be protective only in subgroups of patients or infections. Overall, these data are not sufficient to justify the use of IVIG for the prophylaxis or the treatment of infectious complications in ICU patients [31]. Prospective, randomized, double-blind clinical trials are needed to study the efficacy and address the cost-effectiveness of IVIG therapy in this setting.

The second approach was to focus on infections caused by a limited number of bacterial serotypes, such as *Pseudomonas aeruginosa* infections. While active immunization with *P. aeruginosa* was efficacious [32], passive transfer of anti-*P. aeruginosa* antibodies yielded conflicting results in burned patients [32, 33]. *P. aeruginosa*-hyperimmune IVIG preparations have good opsonic activity *in vitro* and were protective in animal experiments [34–38]. However, the clinical experience with these preparations is limited. Recently, murine or human type-specific anti-*P. aeruginosa* monoclonal antibodies were shown to be protective in animal models [39]. The administration of a combination of monoclonal antibodies to prevent or treat infections caused by a limited number of serotypes is a feasable and interesting therapeutic option. Rapid documentation of infections will be needed if these antibodies are to be used therapeutically.

Core LPS Antibodies

Rough mutants of gram-negative bacilli are characterized by enzymatic deficiencies preventing the attachment of the O-polysaccharide side-chains to the core structure of LPS. The term "rough" refers to the macroscopic aspect of the bacterial colonies on agar plate. The rough aspect is due to the hydrophobicity of the lipidic part of LPS, which is exposed on the surface of these bacteria. By contrast, colonies of gram-negative bacteria with a complete LPS are smooth, because of the hydrophilicity of the external O-side chains. Rough mutants expose on their surface various parts of the core region of LPS, which are usually hidden by the O-side chains and are poorly accessible to immunological reactions. Since the core LPS is made of structures that are common among gram-negative bacilli, an hypothesis formulated during the 1960s was that anti-core LPS antibodies might cross-react between various gram-negative bacteria, and could possibly protect against a wide range of gram-negative infections. The administration of core LPS antibodies was an attractive alternative to the administration of type-specific antibodies for the treatment of gram-negative infections.

The concept of cross-protective anti-core LPS antibodies was supported by the results of experimental studies with antisera from rabbits immunized with rough gram-negative mutants [40–42], and of retrospective human studies, which suggested that high titers of anti-core LPS antibodies were associated with improved survival of patients with gram-negative bacteremia [16, 43, 44]. Two recent articles have reviewed the experimental data obtained with anti-core LPS antibodies [45, 46].

Serum Levels of Anti-Core LPS Antibodies and Survival of Patients with Gram-Negative Bacteremias

The importance of anti-endotoxin antibodies in the host defense against gram-negative infections was suggested by retrospective studies relating patient outcome to titers of core LPS antibodies. The antigens used to detect anti-core LPS antibodies in these patients were rough LPS isolated from the Re mutant of *S. minnesota* [47, 48] and from the J5 mutant of *E. coli* O111B4 [44]. These studies showed the existence of an association between patient survival and anti-core LPS antibody titers at the onset of bloodstream infections due to various gram-negative bacilli [47, 48] or to *P. aeruginosa* [44]. Further analyses showed that this association was independent of anti-O-antibody levels. High levels of IgG or IgM anti-core glycolipid antibody correlated with increased survival. Although these studies did not demonstrate a causal relationship between core LPS antibody and patient outcome, they suggested that core LPS antibodies and specific anti-O antibodies might play a role in the host defense against gram-negative bacteremias.

Serum anti-core LPS antibodies also were measured in 58 patients with documented gram-negative septic shock [6]. Samples were collected near the onset of gram-negative septic shock. Antibodies to J5 LPS, Re LPS, lipid A and to a mixture of 7 smooth LPS were measured by ELISA. With one exception (i.e. anti-lipid A IgM), antibody titers were not different between the 28 survivors and the 30 non-survivors [49]. Surprisingly, median levels of anti-lipid A IgM were higher in non-survivors than in survivors. Therefore, the results obtained in patients with established gram-negative septic shock differed from those obtained in patients with gram-negative bacteremia.

Clinical Studies with E. coli J5 Immune Serum or Hyperimmune Anti-Core LPS Immunoglobulin G

There has been 4 clinical trials conducted with human serum or plasma harvested from volunteers immunized with the J5 mutant of *Escherichia coli* O111:B4 (J5 antiserum), and two studies performed with anti-*E. coli* J5 IgG or with anti-*Salmonella minnesota* Re595 IgG.

E. coli J5 Antiserum

Of 4 clinical studies conducted with J5 immune serum/plasma, 2 were therapeutic and 2 were prophylactic. In 1982, Ziegler et al. [9] published the results of the first randomized, double-blind, multicenter study using J5 antiserum. Three hundred and four patients with a septic syndrome and a suspicion of gram-negative infections were randomized to receive a single intravenous infusion of *E. coli* J5 antiserum or pre-immune (control) serum near the onset of illness. Gram-negative infections were documented in 212 patients (103 patients received J5 antiserum and 109 received control serum), of whom 191 had bloodstream infections (J5 antiserum: 91 patients; control: 100 patients). The 2 treatment groups were similar with respect to age, gender, source of infection, bacteria isolated from blood and appropriateness of antibiotic therapy. Some imbalances existed between the 2 groups regarding underlying conditions. J5 antiserum was found to decrease mortality of patients with gram-negative infections (22 versus 39%, $P=0.011$), gram-negative bacteremia (24 versus 38%, $P=0.04$), and patients with profound shock at study entry (i.e. requiring pressors for more than 6 h) (44 versus 77%, $P=0.003$). Although the antibody titers to J5 LPS were five-fold higher in J5 antiserum than in non-immune serum, there was a wide overlap of the titers between immune and non-immune sera, and protection against death could not be related to J5 antibody titers, regardless of the immune status of the donor. Overall, this study suggested that adjunctive therapy with anti-J5 LPS antibodies reduces mortality of gram-negative bacteremia and septic shock (grade of recommendation A). This study was conducted following standard criteria used for clinical investigation at that time and the results analyzed carefully by a group of experienced investigators. However, clinical data which would be considered essential according to today's criteria were not reported, including an estimation of short-term mortality risk in both treatment groups at study entry, and data on cointerventions such as the administration of other blood-derived products.

In the second, double-blind, multicenter, therapeutic study, children with severe infectious purpura, caused by *Neisseria meningitidis* (in all but 2 cases), were randomized to receive either *E. coli* J5 immune plasma or preimmune plasma in addition to standard therapy [50]. J5 immune plasma was obtained from volunteers immunized with *E. coli* J5 vaccine according to the same immunization schedule used in the pivotal J5 study [9]. This trial was stopped prematurely (i.e. prior to reaching the sample size required by the statistical design of the study) because an intermediate analysis did not show the anticipated reduction of mortality in the J5 plasma treatment group. Forty children were treated with J5 immune plasma and 33 with preimmune plasma. At study entry (i.e. before administration of plasma), clinical and biological parameters were similar in the 2 treatment groups, except for serum concentrations of TNFα and IL-6 (measured in 67% of the children), which were significantly higher in the control group than in the J5 group ($P=0.023$ and $P=0.005$, respectively). Overall mortality was 36% in the control group and 25% in the J5 group (difference 11%, 95% CI: −10 to 32%, P=0.32). By logistic regression analysis, 4 laboratory parameters (fibrinogen level, thrombocyte count, serum levels of TNFα and IL-6) were found to correlate with patient outcome. The trend toward a reduction of mortality with J5 treatment did not persist after adjustments were made for these 4 factors of poor prognosis. Also, there were no statistically significant differences among the 2 treatment groups regarding the occurrence of systemic complications of meningococcemia (duration of hypotension, skin necrosis requiring grafting, amputations) or duration of survival in the non-survivors. Therefore, administration of J5 immune plasma to children with severe infectious purpura did not affect the disease course or reduce mortality (grade of recommendation B). Yet, due to the limited number of patients entered, this study had a low power to detect small differences in mortality between the 2 treatment groups.

In the other two studies, J5 antiserum was administered for the prophylaxis of gram-negative infections. In a randomized, double-blind trial in surgical patients at high risk of developing gram-negative infections, Baumgartner et al. [51] showed that repeated doses of J5 immune plasma did not prevent the acquisition of new focal gram-negative infections (J5 antiserum: 45 of 126, control: 55 of 136, P=0.51), but prevented the development of gram-negative septic shock (15 cases in 136 control patients versus 6 cases in 126 patients treated with J5 immune plasma, P=0.049, one-tailed Fisher's exact test) and its fatal outcome (9 versus 2 deaths, P=0.03) (grade of recommendation B, since the difference would not be significant had two-tailed tests been used for evaluating treatment effect). The incidence of shock and death due to gram-positive bacteria or fungi was not different in the two treatment groups. This study also suffered from a lack of data on cointerventions and of an estimation of short-term mortality in both treatment groups at randomization. In the other prophylactic study, 150 to 200 ml of J5 antiserum or non-immune serum were given to 100 cancer patients at the onset of prolonged chemotherapy-induced granulocytopenia (mean duration 17 days) [52]. One hundred and nine granulocytopenic episodes were included in this trial (J5 group: 52 episodes, control group: 57 episodes). J5 antiserum did not reduce the number of febrile days, gram-negative infections (15 vs 14%, 95% CI: −12 to 15%, P=0.94), or death from these infections (8 vs 4%). With a small number of patient entries, this "negative" study obviously had limited power (i.e. a high false-negative β error) to show a less than dramatic effect of J5 antiserum on the occurrence of gram-negative infections or its complications (grade of recommendation B).

Hyperimmune Immunoglobulins G

The effect of hyperimmune IV immunoglobulins G (IVIG) for the treatment or the prevention of gram-negative infections and septic shock has been studied in 2 randomized, double-blind, multicenter studies. To investigate whether a purified anti-*E. coli* J5 IgG preparation (J5-IVIG), obtained from volunteers immunized with J5 vaccine, would be more suitable for clinical use than the *E. coli* J5 antiserum or plasma, we conducted a randomized, double-blind, multicenter study in patients with established gram-negative septic shock [6]. At study entry, patients received a single dose of 200 mg/kg body weight of either standard IVIG (Sandoglobulin®) or J5-IVIG. Mortality from gram-negative septic shock was 50% (15 of 30) in J5-IVIG recipients, and 49% (20 of 41) in IVIG recipients (95% CI: −22 to 25%, P=0.89). Treatment with J5-IVIG did not reduce the number of systemic complications of shock (57 versus 58%) and did not delay the occurrence of death (median days [range]: 7 [0–32] vs 9 [0–39]). Therefore, J5-IVIG was not superior to standard IVIG in reversing gram-negative septic shock or in reducing mortality (grade of recommendation B). This study also had a limited power to detect less than dramatic differences in mortality between the 2 treatment groups.

In a placebo-controlled study, surgical patients at high-risk of infections were randomized to receive either a standard human IVIG preparation (400 mg/kg of body weight, Gammagard®), or an IVIG preparation enriched in anti-Re LPS antibodies (400 mg/kg of body weight, core-LPS IVIG), or albumin (25% solution, 8 mL/kg of body weight) [25]. Of 352 randomized patients, 329 were evaluable. At study entry, the 3 treatment groups were comparable with respect to age, gender, weight, underlying diseases, APACHE II score, interval between entry to ICU and first infusion of IVIG or placebo, type of surgery, antibiotic therapy or presence of focal infections. The number of patients who acquired infections was lower in the standard-IVIG group (36 of 109 patients, 33%) than in the placebo group (53 of 112 patients, 47%, P=0.03) or core-LPS IVIG group (50 of 108, 46%, P=0.04). The mortality due to infections was not significantly different between the 3 prophylactic groups. Therefore, core-LPS IVIG did not prevent gram-negative infections or their systemic complications (grade of recommendation B).

The clinical trials performed with J5 antiserum for treatment and prophylaxis of gram-negative infections and septic shock have yielded conflicting results (Tables 1 and 2). At face value, J5 antiserum was shown to decrease mortality of patients (mainly adults) with gram-negative bacteremia and septic shock [9] and to prevent the development of gram-negative septic shock and death in high-risk surgical patients [51]. However, in both trials the protective efficacy could not be related to anti-J5 antibody titers. These positive results have not been duplicated since then. In contrast, J5 antiserum did not improve survival of children with fulminant infectious purpura [50]. Administration of J5 antiserum also did not prevent the development of gram-negative infections in cancer patients with granulocytopenia [52]. Even though these studies had been conducted in other types of patients and have included small numbers of patients, limiting their impacts, they have not confirmed the clinical efficacy of J5 antiserum. In addition, anti-J5 immunoglobulin G did not reduce the mortality of gram-negative septic shock [6], and

Table 1. Summary of clinical studies performed with anti-endotoxin antibodies used as adjunctive therapy in patients with gram-negative sepsis

Authors	Ref.	Treatment	Results
Ziegler et al.	[9]	J5 antiserum	Improved survival in patients with gram-negative bacteremia and gram-negative septic shock
J5 Study Group	[50]	J5 antiserum	No improvement in survival of children with severe infectious purpura
Calandra et al.	[6]	J5-IVIG	Not superior to standard IVIG in reducing mortality of patients with gram-negative septic shock
Greenman et al.	[8]	Anti-lipid A monoclonal antibodies (E5)	Improved survival in patients with gram-negative sepsis without shock
Wenzel et al.	[56]	Anti-lipid A monoclonal antibodies (E5)	No improvement in survival of patients with gram-negative sepsis without shock
Ziegler et al.	[64]	Anti-lipid A monoclonal antibodies (HA-1A)	Improved survival in patients with gram-negative bacteremia and shock (*)

IVIG: intravenous immunoglobulin G; (*): results not confirmed by a second HA-1A trial (CHESS Trial)

Table 2. Summary of clinical studies performed with anti-endotoxin antibodies used for the prevention of gram-negative sepsis

Authors	Ref.	Prophylaxis	Results
Baumgartner et al.	[51]	J5 immune plasma	Prevention of gram-negative septic shock and death in surgical patients
McCutchan et al.	[52]	J5 antiserum	No reduction in the frequency of gram-negative infections or their complications in neutropenic cancer patients
The IVIG Collaborative Study Group	[25]	anti-Re595 LPS IVIG	Not superior to human serum albumin in reducing the frequency of gram-negative sepsis and its complications in surgical patients

anti-Re immunoglobulin G did not prevent the occurrence of gram-negative infections and its complications in surgical patients at high risk of infections [25]. Taken together, these results do not support the use of J5 antiserum or anti-core LPS IgG for the prophylaxis or treatment of gram-negative infections.

Anti-lipid A Monoclonal Antibodies

Many monoclonal antibodies have been developed that recognized various epitopes of the core region of endotoxin (for a review see [53]). Two IgM anti-lipid A monoclonal antibodies, one murine (E5) [54] and one human (HA-1A) [55] have been studies extensively *in vitro* and *in vivo*. Recently, these monoclonal antibodies have been used as adjunctive therapy in patients with severe gram-negative infections [7, 8]. Two studies were performed with E5 as well as with HA-1A. In the first randomized, double-blind, multicenter E5 study, 486 patients with suspected gram-negative infection and systemic response were randomly assigned to receive intravenously either E5 murine monoclonal anti-lipid A IgM antibody (2 mg/kg body weight daily × 2) or placebo (5% dextrose in normal saline) [8]. Of the 468 evaluable patients, 316 had confirmed gram-negative sepsis and 179 presented with shock at study entry. Day 30 mortality was similar in both treatment groups when analyzed in all patients (E5: 40%, placebo: 41%) or in those with gram-negative sepsis (38 versus 41%, respectively). E5 was found to reduce mortality in a subgroup of 137 patients with gram-negative sepsis, but without shock at study entry (30 versus 43%, $P=0.01$). Administration of E5 was safe since less than 2% of patients developed allergic side-effects. A second randomized, double-blind, placebo-controlled (human serum albumin) E5 study was conducted in 53 US hospitals [56]. Eight hundred and forty seven patients with suspected gram-negative sepsis syndrome without shock were randomized, 811 were evaluable and 530 had documented gram-negative sepsis. In these 530 patients, day 30 mortality was 70% in the E5 group and 74% in the placebo group (relative risk: 0.8, $P=0.21$). E5 also did not improve survival among 139 patients with gram-negative sepsis and major organ dysfunction at study entry (59 versus 53%, relative risk: 1.3, $P=0.34$). Thus, these results indicate that E5 does not improve survival of patients with gram-negative sepsis syndrome (grade of recommendation B).

In the first double-blind, multicenter HA-1A trial, 543 patients with a presumptive diagnosis of gram-negative infection were randomized to receive intravenously a single dose of 100 mg of a human IgM anti-lipid A monoclonal antibody (in 3.5 g of albumin) or placebo (3.5 g of albumin) [9]. Of 543 patients randomized, 317 had documented gram-negative infections, 200 had a gram-negative bacteremia, and 102 had shock at study entry. In the overall study population, treatment with HA-1A did not reduce 28-day mortality, but it did in patients with gram-negative bacteremia (placebo: 49%; HA-1A: 30%; $P=0.014$), or gram-negative septic shock (57 vs 33%, $P=0.017$) [7], which was reminiscent of the results obtained with J5 antiserum. These results and their clinical implications have been debated extensively [5, 57–61]. Recently, a second, multi-institutional, placebo-controlled HA-1A study (CHESS Trial), which included 2199 patients, was stopped because an interim analysis showed a trend toward an excess mortality among patients without gram-negative bacteremia who had received HA-1A (318 of 785 (41%) versus 292 of 793 patients (37%), $P=0.134$). At the time the study was discontinued, the mortality of patients with documented gram-negative bacteremia (28% of the patients) was 33% (109 of 328) in the HA-1A group and 32% (95 of 293) in the placebo group (P=0.86). Therefore, the second HA-1A study failed to reproduce the results of the first one (grade of recommendation B).

Whereas the first studies performed with E5 or HA-1A suggested some efficacy in subgroups of patients, these results have not been duplicated in subsequent trials. Therefore, clinical data do not support the use of these two anti-lipid A monoclonal antibodies for the treatment of gram-negative sepsis (grade of recommendation B). Recently, a new class of monoclonal antibodies has been described. One of these antibodies, designated WN1 222-5, was shown to recognize a well-characterized epitope of *E. coli* LPS and to cross-react with all *E. coli, Salmonella* and *Shigella* bacterial strains tested [62, 63]. This antibody did not cross-react with *Pseudomonas* species or *Klebsiella* species. *In vivo,* WN1 222-5 afforded cross-protection against challenges with LPS it recognized *in vitro* [63]. The administration of such antibodies, alone or in combinations, deserve further *in vivo* testing.

Conclusions and Recommendations

Over the last 15 years, at least 10 prospective, randomized, double-blind, multicenter trials have tested the role of polyclonal and monoclonal anti-endotoxin antibodies as prophylaxis or adjunctive therapy for gram-negative infections in critically ill patients.

1. *Polyclonal anti-endotoxin antibodies:* Early studies with J5 antiserum or immune plasma demonstrated some beneficial effects in preventing or reducing mortality associated with gram-negative bacteremia or septic shock. However, subsequent studies with either J5 immune plasma or anti-endotoxin immunoglobulin G did not confirm these results. Therefore, the grade of recommendation for polyclonal anti-endotoxin antibodies is A−/B+.
2. *Monoclonal anti-lipid A antibodies:* Most recently, 4 large, multicenter trials of anti-lipid A monoclonal antibodies failed to demonstrate a role for these agents in the treatment of gram-negative bacteremia or septic shock. Thus, the grade of recommendation for monoclonal anti-endotoxin antibodies is B+.

In conclusion, the use of anti-endotoxin antibodies should still be considered experimental today and its efficacy evaluated in double-blind, randomized, prospective studies.

References

1. Increase in National Hospital Discharge Survey Rates for Septicemia, United States, 1979–1987 (1990) MMWR 39:31–34
2. McCabe WR, Jackson GG (1962) Gram-negative bacteremia. I. Etiology and ecology. Arch Intern Med 110:845–855
3. Kreger BE, Craven DE, Carling PC, McCabe WR (1980) Gram-negative bacteremia. III. Reassessment of etiology, epidemiology and ecology in 612 patients. Am J Med 68:332–343
4. Schellekens J, Calandra T (1990) Pathogenesis and treatment of gram-negative septic shock. Cytokines and anti-endotoxin antibodies. Thesis, University of Utrecht, Utrecht, The Netherlands
5. Wenzel RP, Andriole VT, Bartlett JG, et al (1992) Antiendotoxin monoclonal antibodies for gram-negative sepsis: Guidelines from the IDSA. Clin Infect Dis 14:973–976
6. Calandra T, Glauser MP, Schellekens J, Verhoef J, the Swiss-Dutch J5 Immunoglobulin Study Group (1988) Treatment of gram-negative septic shock with human IgG antibody to *Escherichia coli* J5: A prospective, double-blind, randomized study. J Infect Dis 158:312–319
7. Ziegler EJ, Fisher CJ, Sprung CL, et al (1991) Treatment of gram-negative bacteremia and septic shock with HA-1A human monoclonal antibody against endotoxin. A randomized, double-blind, placebo-controlled trial. N Engl J Med 324:429–436
8. Greenman RL, Schein RMH, Martin MA, et al (1991) A controlled clinical trial of E5 murine monoclonal IgM antibody to endotoxin in the treatment of gram-negative sepsis. JAMA 266:1097–1102
9. Ziegler EJ, McCutchan JA, Fierer J, et al (1982) Treatment of gram-negative bacteremia and shock with human antiserum to a mutant *Escherichia coli.* N Engl J Med 307:1225–1230
10. Bone RG, Fisher CJ, Clemmer TP (1987) A controlled clinical trial of high-dose methylprednisolone in the treatment of severe sepsis and septic shock. N Engl J Med 317:653–658
11. The Veterans Administration Systemic Sepsis Cooperative Study Group (1987) Effect of high-dose glucocorticoid therapy on mortality in patients with clinical signs of systemic sepsis. N Engl J Med 317:659–665
12. Parillo JE (1993) Pathogenetic mechanisms of septic shock. N Engl J Med 328:1471–1477
13. Shenep JL, Mogan KA (1984) Kinetics of endotoxin release during antibiotic therapy for experimental gram-negative bacterial sepsis. J Infect Dis 150:380–388
14. Rietschel ET, Seydel U, Zähringer U, et al (1990) Bacterial endotoxin: Molecular relationships between structure and activity. Infect Dis Clin N Am 5:753–779
15. Fuller NA, Wu MC, Wilkinson RG, Heath EC (1973) The biosynthesis of cell wall lipopolysaccharide in *Escherichia coli.* VII. Characterization of heterogenous "core" oligosaccharide structures. J Biol Chem 248:7938–7950
16. Jansson PE, Lindberg AA, Lindberg B, Wollin R (1981) Structural studies on the hexose region of the core in lipopolysaccharides from enterobacteraceae. Eur J Biochem 115:571–577
17. Pollack M, Chia JKS, Koles NL, Miller M, Guelde G (1989) Specificity and cross-reactivity of monoclonal antibodies reactive with the core and lipid A regions of bacterial lipopolysaccharide. J Infect Dis 159:168–188
18. Rietschel ET, Wollenweber HW, Brade H, et al (1984) Structure and conformation of the lipid A component of lipopolysaccharides. In: Proctor RA, Rietschel ET (eds) Handbook of endotoxin. Volume 1: Chemistry of endotoxin. Elsevier, Amsterdam, pp 187–220
19. Pfeiffer R, Kolle W (1896) Ueber die spezifische Immunitaetsreaktion der Typhusbacillen. Z Hyg Infektionskr 21:203–246

20. Tate WJ, Douglas H, Braude AI (1966) Protection against lethality of E. coli endotoxin with "O" antiserum. Ann NY Acad Sci 133:746–762
21. Baker CJ, Melish ME, Hall RT, et al (1992) Intravenous immune globulin for the prevention of nosocomial infection in low-birth-weight neonates. N Engl J Med 327:213–219
22. Chirico G, Rondini G, Plebani A, Chiara A, Massa M, Ugazio AG (1987) Intravenous immunoglobulin therapy for prophylaxis of infection in high-risk neonates. J Pediatr 110:437–442
23. Glinz W, Grob JP, Nydegger UE, et al (1985) Polyvalent immunoglobulins for prophylaxis of bacterial infections in patients with multiple trauma. Intensive Care Med 11:288–294
24. Haque KN, Zaidi MH, Haque SK, Bahakim H, El-Hazmi M, El-Swailam M (1986) Intravenous immunoglobulin for prevention of sepsis in preterm and low birth weight infants. Pediatr Infect Dis 5:622–625
25. The Intravenous Immunoglobulin Collaborative Study Group (1992) Prophylactic intravenous administration of standard immune globulin as compared with core-lipopolysaccharide immune globulin in patients at high-risk of postsurgical infection. N Engl J Med 327:234–240
26. Dominioni L, Dionigi R, Zanello M, et al (1991) Effects of high-dose IgG on survival of surgical patients with sepsis scores of 20 or greater. Arch Surg 126:236–240
27. Duswald KH, Müller K, Seifert J, Ring J (1980) Wirksamkeit von i.v. Gammaglobulin gegen bakterielle Infektionen chirurgischer Patienten. Muench Med Wschr 122:832–836
28. Just HM, Metzger M, Vogel W, Pelka RB (1986) Einfluß einer adjuvanten Immunoglobulintherapie auf Infektionen bei Patienten einer operativen Intensiv-Therapie-Station. Klin Wochenschr 64:245–256
29. Just HM, Vogel W, Metzger M, Pelka RD, Daschner FD (1986) Treatment of intensive care unit patients with severe nosocomial infections. Intensive Care Med 12:345–352
30. Sidiropoulos D, Böhme U, Von Muralt G, Morell A, Barawdum S (1981) Immunoglobulinsubstitution bei der Behandlung der neonatalen Sepsis. Schweiz Med Wochenschr 111:1649–1655
31. Zanetti G, Glauser MP, Baumgartner JD (1991) Review and critique of the use of immunoglobulins in prevention and treatment of infections in critically ill patients. Rev Infect Dis 13:985–992
32. Young LS (1984) Immunoprophylaxis and serotherapy of bacterial infections. Am J Med 76:664–671
33. Baumgartner JD, Glauser MP (1987) Controversies in the passive immunotherapy of bacterial infections in the critically ill patients. Rev Infect Dis 9:194–205
34. Collins MS, Dorsey JH (1984) Comparative anti-Pseudomonas aeruginosa activity of chemically modified and native immunoglobulins G (human), and potentiation of antibiotic protection against Pseudomonas aeruginosa and group B streptococcus in vivo. Am J Med 76:155–160
35. Holder IA, Naglich JG (1984) Experimental studies of the pathogenesis of infections due to Pseudomonas aeruginosa. Treatment with intravenous immune globulin. Am J Med 76:161–167
36. Collins MS, Roby RE (1984) Protective activity of an intravenous immune globulin (human) enriched in antibody against lipopolysaccharide antigens of Pseudomonas aeruginosa. Am J Med 76:168–174
37. Pennington JE, Menkes E (1981) Type-specific versus cross-protective vaccination for gram-negative pneumonia. J Infect Dis 144:599–603
38. Pollack M (1983) Antibody activity against Pseudomonas aeruginosa in immune globulins prepared for intravenous use in humans. J Infect Dis 147:1090–1098
39. Pennington JE (1988) Impact of molecular biology on Pseudomonas aeruginosa immunization. J Hosp Inf 11 (Suppl):96–102

40. Chedid L, Parant M, Parant F, Boyer F (1968) A proposed mechanism for natural immunity to enterobacterial pathogens. J Immunol 100:292–301
41. Braude AI, Douglas H (1972) Passive immunization against the local Schwartzman reaction. J Immunol 108:505–512
42. McCabe WR (1972) Immunization with R mutants of S. minnesota. I. Protection against challenge with heterologous gram-negative bacilli. J Immunol 108:601–610
43. Pollack M, Young LS (1979) Protective activity of antibodies to exotovin A and lipopolysaccharide at the onset of Pseudomonas aeruginosa septicemia in man. J Clin Invest 63:276–286
44. Pollack M, Huang AI, Prescott RK, et al (1983) Enhanced survival in Pseudomonas aeruginosa septicemia associated with high levels of circulating antibody to Escherichia coli endotoxin core. J Clin Invest 72:1874–1881
45. Baumgartner JD (1990) Immunotherapy with antibodies to core lipopolysaccharide: A critical appraisal. Infect Dis Clin N Am 5:915–927
46. Baumgartner JD, Glauser MP (1993) Immunotherapy of endotoxemia and septicemia. Immunobiol 187:464–477
47. McCabe WR, Kreger BE, Johns M (1972) Type-specific and cross-reactive antibodies in gram-negative bacteremia. N Engl J Med 287:261–267
48. Zinner SH, McCabe WR (1976) Effects of IgM and IgG antibody in patients with bacteremia due to gram-negative bacilli. J Infect Dis 133:37–45
49. Baumgartner JD, Heumann D, Calandra T, Glauser MP, and the Swiss-Dutch J5 study group (1989) Antibodies to core LPS in patients with gram-negative septic shock: Absence of correlation with outcome. 29th Interscience Conference on Antimicrobial Agents and Chemotherapy, Houston. Am Soc Microbiol, Washington, p 175 (Abst)
50. J5 Study group (1992) Treatment of severe infectious purpura in children with human plasma from donors immunized with Escherichia coli J5: A prospective double-blind study. J Infect Dis 165:695–701
51. Baumgartner JD, Glauser MP, McCutchan JA, et al (1985) Prevention of gram-negative shock and death in surgical patients by prophylactic antibody to endotoxin core glycolipid. Lancet 2:59–63
52. McCutchan JA, Wolf JL, Ziegler EJ, Braude AI (1983) Ineffectiveness of single-dose human antiserum to core glycolipid (E. coli J5) for prophylaxis of bacteremic, gram-negative infection in patients with prolonged neutropenia. Schweiz Med Wsch 113 (Suppl) 14:40–45
53. Baumgartner JD (1990) Monoclonal anti-endotoxin antibodies for the treatment of gram-negative bacteremia and septic shock. Eur J Clin Micro Inf Dis 9:711–716
54. Young LS (1984) Functional activity of monoclonal antibodies against lipopolysaccharide (LPS) antigens of gram-negative bacilli. Clin Res 32:518A (Abst)
55. Teng NNH, Kaplan HS, Hebert JM (1985) Protection against gram-negative bacteremia and endotoxemia with human monoclonal IgM antibodies. Proc Natl Acad Sci USA 82:1790–1794
56. Wenzel RP, Bone RC, Fein AM, et al (1991) Results of a second double-blind, randomized, controlled trial of antiendotoxin antibody E5 in gram-negative sepsis. 31st Interscience Conference on Antimicrobial Agents and Chemotherapy 294 (Abst)
57. Baumgartner JD, Heumann D, Glauser MP (1991) The HA-1A monoclonal antibody for gram-negative sepsis. N Engl J Med (Lett) 325:281–282
58. Warren HS, Danner RL, Munford RS (1992) Anti-endotoxin monoclonal antibodies. N Engl J Med 326:1153–1157
59. Wenzel RP (1992) Anti-endotoxin monoclonal antibodies – A second look. N Engl J Med 326:1151–1153
60. Ziegler EJ, Smith CR (1992) Anti-endotoxin monoclonal antibodies. N Engl J Med 326:1165 (Lett)
61. Bone RC (1991) A critical evaluation of new agents for the treatment of sepsis. JAMA 266:1686–1691

62. Saxen H, Vuopio-Varkila J, Luk J, et al (1993) Detection of enterobacterial lipopolysaccharides and experimental endotoxemia by means of an immunolimulus assay using both serotype-specific and cross-reactive antibodies. J Infect Dis 168:393–399
63. Di Padova FE, Brade H, Barclay GR, et al (1993) A broadly cross-protective monoclonal antibody binding to *Escherichia coli* and *Salmonella* lipopolysaccharides. Infect Immun 61:3863–3872
64. Hogg N, Ross GD, Jones DB, Slusarenko M, Walport MJ, Lachmann PJ (1984) Identification of an anti-monocyte monoclonal antibody that is specific for membrane complement receptor type one (CR1). Eur J Immunol 14:236–243

Critical Reappraisal of Steroids and Other Anti-Inflammatory Agents

J. Carlet and L. Cronin

Introduction

Severe sepsis, septic shock, and adult respiratory distress syndrome (ARDS) remain a challenge for intensivists since the mortality of these syndromes appears to remain unchanged (around 50%) over the past two decades despite dramatic improvements in the overall management of ICU patients [1–2]. A number of therapeutic approaches have followed step by step improvements in our understanding of the pathophysiology of severe sepsis and ARDS.

Unfortunately, most of these therapeutic trials failed to decrease mortality. As anti-inflammatory agents, corticosteroids are one of the therapies which have been used extensively and empirically in ICU setting, before a couple of human studies gave negative results [1–6]. Since that time, most ICU practitioners abandoned the use of corticosteroids in the management of septic shock and ARDS, except for some very rare and still empiric indications of severe hypoxemia due to extensive fibrosis during the evolution of ARDS patients [7].

However, recent editorials and position papers still challenge those negative results and perpetuate the dream that corticosteroids might be effective in some subgroups of patients [8–9].

Rationale for the Use of Anti-Inflammatory Agents

Pathophysiology of Severe Sepsis

Severe sepsis and ARDS are considered to be due to an uncontrolled inflammatory process induced by components of bacteria, mainly endotoxin of gram-negative bacteria, but also techoic acid or superantigens of gram-positive cocci [10]. As a consequence, a massive production of cytokines (mainly TNF) by monocytes and macrophages occurs which is responsible for the stimulation of polymorphonuclear leukocytes, the adhesion of those leukocytes to the endothelium of vascular vessels (via adhesins), and an intense vasodilatation due at least partly to the increased production of nitric oxide (NO). Activation of the complement system with liberation of anaphylatoxins (C3a, C5a) and the activation of coagulation system is also usual. Coagulation abnormalities are due to several different mechanisms including the liberation of platelet activating factor (PAF) by macrophages and leukocytes.

The activation of the arachidonic cascade is obviously a key process in this inflammatory cascade (Fig. 1) [11–12]. Both the cyclooxygenase and the lipoxygenase pathways are activated during septic shock leading to the production of prostaglandins (prostacyclin, PGI_2, PGF_2 α...) and leukotrienes. These compounds possess inflammatory effects. Some have an important vasoconstrictive effect, while PGI_2 has vasodilating and anti-inflammatory effects.

Effects of Anti-Inflammatory Agents

Effects on Arachidonic Cascade: Corticosteroids have some important effects upon phospholipase A2, and act on both cyclooxygenase and lipoxygenase pathways [13]. Cyclooxygenase inhibitors like indomethacin, ibuprofen and meclofenamate reduce the production of TXA_2 and PGI_2. Selective thromboxane synthase inhibitors such as ketoconazole [14–15], and lipoxygenase inhibitors as diethylcarbamazine (DEC) and LY 255283, a leukotriene B4 inhibitor [16] are available. Aspirin has also some anti-inflammatory and antithrombotic effect due to the inhibition of cyclooxygenase 2 [17–18].

Other Effects of Corticosteroids: At high dose (30 mg/kg), corticosteroids prevent the activation of the complement cascade [19], prevent the hyperaggregation and adhesion of leukocytes induced by endotoxin [20–22], suppress

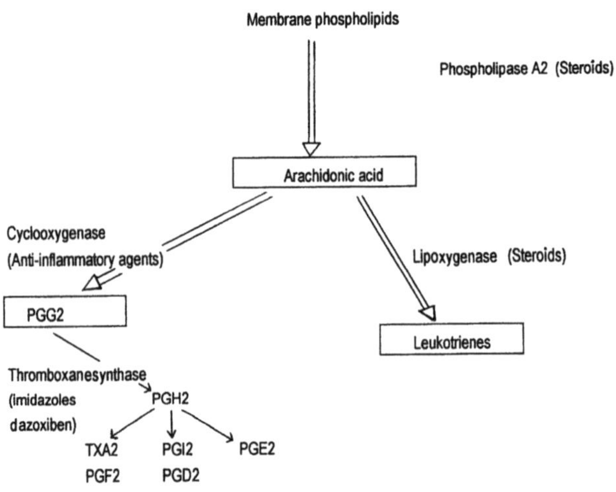

Fig. 1. Arachidonic metabolites. Cyclooxygenase and lipoxygenase pathways

histamine release [23], inhibit endorphin release by a negative feed back upon ACTH release [23], decrease PAF release during endotoxin challenge [24], and inhibit exogenous NO synthase [25]. They also prevent TNF and IL-1 release from mononuclear cells [26–31], by a pretranscriptional blockade of messenger RNA [32]. Most of those effects, as well as the decrease of vascular permeability, are observed only if corticosteroids are given before or immediately after the inflammatory challenge. In some experiments [33–34], steroids maintain some activity even if injected after the inflammatory challenge.

Effects of Prostaglandin E1: Apart from its vasodilatory effect [35], PGE_1 is known to have some anti-inflammatory effects. It reduces platelet aggregation [36], macrophage activation [37], neutrophil chemotaxis [38], neutrophil release of oxygen radicals and lysosomal enzymes [39].

Experimental Data

A large amount of experimental data, in some cases controversial, is available on the use of corticosteroids and non-steroidal anti-inflammatory agents such as indomethacin, and more recently ibuprofen.

Corticosteroids

Corticosteroids are able to prevent septic shock and multiple organ failure (MOF) in animals challenged with live gram-negative bacteria, endotoxin, gram-positive cocci or cell wall extracts [40–46]. However, in most studies, the effect occurs only if the animals are pretreated, and each hour of delay in steroid administration can result in increased morbidity and mortality. In the study from Hinshaw et al. [47], some protective effects were noted up to 4 h after endotoxin challenge. Both dexamethasone and methylprednisolone have been used in canine, murine or baboons models. Lung injury and vascular permeability have also been prevented in ARDS animal models [43, 48, 49]. In some experiments, combination of steroids and antibiotics have been used successfully [45–50].

Non-Steroidal Anti-Inflammatory Agents

Results in animal experimental studies are still controversial. In dogs [51], ibuprofen does not reduce the initial hypotension induced by endotoxin but more rapidly restores cardiac output and prevents acidosis. It does not prevent the permeability abnormalities [52]. The effect is more pronounced when the drug is given before endotoxin challenge [53].

The combination of ibuprofen and corticosteroids has resulted in a modification of pulmonary responses to endotoxemia [49] but has also increased mortality in one study during experimental peritonitis in rats [54].

Inhibitors of thromboxane synthase do not prevent pulmonary leukostasis, leukopenia [55–56] and do not decrease mortality [57]. However, mortality in rats challenged with *Salmonella* endotoxin was reduced by imidazole [57] and regional blood flow was maintained compared to control [58].

Ibuprofen protects the lung microvascular integrity in different experimental models of ARDS [59–61], and has been shown to improve systemic blood flow and systemic vascular resistance, and to decrease lactic acidosis during endotoxin models in pigs [62], dogs [63] and sheep [64]. Finally, ibuprofen reduces TNF activity during sepsis-induced acute lung injury [29].

Possible Side Effects of Anti-Inflammatory Agents

Both **steroids** and **non-steroidal agents** dramatically reduce inflammation via a decrease in leukocyte influx, aggregation and adherence, and TNF production. Hence, they should have deleterious side effects by reducing the natural defenses against infection.

Corticosteroids have an important depressant action upon immunity [65]. They decrease phagocytosis and bactericidal activity of phagocytes [65, 66] and macrophages [65], reduce the number and activity of T lymphocytes [67], and impair opsonization of particles by reticulo-endothelial system [68]. Therefore, they may increase the risk of nosocomial infections, mainly pneumonia [69, 70].

Human Experience with Anti-Inflammatory Agents

Prostaglandin E1: A preliminary study with PGE_1 have been conducted a few years ago by Holcroft et al. [35]. This randomized, prospective, placebo-controlled, double blind study including only 41 patients with ARDS, showed a significantly greater survival at day 30 in treated patients (71% alive), than in placebo patients (35% alive) ($p=0.03$). However, hospital mortality was not different. This study had a lot of methodological pitfalls, including the lack of assessment of underlying diseases, of the severity of the patients studied, the absence of any comparison between treated- and placebo-patients, and a very low number of patients. A second double blind study coordinated by Bone et al. [71] failed to demonstrate any effect of the drug in patients with ARDS. A third study performed in Europe but never published confirmed those negative results.

Non-Steroidal Anti-Inflammatory Agents: Very few studies with non-steroidal anti-inflammatory agents have been available in humans. In a pilot study in 10 patients treated with indomethacin (1 mg/kg), Hanly et al. [72] found some increase in PaO_2/FiO_2 ratio in patients requiring mechanical ventilation for acute respiratory failure.

A randomized, double blind multicenter study has been performed in 52 patients, using a rectal route, looking at physiologic effects and side effects [73]. This study showed that the drug was well tolerated, with a significant decrease in temperature but no other physiological effects.

A pilot study performed using ibuprofen (IV route) in "sepsis syndrome" patients [74] showed that the treated patients experienced a significant decrease in heart rate, body temperature, peak airway pressure and minute ventilation with a decrease in urinary metabolites of prostaglandins (prostacyclin and thromboxane). The drug was well tolerated. A multicenter study in patients with sepsis and ARDS is presently on going in North America.

Corticosteroids: There have been so far 126 citations in the literature during severe sepsis on the use of steroids in ICU patients, especially during septic shock [75–81] and ARDS due to aspiration [82], fat embolism [83–85] and trauma. These studies without control groups did not reach the minimal methodological standard and are not contributary. A review from Weizman et al. in 1974 [88] pointed out that no firm conclusions were possible at that time.

In a meta-analysis which is presently ongoing (Cronin L, manuscript in preparation), 12 papers were identified as methodologically relevant by three independent reviewers. Excluding duplicate publications, 8 published studies [1, 3–6, 69, 87, 88] and one unpublished [89], gathering a total of 1358 patients are available in patients with severe sepsis.

Additional studies are available in severely infected patients, mainly with typhoid fever [90] and in children with meningococcal and pneumococcal meningitis [91].

A lot of studies have been performed in patients with ARDS [92], looking either at lung water and vascular permeability [93] or at mortality [94–96]. Some studies in patients with severe acute lung injuries due to *Pneumocystis carinii* have been recently published [97–99].

Studies Performed in Severe Sepsis

The characteristics of the 8 available studies are presented in Table 1, and the effects of the drug upon mortality in Table 2. The only study in which mortality was significantly improved was the study by Shumer et al. [88], indicating that mortality was decreased from 38.3% in the control group down to 9.3% and 11.6% in the two treated groups. The other studies showed very little effect of corticosteroids on mortality so that the meta-analysis of those 8 studies (1250 pts) gave an overall odd ratio of 0.96 (0.752–1.216) which represents a small and non-significant reduction in mortality. However, this effect disappears totally after withdrawal of the studies with a

Table 1. Summary of study design in the 8 randomized studies

Authors	Ref.	Years	Number of patients	Inclusion criteria	Severity of underlying disease	Severity Indexes	Adjustments with confounding variables	Treatment	Outcome Endpoint
Cooperative study group	[87]	1985	194	Life-threating infections with hypotension	Not reported	Not reported	NO	Hydrocortisone 30 mg/kg on day 1 50 mg/6 days	Mortality Complications
Klastersky et al.	[69]	1971	85	Severe sepsis with positive blood cultures. Cancer patients and leukemias	Not reported	Not reported	NO	Betamethasone 1 mg/kg/day	Mortality Complications
Lucas et al.	[3]	1984	48	Severe sepsis, bacteremia and shock (BP < 80 mm Hg)	Not reported "Severity was similar for both groups"		NO	Dexamethasone 2 mg/kg 2 days	Mortality Complications
Schumer et al.	[88]	1976	172	Bacteremia, hypotension	Not reported	Not reported	NO	Methylprednisolone 30 mg/kg Dexamethasone 3 mg/kg 1 dose	Mortality Complications
Sprung et al.	[4]	1984	59	Septic shock, bacteremia	McCabe comparable	Not reported but some assessment of severity	NO	Methylprednisolone 30 mg/kg Dexamethasone 6 mg/kg 1 dose ± second dose	Hospital mortality Complications
Bone et al.	[1]	1987	382	Sepsis syndrome	McCabe comparable	Not reported	NO	Methylprednisolone 30 mg/kg 24 h	14-day mortality Complications
VASSCS Group	[5]	1987	223	Septic shock	Not reported	No severity index but criteria well described	NO	Methylprednisolone 30 mg/kg + 5 mg/kg 9 h	14-day mortality Complications
Luce et al.	[6]	1988	56	Septic shock	Not reported	Not reported Some assessment of severity	NO	Methylprednisolone 30 mg/kg 4 times 24 h	ARDS Hospital mortality Complications

Table 2. Mortality in the randomized studies

Authors	Ref.	Mortality					
		Treated patients			Control patients		
		N	Deaths	Mortality (%)	N	Deaths	Mortality (%)
Klasterky	[96]	46	24	52	39	21	53
Shumer	[88]	43	4	9.3	86	33	38.3
		43	5	11.6			
Lucas	[3]	23	5	21.7	25	5	20
Sprung	[4]	21	16	76	16	11	69
		22	17	77			
Bone	[1]	191	65	34	190	48	25
VASSCS	[5]	112	23	20.5	111	24	21.6
Luce	[6]	38	22	58	37	20	54

poor methodological score (751 pts remain): odd ratio = 1.30 (95% CI=0.946–1.797), p=0.80.

The study from Schumer et al. [88] is difficult to analyze since it has a lot of methodological problems. The overall duration of the study is 8 years with a retrospective and a prospective part. The study assessed neither the type of severity of the underlying diseases nor the comparability of the groups. The type of infections was not described and the population was extremely heterogeneous. However, there are also a lot of methodological problems in the 4 more recent randomized, placebo-controlled, double blind studies (Table 1 and 2).

In a study by Sprung et al. [4], the size of the population (59 pts) was rather small. There was some assessment of the underlying disease (Mc Cabe score) and of the severity of the acute disease, even if no score was used. The treated group and the placebo groups appeared comparable. There was some early beneficial effect of steroids on the incidence of shock and mortality, but this effect disappeared later on. Superinfections were significantly more frequent in the treated group (36 and 14%) than in the control one (6%).

In the study by Bone et al. [1], the population studied was large enough (382 pts), the diagnoses were presented in detail, and properly balanced between both groups. The McCabe Score had been recorded and was stated to be comparable in both groups, but was not given. The severity of the patients was assessed, but no severity score was provided. The comparison between groups was difficult because the data were incomplete. The placebo group included more patients with multiple sites of infection and more patients with creatinine levels >2 mg/dL (42 vs 31% for treated group). The drug had no significant effect on mortality. In the patients with a creatinine level

>2 mg/dL (stratification made *a posteriori*), mortality was even higher in treated patients (55 versus 40% in placebo patients, $p<0.05$). The crude incidence of secondary infections was the same (19 versus 20%) but the mortality due to infection was higher in treated patients (34 versus 7%, $p<0.015$). It was however difficult to know if this analysis was planned in the initial protocol.

In the VA study [5], 233 patients were evaluated in a rather well designed trial. There was a good assessment of the comparability of the groups. Even though the McCabe score was not provided, all variables to calculate the score were presented, as well as a severity score, the site of infection and the micro-organisms responsible for infection. Adequacy of antibiotherapy was also assessed. The main endpoint, 14 days mortality, was analyzed in a sequential fashion, and was not significantly influenced by steroid therapy. However, the placebo patients were probably less severely ill. There were fewer patients with hypotension (39 versus 51%, $p=0.08$), thrombocytopenia (8 versus 16%, $p=0.07$), hypocapnia (56 versus 73%, $p=0.02$). Mean blood glucose was lower in the placebo group than in the treated group ($p=0.01$). A calculated Apache II or SAPS score could have been lower in the placebo patients. Unfortunately there was no multivariate analysis with adjustments for those confounding variables.

In patients with evidence of infection, mortality was 21.4% in the placebo group and 17.4% in the treated group. In patients with appropriate antibiotherapy, mortality was 21.7% in the placebo group and 13.9% in the treated group ($p=0.32$). A trend was also obvious in patients with gram-negative infections (25.4 vs 17.4%, $p=0.35$) or gram-negative bacteremia (27.3 vs 6.9%, $p=0.11$). Progression of initial infection was more frequent in the steroid group than in the placebo group (17 versus 11%). Secondary infections were however more frequent in placebo group than in the treated group (21 vs 15%, $p=0.20$). The incidence of respiratory failure was lower in the treated group, especially in the patients with gram-negative bacteremia (36 vs 10%, $p=0.03$).

In conclusion, in this well designed study, there was no effect of glucocorticoids in the overall population, but some imbalance was noted in the severity of the patients, favoring the placebo group. Furthermore, some trend was apparent in subgroups in favor of the steroid group.

Finally, the study from Luce et al. [6], gathering 87 patients with septic shock, looked not only at mortality but also the occurrence of ARDS in septic shock patients. The main problem in this study was that the small size of the population precluded any firm conclusions. Moreover, the two groups were not comparable. In particular mechanical ventilation was used in 68% of the treated patients but only in 40% of the placebo patients. Neither the mortality or the incidence of ARDS were affected by the therapy. The occurrence of secondary infections was similar in both groups.

Studies Performed during Severe Infections without Sepsis Syndrome

Infections without Respiratory Insufficiency: In patients with severe typhoid fever [90], steroid therapy was shown to significantly reduce mortality from 55.6% in the placebo group down to 10% in the treated group ($p=0.003$). Patients were rather severely ill with 10% of patients in shock and 30% of patients with some hemodynamic abnormalities (mild shock). However, the size of the study was far too small to allow any firm conclusions.

A double blind study performed by Lebel et al. [91] in 200 children with meningitis showed that the incidence of sequellae was significantly prevented by steroid therapy ($p<0.001$). Mortality was very low in both groups.

Infections with Acute Respiratory Insufficiency: Steroids appeared to be effective during severe *Pneumocystis carinii* pneumonia with either severe [98, 99] or moderate acute respiratory failure [97]. Mortality, incidence of ARDS or worsening of the pulmonary function were all reduced. No side effects were noted in treated patients. The doses of steroids were far lower than those used in severe sepsis or ARDS but the treatment was prolonged for 7 to 14 days. A US consensus statement [100] proposed to use steroids during severe *Pneumocystis* pneumonia, and these agents have been now widely used in this setting.

Studies Performed in ARDS Patients

Initial studies by Sibbald et al. [93] demonstrated that high dosc corticosteroid therapy was able to reduce alveolo-capillary permeability in human septic ARDS patients ($n=14$), but only if used early in the course of the illness. A subgroup of 5 patients were non-responders.

Three randomized, comparative, placebo-controlled, double blind studies have been performed in ARDS patients [92, 94, 95].

The first study, by Weigelt et al. [92], included 81 patients at risk for ARDS. Steroids failed to improve pulmonary function or to prevent ARDS (64% steroids, 33% placebo), and even increased the rate of infectious complications (77 vs 43%, respectively).

The second study [94] included the population of the "Methylprednisolone severe sepsis study group" [1], but evaluated the incidence and the reversal of ARDS to the 14-day mortality. ARDS was reversed in less often than placebo patients (31 vs 61%, $p=0.005$). The 14-day mortality rate was higher in the treated than the placebo patients (51 vs 22%, $p=0.004$), however, the comparability of the groups was not shown in this paper.

The third study by Bernard et al. [95] included 99 patients, 49% of whom were septic. The two groups were well balanced in terms of severity, apart from the bilirubin level which was higher in the placebo patients ($r=0.29$, $p<0.05$). Even after controlling for the bilirubin level (which was a prognostic factor: $r=0.29$, $p<0.05$), no significant effect of steroids on the mortality was observed: the 45-day mortality was 60% in the treated group (95%, CI 49 to 77, p=0.74) and 63% in placebo group (95%, CI 49 to 77). Results were similar in the subgroup of septic patients with ARDS. The reversal of ARDS was also similar in both groups. Infectious complications were also similar.

Finally, some recent data were presented in non-infectious ARDS, showing for example a decrease of IL-8 production in patients receiving prednisolone prior to extracorporeal bypass [101].

Critical Reappraisal

In view of the pathophysiology of sepsis and ARDS, the known effects of corticosteroids and other anti-inflammatory compounds and the results of numerous animal studies, these drugs may be excepted to be effective in humans. Therefore the results of the human studies are very disappointing. Meta-analysis of the data showed some no substantial benefit of the drug in the overall population (OD=0.94), and the possibility of harm is raised after withdrawing the studies with a poor level of pertinence. Except for the study from Shumer et al. [88], the studies gave negative results. There are several explanations for that.

The first point is that, even though the studies were reasonably well designed, and double-blind, they raise a lot of methodological problems. In most of them, underlying diseases were not assessed properly. No severity score was available, the comparability of the 2 groups was not properly addressed and there was no adjustment of the data according to possible confounding factors known to influence mortality (except one study), and adequacy of antibiotherapy was not assessed. Furthermore, those studies were too inhomogeneous. Definitions, delays between onset of the disease and therapy, doses of steroids were all different. Mortality was also very different from one study to another. In some studies, the delay between therapy and the onset of sepsis was very long, and animal studies showed that steroids are more effective when injected before or immediately after the septic challenge. This difference is probably crucial.

Another explanation could be that some beneficial effect of the drug might be balanced by negative side effects, mainly infections. However, the meta-analysis did not show any significant increase in side effects, especially nosocomial infections and bleeding. Some detrimental effects of steroids have also been shown on hepatic and renal blood flow during sepsis syndrome and shock [102].

Finally, the entry criteria used for the sepsis syndrome might account for those negative results not only for steroid trials but also for other drugs such as anti-endotoxin antibodies, anti-TNF or other anti-cytokine therapies. The effects of those drugs could be different in systemic infections and in focal infections such as peritonitis. The effects could also be different in patients with gram-negative or gram-positive infections. Platelet activating factor

(PAF) for example seems to be more effective in patients with gram-negative infections. In the study from the Veteran Administration [5], some trend was noted in patients with gram-negative infections. On the contrary, mortality due to gram-positive cocci is not influenced, or was even increased in treated patients.

Steroids seem to be effective in some specific infectious diseases such as typhoid fever and severe *Pneumocystis carinii* pneumonia. This might be due to the fact that those diseases are homogeneous in contrast to sepsis syndrome (despite the fact that patients with infections due to *Pneumocystis* may have a hyperdynamic profile quite similar to bacterial pneumonia and sepsis) [103]. This also may be due to the fact that steroid therapy is in this case prolonged (7 to 14 days in *Pneumocystis carinii* pneumonia). Some prolonged treatments with steroids have been used in fibrosis due to ARDS, with some interesting results [7, 104], but this has to be confirmed in well designed, prospective and controlled studies.

Conclusion

The results of the studies comparing high dose steroids and placebo during severe sepsis are extremely disappointing, since the rationale for the use of steroids was very strong [105]. However, a lot of methodological problems can be raised in the available trials. Well designed studies, in homogeneous groups of patients using an accurate illness severity score would be of great interest, and should be considered, before abandoning these inexpensive drugs for new, far more expensive experimental therapies.

Recommendations

1. Corticosteroids are not recommended for the management of severe sepsis, especially septic shock, and ARDS (Grade B recommendation).
2. Prostaglandin E1 is not recommended in the treatment of ARDS (Grade B recommendation).
3. Anti-inflammatory agents, such as indomethacin and ibuprofen, are not recommended for the treatment of severe sepsis or ARDS (Grade A recommendation).
4. In view of the attractive pathophysiologic rationale of steroids and other anti-inflammatory agents, and because of their low cost, further studies of steroids and anti-inflammatory agents are warranted in homogeneous populations, with an adequate stratification according to underlying disease and severity (Grade A recommendation).

References

1. Bone RC, Fisher C, Clemmer T, et al (1987) A controlled clinical trial of high-dose methylprednisolone in the treatment of severe sepsis and septic shock. N Engl J Med 317:653–658
2. Reinhart K, Eyrich K, Sprung C (1994) Sepsis: Current perspectives in pathophysiology and therapy. In: Vincent JL (ed) Update in Intensive Care and Emergency Medicine. Springer Verlag, Vol 18, 570 pages
3. Lucas C, Ledgerwood A (1984) The cardiopulmonary response to massive doses of steroids in patients with septic shock. Arch Surg 119:537–541
4. Sprung CL, Caralis PV, Marcial EH, et al (1984) The effect of high-dose corticosteroids in patients with septic shock. N Engl Med 311:1137–1143
5. The Veterans Administration Systemic Sepsis Cooperative Study Group (1987) Effect of high-dose glucocorticosteroid therapy on mortality in patients with clinical signs of systemic sepsis. N Engl J Med 317:659–665
6. Luce J, Montgomery BA, Marks JD, et al (1988) Ineffectiveness of high-dose methylprednisolone in preventing parenchymal lung injury and improving mortality in patients with septic shock. Am Rev Respir Dis 138:62–68
7. Ashbaugh DG, Maier RV (1985) Idiopathic pulmonary fibrosis in Adult Respiratory Distress Syndrome: Diagnosis and treatment. Arch Surg 120:530–535
8. Putterman C (1989) Corticosteroids in sepsis and septic shock: Has the jury reached a verdict? Isr J Med Sci 25:332–338
9. Sjolin J (1991) High-dose corticosteroid therapy in human septic shock: Has the jury reached a correct verdict? Circ Shock 35:139–151
10. Casey LC, Back RA, Bone RC (1993) Plasma cytokine and endotoxin levels correlate with survival in patients with the sepsis syndrome. Ann Intern Med 119:771–778
11. Fink MP (1993) Phospholipases A2: Potential mediators of systemic inflammatory response syndrome and the multiple organ dysfunction syndrome. Crit Care Med 21:957–959
12. Vadas P, Schouten BD, Stefanski E, Scott K, Pruzanski W (1993) Association of hyperphospholipasemia A2 with multiple system organ dysfunction due to salicylate intoxication. Crit Care Med 21:1087–1091
13. Flower RJ, Blakwell GJ (1979) Anti-inflammatory steroids induce biosynthesis of a phospholipase A2 inhibitor which prevents prostaglandin generation. Nature 278:456–459
14. Watkins W, Huttemeier P, Kong D (1982) Thromboxan and pulmonary hypertension following E. coli endotoxin infusion in sheep: Effect of an imidazole derivate. Prostaglandins 23:273–281
15. Yu M, Tomasa G (1993) A double-blind, prospective, randomized trial of ketoconazole, a thromboxane synthase inhibitor in the prophylaxis of the adult respiratory distress syndrome. Crit Care Med 21:1635–1644
16. Fink MP, O'Sullivan BP, Menconi MJ, et al (1993) A novel leukotriene-B4-receptor antagonist in endotoxin shock: A prospective, controlled trial in a porcine model. Crit Care Med 12:1825–1837
17. Vane J (1994) Towards a better aspirin. Nature 367:215–216
18. Picot D, Loll PJ, Garavito M (1994) The X-ray crystal structure of the membrane protein prostaglandin H2 synthase-1. Nature 367:243–249
19. Packard BD, Weiler JM (1983) Steroids inhibitor activation of the alternative amplification pathway of complement. Infect Immunol 40:1011–1019
20. Jacob HS, Craddock RP, Hammerschmidt DE, Moldow CF (1980) Complement-induced granulocyte aggregation: An unsuspected mechanism of disease. N Engl J Med 302:789–794
21. Hammerschmidt DE, White JG, Craddock PR, Jacobs HS (1979) Corticosteroids inhibit complement-induced granulocyte aggregation: A possible mechanism for their efficacy in shock states. J Clin Invest 63:798–803

22. Skubitz KH, Craddock PR, Hammerschmidt DE, August JT (1981) Corticosteroids block binding of chemotactic peptid to its receptor or granulocytes and cause disaggregation of granulocytes aggregates in vitro. J Clin Invest 68:13–20
23. Sheagren JN (1994) Corticosteroids for the treatment of septic shock in "gram-negative septicemia and septic shock". Infect Dis Clin N Am 5:875–882
24. Dhainaut JF, Mira JP (1993) The role of platelet activating factor in sepsis. In: Baumgartner JD, Calandra T, Carlet J (eds) Mediators of Sepsis: From pathophysiology to therapeutic approaches. Flammarion, Paris, pp 147–165
25. Moncada S, Higgs A (1993) The L-Arginine-Nitric oxide pathway. New Engl J Med 329:2002–2012
26. Snyder DS, Unarrue ER (1982) Corticosteroids inhibit murine macrophage 1a expression and interleukin-1 production. J Immunol 129:1803–1809
27. Beutler B, Krochin N, Milsark IN et al (1986) Control of cachectin synthesis-mechanisms of endotoxin resistant. Science 232:977–989
28. Parant M, Le Contel C, Parant F, Chedid L (1991) Influence of endogenous glucocorticoid on endotoxin induced production of circulating TNF-α. Lymph Cytok Res 10:267–271
29. Leeper-Woodford SK, Carey PD, Byrne K, et al (1991) Ibuprofen attenuates plasma tumor necrosis factor activity during sepsis-induced acute lung injury. J Appl Physiol 71:915–923
30. Barber AE, Coyle SM, Marano MA, Fischer E, Calvano SE, Fong Y (1993) Glycocorticoid therapy alters hormonal and cytokine responses to endotoxin in man. J Immunol 150:1999–2006
31. Han J, Thompson P, Bentler B (1990) Dexamethasone and pentoxifylline inhibit endotoxin-induced cachectin/tumor necrosis factor synthesis at separate points in the signaling pathway. J Exp Med 172:391–397
32. Knudsen PJ, Dinarello CA, Strom TB (1987) Glucocorticoids inhibit transcriptional and post-transcriptional expression of interleukin-1 in U 937 cells. J Immunol 139:4129–4134
33. Hubbard JD, Janssen HF (1986) Effects of methylprednisolone upon vascular permeability changes in endotoxic shock. Circ Shock 18:179–192
34. Cintora I, Bessa S, Goodale RL, Motsay GW, Borner JW (1974) Further studies of endotoxin and alveolocapillary permeability: Effect of steroid pretreatment and complement depletion. Ann Surg 179:372–375
35. Holcroft JW, Vassar MJ, Weber CJ (1986) Prostaglandin E1 and survival in patients with the Adult Respiratory Distress Syndrome. Ann Surg 203:371–378
36. De Gaetano G, Bertele V, Cerletti C, Di Minno G (1982) Prostaglandin effects on platelets. In: Wu KK, Rossi EC (eds) Prostaglandins in clinical medicine: Cardiovascular and thromboxane disorders. Yearbook Medical Publishers, Chicago
37. Stenson WF, Parker CW (1980) Prostaglandins, macrophages, and immunity. J Immunol 125:1–5
38. Fantone JC, Marasco WA, Elgas LJ, Ward PA (1984) Stimulus specificity of prostaglandin inhibition of rabbit polymorphonuclear leukocyte lysosomal enzyme release and superoxide anion production. Am J Pathol 115:9–16
39. Weissmann G, Smolen JE, Korchak H (1980) Prostaglandins and inflammation: Receptor/cyclase coupling as an explanation of why PGE2 and PGI1 inhibit functions of inflammatory cells. Adv Prostagl Thromb Res 8:1637–1653
40. Geller P, Merrill ER, Jawetz E (1954) Effects of cortisone and antibiotics on the lethal action of endotoxins in mice. Proc Soc Exp Biol Med 86:716–721
41. Ottosson J, Brandberg A, Erikson B, Hedman L, Davidson I, Soderberg R (1982) Experimental septic shock: Effects of corticosteroids. Circ Shock 9:571–577
42. Demling RH, Smith M, Gunther R, Wandzilq KT (1981) Endotoxin-induced lung injury in unanesthetized sheep: Effect of methylprednisolone. Circ Shock 8:351–360
43. Payne JG, Bowen JC (1981) Hypoxia of canine gastric mucosa caused by E. coli sepsis is prevented with methylprednisolone therapy. Gastroenterology 80:84–93

44. Sable CA, Wispelwey B (1994) Pharmacologic interventions aimed at preventing the biologic effects of endotoxin in gram-negative septicemia and septic shock. Infect Dis Clin N Am 5:883–898
45. Pitcairin M, Schuler J, Erne P, Holtzman S, Schumer W (1975) Glucocorticoids and antibiotic effects on experimental gram-negative bacteremic shock. Arch Surg 110:1012–1017
46. Hinshaw LB, Beller BK, Ardier LT, Flournoy DJ, White BL, Philipps RW (1979) Recovery from lethal Escherichia coli shock in dogs. Surg Gynecol Obstet 149:545–553
47. Hinshaw LB, Archer LT, Beller Todd BK, Benjamin B, Flournoy DJ, Passey R (1981) Survival in primates in lethal septic shock following delayed treatment with steroid. Circulatory Shock 8:291–300
48. Brigham KL, Bowers RE, Mc Keen CR (1981) Methylprednisolone prevention of increased lung vascular permeability following endotoxemia in sheep. J Clin Invest 67:1103–1110
49. Begley CJ, Ogletree ML, Meyrick BO, Brigham K (1984) Modification of pulmonary responses to endotoxemia in awake sheep by steroidal and non-steroidal anti-inflammatory agents. Am Rev Respir Dis 130:1140–1146
50. Wise WC, Malushka PV, Knapp PG, et al (1985) Ibuprofen, methylprednisolone and gentamicin as conjoint treatment in septic shock. Circ Shock 17:59–68
51. Jacobs ER, Soulsky ME, Bone RC, Wilson FJ, Miller FC (1982) Ibuprofen in canine endotoxin shock. J Clin Invest 70:536–541
52. Snapper JR, Hutchison AA, Obletree ML, Brigham KL (1983) Effects of cyclooxygenase inhibitors on the alterations of lung mechanics caused by endotoxemia in unanesthetized sheep. J Clin Invest 72:63–76
53. Balk RA, Tryka F, Bone RC, et al (1986) The effect of ibuprofen on endotoxin induced injury in sheep. J Crit Care 1:230–240
54. Elinger JH, Seyde WC, Longnecker DE (1984) Methylprednisolone plus ibuprofen increases mortality in septic rats. Circ Shock 14:203–208
55. Goldblum SE, Wu KM, Tai HH (1986) Streptococcus pneumoniae-induced alterations of levels of circulating thromboxane and prostacyclin. Dissociation from granulocytopenia, thrombocytopenia and pulmonary leukostasis. J Infect Dis 153:71–77
56. Webb PJ, Westwick J, Scully MF, et al (1981) Do prostacyclin and thromboxane play a role in endotoxin shock? Br J Surg 68:720–724
57. Butler RR, Wise WC, Halushka PV, et al (1983) Gentamicin and indomethacin in the treatment of septic shock: Effects on prostacyclin and thromboxane A2 production. J Pharmacol Exp Ther 225:94–101
58. Cook JA, Wise WC, Halushka PV (1980) Elevated thromboxane levels in the rat during endotoxic essential fatty acid deficiency. J Clin Invest 65:227–230
59. Tempel GE, Cook JA, Wise WC, Halushka PV, Corral D (1983) Improvement of organ blood flow by inhibitor of thromboxane synthase during endotoxic shock in rat. J Cardiovasc Pharmacol 8:514–519
60. Kopolovic R, Thraikill KM, Martin DT, et al (1984) Effects of ibuprofen on a porcine model of acute respiratory failure. J Surg Res 36:300–305
61. Jacobs ER, Soulsby ME, Bone RC, Wilson FJ Jr, Hiller FC (1987) Ibuprofen in canine endotoxin shock. J Clin Invest 70:536–541
62. Gnidec AG, Sibbald W, Cheung H, Metz CA (1988) Ibuprofen ameliorates an increase in pulmonary microvascular fluid flux in a sheep model of surgically-induced peritonitis and permeability edema. J Appl Physiol 65:1024–1032
63. Rinaldo JE, Pennock B (1986) Effects of ibuprofen on endotoxin-induced alveolitis. Am J Med Sci 291:29–38
64. Shinozawa Y, Hales C, Jung W, Burke J (1986) Ibuprofen prevents synthetic smoke-induced pulmonary edema. Am Rev Respir Dis 134:1145–1148
65. Fauci AS, Dale DC, Balow JE (1976) Glucocorticosteroid therapy: Mechanisms of action and clinical considerations. Ann Intern Med 84:304–309
66. Thompson J, Vanfurth R (1970) The effect of glucocorticoids on the kinetics of mononuclear phagocytes. J Exp Med 131:429

67. Balow JE, Rosenthal AS (1973) Glucocorticoid suppression of macrophage migration inhibitory factor. J Exp Med 137:1031
68. Atkinson JP, Schreiber AD, Frank MM (1973) Effects of corticosteroids and splenectomy on the immune clearance and destruction of erythrocytes. J Clin Invest 52:1509
69. Klastersky J, Cappel R, Debuscher L (1971) Effectiveness of betamethasone in management of severe infections. N Engl J Med 22:1248–1250
70. Wolfe JE, Bone RC, Ruth WE (1977) Effect of corticosteroids in the treatment of patients with gastric aspiration. Am J Med 63:179–187
71. Bone RC, Slotman G, Maunder R, et al (1989) Randomized, double-blind, multicentric study of prostaglandin E1 in patients with the adult respiratory distress syndrome. Chest 96:114–119
72. Hanly PJ, Roberts D, Dobson K, Light RB (1987) Effect of indomethacin on arterial oxygenation in critically ill patients with severe bacterial pneumonia. Lancet 1:351–354
73. Haupt MT, Jastremski MS, Clemmer TP, Metz CA, Goris GB, and the Ibuprofen study group (1991) Effect of ibuprofen in patients with severe sepsis. A randomized double blind multicenter study. Crit Care Med 19:1339–1347
74. Bernard GR, Reines HD, Harushka PV, et al (1991) Prostacyclin and thromboxan A2 formation is increased in human sepsis syndrome effect of cyclooxygenase inhibition. Am Rev Respir Dis 144:1095–1101
75. Bihari DJ, Tinker J (1982) Steroids in intensive care. Br J Hosp Med 28:323–331
76. Lederer V (1984) Betamethasone sodium phosphate injection: High-dose regimen in septic shock. Clin Ther 6:719–726
77. Hughes GS Jr (1984) Naloxone and methylprednisolone sodium succinate enhance symphatomedullary discharge in patients with septic shock. Life-Science 35:2319–2326
78. Sheagren JN (1981) Septic shock and corticosteroids. N Engl J Med 8:456–457
79. Blaisdell FW (1981) Controversy in shock research; Con: The role of steroids in septic shock. Circ Shock 8:667–671
80. Kass EH (1984) High-dose corticosteroids for septic shock. N Engl J Med 311:1178–1179
81. Nicholson DP (1983) Corticosteroids in the treatment of septic shock and the Adult Respiratory Distress Syndrome. Med Clin N Am 67:717–724
82. Flick MR, Murray JF (1984) High-dose corticosteroids therapy in the Adult Respiratory Distress Syndrome. JAMA 251:1054–1056
83. Ashbaugh DG, Petty TL (1966) The use of corticosteroids in the treatment of respiratory failure associate with massive fat embolism. Surg Gynecol Obstet 123:493–502
84. Fisher SE, Turner RH, Herndon JH, Riseborough FJ (1970) Massive steroid therapy in severe fat embolism. Surg Gynecol Obstet 172:805–811
85. Broe PJ, Toung TJK, Margolis S, Permutt S, Cameron JL (1981) Pulmonary injury caused by free fatty acids evaluation of steroid and albumin therapy. Surgery 89:582–592
86. Weitzman S, Berger S (1974) Clinical trial design in studies of corticosteroids for bacterial infections. Ann Intern Med 81:36–42
87. Cooperative Study Group (1963) The effectiveness of hydrocortisone in the management of severe infections. JAMA 183:462–465
88. Schumer W (1976) Steroids in the treatment of clinical septic shock. Ann Surg 184:333–341
89. Thompson W, Gurley H, Lutz B, et al (1976) Inefficacy of glucocorticosteroids in shock. Clin Res 8A:24–25 (Abst)
90. Hoffman SL, Pun Jabi NH, Kumala S, et al (1984) Reduction of mortality in chloramphenicol-treated severe typhoid fever by high-dose dexamethasone. N Engl J Med 310:82–88
91. Lebel MH, Bishara JR, Syrogiannopoulos GA, et al (1988) Dexamethasone therapy of bacterial meningitis: Results of two double-blind, placebo-controlled trials. N Engl J Med 13:964–971

92. Weigelt JA, Norcross JF, Borman KR, Shyder WH (1985) Early steroid therapy for respiratory failure. Arch Surg 120:536–540
93. Sibbald WJ, Anderson RR, Reid B, Holliday RL, Driedger AA (1981) Alveolo-capillary permeability in human septic ARDS. Chest 79:133–142
94. Bone RC, Fisher C, Clemmer T, et al (1987) Early methylprednisolone treatment for septic syndrome and the adult respiratory distress syndrome. Chest 92:1032–1036
95. Bernard GR, Luce JM, Sprung CL, et al (1987) High-dose corticosteroids in patients with the Adult Respiratory Distress Syndrome. N Engl J Med 317:1565–1570
96. Luce JM, Montgomery BA, Mark SJD, Turner J, Metz CA, Murray JF (1988) Ineffectiveness of high-dose methylprednisolone in preventing parenchymal lung injury and improving mortality in patients with septic shock. Am Rev Respir Dis 138:62–68
97. Montaner JSG, Lawson LM, Levitt N, et al (1990) Corticosteroids prevent early deterioration in patients with moderately severe Pneumocystis carinii pneumonia and the acquired immunodeficiency syndrome. Ann Intern Med 113:14–20
98. Bozzette SA, Sattler FR, Chiu J, et al (1990) A controlled trial of early adjunctive treatment with corticosteroids for Pneumocystis carinii pneumonia in the acquired immunodeficiency syndrome. N Engl J Med 323:1451–1457
99. Gagnon S, Boota AM, Fishi MA, et al (1990) Corticosteroids as adjunctive therapy for severe Pneumocystis carinii pneumonia in the acquired immunodeficiency syndrome. A double blind, placebo controlled trial. N Engl J Med 323:1444–1450
100. The National Institutes of Health-University of California (1990) Consensus statement on the use of corticosteroids as adjunctive therapy for Pneumocystis pneumonia in the acquired immunodeficiency syndrome. N Engl J Med 22:1500–1504
101. Jorens PG, De Jongh R, De Backer W, et al (1993) Interleukin-8 production in patients undergoing cardiopulmonary bypass. Effect of methylprednisolone. Am Rev Respir Dis 148:890–895
102. Lotman G, Fisher C, Bone R (1993) Detrimental effects of high-dose methylprednisolone sodium succinate on serum concentration of hepatic and renal function indicators in severe sepsis and septic shock. Crit Care Med 21:191–195
103. Parker MM, Ognibene FP, Rogers P, et al (1994) Severe Pneumocystis carinii pneumonia procedures: A hyperdynamic profile similar to bacterial pneumonia with sepsis. Crit Care Med 22:50–54
104. Meduri GN, Belenchia JM, Este RJ, et al (1991) Fibroproliferative phase of ARDS: Clinical finding and effects of corticosteroids. Chest 100:943–952
105. Mela L, Miller LD (1983) Efficacy of glucorticoid in preventing mitochondiral metabolic failure in endotoxemia. Circ Shock 10:371–381

Investigational Therapy of Sepsis: Anti-TNF, IL-1ra, Anti-PAF and G-CSF

J.-F. Dhainaut, J. P. Mira, and F. Brunet

Introduction

Severe sepsis and septic shock are widely recognized as serious clinical problems causing substantial morbidity and mortality [1]. Despite modern antibiotics, state-of-the-art intensive care, and timely surgery, the sequelae of severe sepsis are seemingly dissociated in time from the underlying infection. Recent advances in the biology of inflammatory response to infection shed light on this apparent dissociation of tissue injury from the underlying infection [2]. Indeed, the host-derived factors of the inflammatory response that result in an effective defense against infection, may become exaggerated, causing severe sepsis and organ dysfunction syndrome [3–4]. These mediators of this response to infection could be ultimately responsible for the progression of the lethal sepsis.

Among these mediators, cytokines occupy a pivotal role in the pathogenesis of severe sepsis. Cytokines are small proteins, active in low concentrations, and possess multiple biological activities [5]. There are now over 30 different cytokines, but two of them play a major role: tumor necrosis factor (TNF) and interleukin-1 (IL-1). TNF and IL-1 (with IL-8 family) are grouped together and called "pro-inflammatory cytokines" to distinguish them from the anti-inflammatory cytokines IL-4 and IL-10 (with TGFβ); when injected into animals, they reduce the severity of the disease and the production of pro-inflammatory cytokines. When administered into animals, either TNF or IL-1 induces hypotension and shock; however, when injected together, these pro-inflammatory cytokines act synergistically [5].

Bioactive lipids, especially platelet activating factor (PAF), also play an important role. Although initially named for its effects on platelets, PAF is now known to be a potent phospholipid autacoid mediator involved in sepsis [6]. It is produced by a variety of cells, including endothelial cells, platelets, leukocytes, monocytes, and lymphocytes. PAF, as an important trigger of cell-to-cell interaction, leads to the release of important inflammatory mediators [7].

The evidence is derived from studies showing that 1) injection of TNF, IL-1, or PAF into animals or humans causes a fall in systemic arterial pressure and coagulopathy often observed in sepsis [8–9]; 2) plasma levels of these mediators often are elevated in patients with this syndrome [9–12]; and

3) specific blockade of the action of these mediators in animals with a sepsis-like syndrome reduces mortality [2, 4–7, 9, 13–14]. Because TNF, IL-1, and PAF may be released not only by endotoxin but also by other bacterial and fungi stimuli [15–18], it seems attractive to consider the use of therapy directed at these circulatory mediators in patients with severe sepsis.

Lastly, many cytokines are growth factors, such as fibroblast, endothelial cells, and hematopoietic growth factors. Among them, granulocyte-colony stimulating factor (G-CSF) seems able to augment host defenses by increasing the number and function of neutrophils [19].

This chapter provides a critical review of the clinical trials devoted to anti-TNF, IL-1 receptor antagonist (IL-1ra), anti-PAF, and G-CSF in patients with severe sepsis or septic shock. However, several trials are in progress or the results of these trials are not published yet.

Strategies for TNF Antagonism

Whether the administration of some other putative mediators of severe sepsis (IL-1, PAF) may trigger individual components of this syndrome, TNF is the only endogenous mediator that is sufficient to trigger the entire spectrum of hemodynamic, metabolic, organ dysfunction, tissue injury, and cytokine cascade response [8, 20–22]. A recent study suggests lethal TNF toxicity is primary the result of the TNF receptor 1 (TNF-R1) stimulation, since transgenic mice made deficient for TNF-R1 (but with intact TNF-R2) are resistant to endotoxin challenge [23]. This study offers support for the theory that severe sepsis has its origins in a singular receptor-ligand interaction, and offers caution hope for the development of drugs that act by neutralizing TNF in this syndrome.

Strategies for TNF antagonism include anti-TNF monoclonal antibodies and soluble TNF receptors. With few exceptions, animal studies have demonstrated that these strategies prevent shock and death due to septic challenge.

Monoclonal Antibodies to TNF

Preclinical testing of anti-TNF monoclonal antibodies suggests that passive immunization has protective effects in different models of bacterial sepsis. The first evidence that neutralizing antibodies to TNF prevented death following injection of endotoxin was a Beutler et al. study in mice [13]. This protection was confirmed in a model of lethal septic shock in bacteremic primates, despite the presence of replicating bacteria in the blood for up to 8 h [24]. Although increased concentrations of TNF were only detectable for several hours after the infusion of bacteria, the anti-TNF therapy also prevented the later increase of IL-1 and IL-6 [25]. Subsequent studies showed that blocking TNF with monoclonal antibodies reduced death in different models of endotoxin challenge and bacterial (either gram-negative or gram-positive) septic shock [26–30].

The efficacy of anti-TNF antibodies may rest, in part, on their ability to interrupt the cycle of TNF production that results from macrophage stimulation. In mice infected with *P. berghei*, anti-TNF not only abolished the biological activity of TNF in the circulation, but also prevented TNFmRNA accumulation in the brain and lymphoid organs. A similar finding was observed in mice infected with Calmette-Guérin bacillus [31]. Neutralizing monoclonal antibodies against TNF affects blockade of TNF activity by steric inhibition of receptor binding, or by distortion of the trimer, such that the receptor no longer recognizes the binding sites.

Based on these studies, humans have received either mouse-derived anti-human monoclonal anti-TNF antibodies or "humanized" forms of these antibodies for the treatment of severe sepsis.

CB0006: A murine immunoglobulin (IgG) monoclonal antibody to human TNF: CB0006 (Celltech) was the first antibody evaluated in septic patients. A phase I, devoted to safety and pharmacokinetics, have enrolled 14 patients with hypotension, severe organ dysfunction and a lack of therapeutic responses to conventional therapy [32]. Anti-TNF antibodies in doses ranging from 0.4 to 10.0 mg/kg were well tolerated with a half-life of 42 h.

A phase II multicenter trial was subsequently performed in 80 patients with severe sepsis who received one of four dosing regimens: 0.1, 1.0, 10 mg/kg or two doses of 1 mg/kg 24 h apart [15]. The study confirmed the good tolerability of this antibody, and a half-life of 42 h. Increased IL-6 levels or a failure of IL-6 to decline over the first 24 h of treatment predicted a fatal outcome, but TNF levels were not found to be a reliable prognostic indicator. IL-6 levels were markedly affected by the dose of CB0006 (Fig. 1). No survival benefit was found for the total population, but there were only 20 patients per treatment arm. However, patients with increased circulating TNF concentrations at entry appeared to benefit from the high dose of anti-TNF antibody. In both the phase I and II trials, antibody formation against murine anti-TNF was seen in the majority of patients, but this was not correlated with any adverse event.

Bay x1351: Another murine monoclonal antibody: Bay x1351 (Miles) was evaluated in a phase I study and two phase III studies. The phase I study enrolled 20 patients at risk of sepsis who received single doses of 1 to 15 mg/kg anti-TNF monoclonal antibody or two doses of 15 mg/kg, and 16 patients with sepsis syndrome who received a single dose of 15 mg/kg anti-TNF monoclonal antibodies [33]. This antibody was well tolerated and had a serum half-life of 50 to 54 h. A positive human anti-mouse antibody response was detected in the majority of patients. There were no serum sickness-like reactions, skin reactions, nor evidence of systemic hypersensitivity in any patients. The relatively long half-life of the anti-TNF monoclonal antibodies in

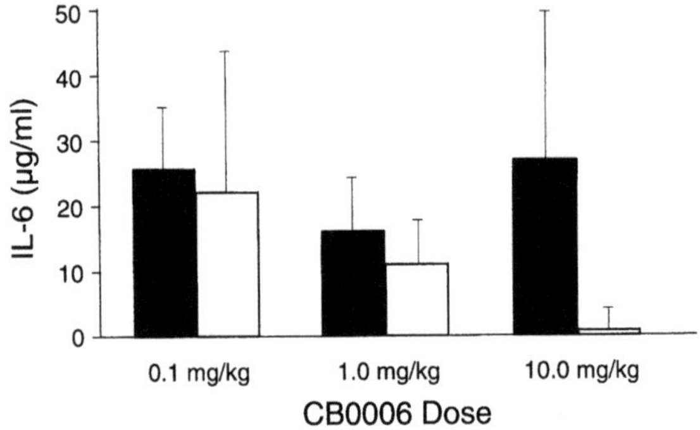

Fig. 1. Plasma IL-6 levels at study entry and at 24 h after CB0006 in those patients with increased (>50 pg/mL) TNF levels at study entry (n=35). Closed bars represent pre-treatment; shaded bars represent 24 h post-treatment. The numbers of patients in each group are as follows: 0.1 mg/kg (n=8); 1.0 mg/kg (n=20) including patients who received a single 1.0 mg/kg of CB0006 and patients who subsequently received a second dose of 1.0 mg/kg 24 h later (n=10); 10 mg/kg (n=7). * p=0.01 for 10 mg/kg dose by analysis of variance. (From [15] with permission)

comparison to that of receptor antagonists lends itself to evaluation of single dose therapy for the treatment of severe sepsis.

Two phase III placebo-controlled, three-arm studies were conducted in the US and Europe. Patients with sepsis syndrome were enrolled within 12 h of the onset of this syndrome, were stratified by shock/non-shock status, and were randomized to receive a single IV infusion of either 7.5 mg/kg, 15 mg/kg of the anti-TNF monoclonal antibody, or placebo. Patients were infused with the study drug within 4 h after randomization. The primary endpoint was time to death over the 28-day postdosing period. The preliminary results of the phase III trial conducted in the US [34] showed that the three treatment arms were well balanced with respect to demographics, APACHE II score and other parameters. For all infused patients with sepsis syndrome, those who received anti-TNF monoclonal antibodies had slightly reduced 28-day all cause mortality compared to placebo. Among shock patients, there was a more pronounced trend toward efficacy at day 28 with lower mortality rate in both active treatment arms. Among non-shock patients, anti-TNF monoclonal antibody did not appear beneficial and may even worsen the prognosis of the subgroup of patients. The final analyses of these studies are ongoing.

cA2: The first chimeric anti-TNF monoclonal antibody evaluated in septic patients was an anti-TNF monoclonal antibody, cA2 (Centocor). A phase I–II trial was conducted in three stages (141 patients). Stage 1 was an open label trial in which 4 groups of 5 septic patients each with the clinical diagnosis of sepsis received ascending doses of cA2 (0.1, 1, 5, 10 mg/kg). Stage 2 was a randomized, double-blind study in which patients received a single dose of HA-1A (100 mg) and placebo, or one of 3 doses of cA2 (1, 5, 10 mg/kg).

Stage 3 was a randomized, double-blind study in which patients received a single dose of placebo or one of 3 doses of cA2 (0.1, 1, 10 mg/kg).

Primary analyses were devoted to patients of the stages 1 and 3. There were 65 patients who received cA2 exclusively and 16 patients who received placebo. Administration of cA2 was well tolerated. Human anti-chimeric antibody responses were positive in 61%. The mean half-life was 70 h. A dose-related decrease in TNF concentration was observed one hour after infusion of this antibody [35].

CDP571: Another humanized antibody to human TNF: CDP571 (Celltech) was recently evaluated during a phase II trial which enrolled 42 patients with rapidly evolving septic shock who received intravenously either placebo or one of 4 single doses of this antibody (0.1, 0.3, 1.0 or 3.0 mg/kg). The humanized anti-TNFα antibody was well tolerated. The immune response detected had little effect on the ability of circulating CDP571 to bind TNF and on the pharmacokinetics of the antibody.

CDP571 was followed by a dose-dependent reduction in circulating TNF concentration. IL-1 and IL-6 plasma concentrations decreased with time in all dosage groups, and this decrease was higher during the initial 24 h in the treatment groups than in the placebo group [36]. Further studies are needed to determine the efficacy of the antibody to improve survival of severe sepsis.

MAK 195F: Lastly, a F(ab′)2 fragment of a murine monoclonal anti-TNF antibody: MAK 195F (Knoll) was developed to reduce the potential immunogenicity and to facilitate tissue penetration. A phase II study enrolled 122 patients with severe sepsis who received one of the three different doses of MAK 195F (0.1; 0.3 and 1 mg/kg) or placebo over a period of 72 h in random order. At this time, only an interim analysis of 60 patients is available indicating that MAK 195F in all 3 dosage groups resulted in a decrease in IL-6. This contrasted with a further increase of IL-6 in the placebo patients. No serious side effects have been reported [37].

Monoclonal Antibodies to TNF: After the reduction of circulating TNF concentrations related to anti-TNF antibodies (CDP571) administration, TNF concentrations tended to progressively increase with time [36]. This observation has previously been noted using Medgenix assay measurement of TNF following administration of other TNF antibodies. Indeed, a clinical trial of the safety of an anti-TNF antibody (CB0006) in African children with *Plasmodium falciparum* infection showed that circulating TNF levels actually increased after treatment with this anti-TNF antibody, although the clinical effects of TNF seemed inhibited, as indicated by a significant dose-dependent reduction of fever [38]. Another clinical trial, using the same antibody in patients with severe sepsis, also demonstrated a progressive rise of plasma TNF levels after the initial fall; by contrast, no bioactive TNF was detected in the plasma of any patient after anti-TNF therapy [15]. In the present study, using a humanized anti-TNF monoclonal antibody, a modified ELISA which utilized a polyclonal antibody was unable to demonstrate the rebound rise in TNF levels. The rebound rise observed when using the Medgenix assay may be the result of immunoactive but not bioactive forms of TNF being detected, possibly TNF fragments.

While free TNF is rapidly cleared from the circulation [39] as the result of its association with plasma membrane receptors, TNF that is maintained as a complex with anti-TNF monoclonal antibodies may circulate for a prolonged period of time [15, 36] and is ultimately disposed of in a different manner.

While very effective in blocking the activity of TNF, monoclonal antibodies might conceivably pose problems related to their antigenicity (particularly in the event that murine reagents are employed) and might also prove injurious, because they form circulating immune complexes with the target protein. These considerations may be of minimal importance given the emergency of the threat posed by excessive TNF production in severe sepsis.

Soluble TNF Receptors

There are two types of soluble TNF receptors: type I and type II. The soluble forms of both receptors were initially discovered in and purified from the urine of healthy humans [40]. The soluble TNF receptors are proteolytic cleavage products of the cell-bound TNF receptors. The soluble receptors to the TNF type I receptor were able to reduce the severity of the *E. coli*-induced shock in baboons [41]. In order to prolong the half-life of soluble TNF receptors in the circulation, molecules have been constructed consisting of two extracellular portions of TNF type I receptors linked covalently to the complement-binding portion of IgG. This results in a molecule with the ability to bind two TNF molecules. The recombinant proteins circulate with a half-life that varies depending on the cellular source and purification technique, but that exceeds 48 h [42].

TNF inhibitors of this sort offer a potential approach to the therapy of diseases in which TNF is produced over a long period of time. They have the advantage of being nearly or entirely non-antigenic. Of theoretical concern, however, is the possibility that auto-antibodies against the TNF receptor, some of which may have agonist potential, might be generated in response to the administration of recombinant material.

Unfortunately, the preliminary results of a phase II clinical trial using this TNF inhibitor (rsTNFR-p75-IgG: Immunex) are quite disappointing [43]. It is possible that much of the TNF that becomes bound to this molecule is not cleared, but is merely stored in a circulating form and later released. A new bivalent TNF-binding protein was produced with another recombinant TNF receptor extracellular domain: rsTNFR-p55 (Ro 45-2088; Hoffmann-La Roche). When the exchange rates of TNF in the complexes with the receptor-IgG constructs were compared in radiotracer studies, a significantly higher kinetic stability was found in the complex with the fusion proteins containing the 55 kDa than with that containing the 77 kDa TNF receptor sequence. Because of these different pharmacologic properties, the fusion protein with 55 kDa TNF receptor was selected for a phase II clinical trial with the agreement of the FDA.

Anti-TNF Strategies

TNF has both helpful and harmful immunologic and inflammatory functions. Although TNF in large concentrations is clearly harmful to the infected host, there is also evidence that TNF in lower concentrations may be useful in suppressing granulomatous infections (tuberculosis, leishmaniasis) and infections caused by intracellular pathogens such as *Listeria monocytogenes* and *Legionella pneumophila* [44]. Strategies designed to avoid or closely monitor patients with infections due to intracellular parasites or other facultative pathogens are important. Fortunately, such patients represent a very small percentage of the septic patients.

Perhaps it is not surprising to learn that the "good" and "bad" effects of TNF are really one and the same, that a good medicine can be harmful if applied either at the wrong time, or at an improper dose [44].

Strategies for Preventing IL-1 Activity

Naturally occurring substances that specifically inhibit IL-1 have been detected in various human body fluids. Among these substances, the most studied and well-characterized has been the IL-1 receptor antagonist (IL-1ra). IL-1ra is produced by macrophages in response to different microbial products. This antagonist recognizes and binds to both types of IL-1 receptors; it possesses no IL-1 agonist activity [45–46]. IL-1ra is bound to its receptor; it sterically inhibits IL-1 from binding and thereby disrupts signal transduction and cellular responses induced by IL-1 [46–47]. The non-glycosolated form of IL-1ra has been isolated, purified, and produced by recombinant DNA technology using *E. coli* fermentation. Human recombinant IL-1ra is identical to the naturally occurring non-glycosolated human form of IL-1ra with the exception of the addition of one N-terminal methionine. IL-1ra prevents mortality in animal models of endotoxemia [48] and *E. coli* bacteremia [49] and attenuates the decrease in mean arterial pressure resulting from challenge with endotoxin, gram-negative and gram-positive bacteria [49–51].

Recently, IL-1ra has been observed to be elevated in the plasma of patients in septic shock [52]. In human volunteers, IL-1ra plasma concentration increased in parallel with the increase in IL-1 plasma concentration, following injection of small doses of endotoxin [53]. Human recombinant IL-1ra has been shown to attenuate IL-6 production from peripheral blood mononuclear cells after stimulation with endotoxin *ex vivo* in human volunteers

[54]. Due to the potent intrinsic activity of IL-1 on target tissue, it is necessary to administer human recombinant IL-1ra as a continuous infusion at a dose that creates a large molar excess over measured IL-1 concentration: 10000-fold molar excess of IL-1ra was necessary to ablate the effects of exogenous IL-1 infusion in animals [55].

Based on these observations, a phase II clinical trial (Synergen) was performed in 99 patients with sepsis syndrome who received an IV loading dose of either human recombinant (rh) IL-1ra (100 mg) or placebo, followed by a 72-h IV infusion of either one of the three doses of rhIL-1ra (17, 67, or 133 mg/h) or placebo [56]. All patients were evaluated for 28-day all cause mortality. This first clinical trial showed that human recombinant IL-1ra was well tolerated and provided a dose-related survival advantage in patients with sepsis syndrome, as indicated by the following mortality rate: 44% in the 25 placebo patients, 32% for the 25 patients receiving rhIL-1ra 17 mg/h, 25% for the 24 patients receiving rhIL-1ra 67 mg/h, and 18% for the 25 patients receiving rhIL-1ra 133 mg/h (Fig. 2). In patients with an increased IL-6 concentration at study entry, the magnitude of the decrease in IL-6 concentra-

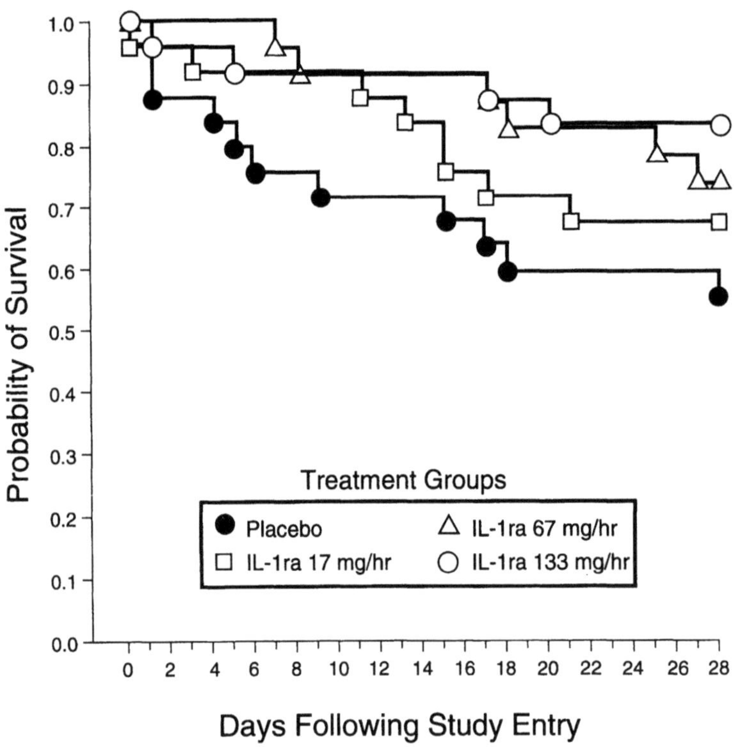

Fig. 2. Probability of survival in patients with sepsis syndrome. Comparison of the cumulative survival estimates over a 28-day period for patients (n=99) who received either IL-1ra: 17, 67, or 133 mg/h, or placebo. (From [56] with permission)

tion 24 h after the initiation of therapy was correlated with increasing the rhIL-1ra treatment dose (Fig. 3). A renal elimination mechanism was suggested by the positive correlation between IL-1ra plasma clearance and estimated creatinine clearance.

In a recent phase III clinical trial, 893 patients were randomized to receive either an IV loading dose of rhIL-1ra 100 mg or placebo, followed by a continuous 72 h IV infusion of either one of the two doses of rhIL-1ra (1.0 or 2.0 mg/kg/h), or placebo [57]. All patients were evaluated for 28-day all cause mortality. Treatment groups were well balanced at entry for predicted risk of mortality as determined by a risk assessment model developed independently of the clinical trial database [58]. A comparison of mortality at 28 days revealed a 15% reduction with rhIL-1ra treatment compared to placebo ($p=0.22$); while the magnitude of the reduction in mortality rate with rhIL-1ra treatment was less than that observed in the phase II trial, these findings are within the 95% confidence intervals from the last trial. In patients with one organ failure or more, a 23% reduction in mortality at 28 days was observed with rhIL-1ra 2.0 mg/kg/h treatment compared to placebo ($p=0.009$). For patients with a predicted risk of mortality higher than 24%, a retrospective analysis demonstrated a 22% reduction in 28-day mortality rhIL-1ra 2.0 mg/kg/h treatment ($p=0.005$) and a 31% reduction in mortality in patients with both one organ failure or more and a predicted risk of mortality higher than 24% compared to placebo ($p=0.002$). rhIL-1ra was well tolerated.

The results from this phase III clinical trial using several different measures of disease severity, including organ failure and a predicted risk of mortality model, suggest a survival benefit with rhIL-1ra treatment with increasing severity of illness. The potential therapeutic use of human recombinant IL-1ra in patients with severe sepsis should be confirmed in a large phase III clinical trial.

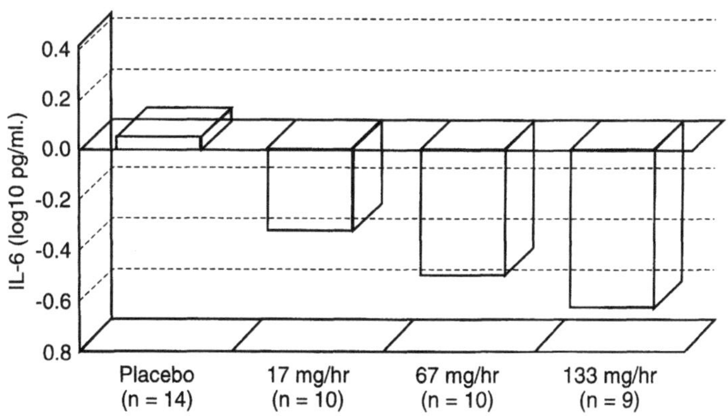

Fig. 3. Change in plasma IL-6 concentration 24 h after study entry for patients who received either IL-1ra: 17, 67, or 133 mg/h, or placebo. (From [56] with permission)

Strategies for PAF Antagonism

Several structurally different PAF antagonists have been reported to reduce mortality caused by gram-negative [14] and fungi [12] sepsis in animals, whereas their efficacy in gram-positive infection remains to be proved.

Studies on the pathophysiological role of PAF have been facilitated by a variety of compounds which can specifically inhibit the binding of PAF to its receptors in various cells and tissues. These several structurally different PAF antagonists have been reported to inhibit sepsis-induced hypotension, organ injury, and mortality [14].

In endotoxin shock, PAF antagonists provide significant protection [9, 59–61]. The role of PAF in endotoxin shock has been substantiated by the beneficial effects of the highly selective and potent PAF antagonist, BN-52021 which was shown to markedly reduce the hypotensive response as well as the thrombocytopenia produced by *S. typhimurium* endotoxin in guinea pig [62], and a significant dose-dependent inhibition of the lethality was observed [63, 64]. A prophylactic effect of a novel PAF receptor antagonist (BN 50739) on endotoxin-induced hypotension, hemoconcentration, TXB2 and TNF production in rats has been recently reported [65]; an improvement of survival in rats exposed to sublethal and lethal endotoxin challenge was also observed. Conversely, few studies have been devoted to gram-positive sepsis, and the preliminary results are not convincing [6].

Recently, Graham et al. [66] demonstrated a prolonged PAF half-life in septic patients with the worst outcome, due to depression of acetylhydrolase activity. The authors suggested that the breakdown in plasma degradation of PAF could have contributed to pathophysiology in these patients.

Based on these preclinical studies, an open-label, prospective, clinical trial with single doses of a natural PAF antagonist, BN 52021, recently demonstrated its safety in 22 patients with septic shock. An IV injection of 0.5 mg/kg was first tested in 7 patients, 4 mg/kg was then used in the 15 last patients. Thirteen men and 9 women (mean age, 63 ± 18 years; SAPS, 18 ± 5, systolic blood pressure 69 ± 12 mm Hg) were enrolled in the study. Intensive care mortality was 66%. Eight out of the 13 patients with documented gram-negative infections were bacteremic. Gram-positive infections occurred in 8 patients while 3 patients had mixed infections. No clinical (bronchospasm, skin rashes ...), hemodynamic (hypotension, cardiac failure ...) or laboratory evidence of BN 52021-related toxicity was observed at any dose (unpublished data). Thus, the PAF antagonist BN 52021 has proven to be safe in patients with septic shock.

A randomized, placebo-controlled, double blind, multicenter clinical trial on efficacy (mortality at day 28) of BN 52021 (240 mg/day over 4 days) in severe sepsis has enrolled 262 patients. For the entire population, no significant difference was observed between the two groups. However, there was a 42% decrease of mortality (57 vs 33% in the treated group, $p < 0.01$) in 119 patients with documented gram-negative sepsis [67]. At inclusion, among the patients with gram-negative sepsis, the treatment and placebo groups were well balanced with respect to demographic characteristics, underlying diseases, infection sites, causative organisms, severity of the disease, shock, and organ failures except for liver dysfunction. After statistical adjustment for the major independent prognostic factors, $p = 0.09$. In the absence of documented gram-negative infection, no difference was observed. There were no differences in adverse events between the placebo and the treated groups. PAF antagonist BN 52021 seems a safe and promising treatment in gram-negative severe sepsis.

Strong evidence has been accumulated to support that PAF plays a major role in priming, amplification, and downregulation of inflammatory mediator release in sepsis. PAF antagonists appear to be effective in animal and human severe sepsis. PAF antagonist seems of great interest in gram-negative severe sepsis, and a confirming study is in progress.

Strategies for Improving Host Defenses: G-CSF

Manipulating the production and function of phagocytic cells to improve host defenses against severe sepsis may be beneficial in critically ill patients. The proliferation and differentiation of granulocytes and macrophages are controlled by a group of colony-stimulating factors. Among them, G-CSF not only stimulates the growth and differentiation of neutrophils, but also stimulates the fully differentiated progeny for enhanced functional capacity, improves chemotactic peptide binding on peripheral blood neutrophils and increases antibody dependent cellular cytotoxicity [68].

Clinical trials in patients who received rhG-CSF following chemotherapy for transitional-cell carcinoma demonstrate significantly shorter periods of neutropenia and fewer days requiring antibiotic coverage. In patients receiving chemotherapy for small-cell lung cancer, G-CSF administration resulted in a decreased number of septic episodes [69]. More interestingly, several studies showed that G-CSF can improve survival in number of infection models in neutropenic and non-neutropenic animals [19]. Several pilot studies are encouraging, and a phase II study in patients with peritonitis is in progress.

The availability of rhG-CSF to augment host defense by increasing the numbers and function of neutrophils offers a new possibility for therapeutic intervention to reduce the morbidity and mortality of severe sepsis.

Conclusion and Recommendations

The strategies for modulating the immuno-inflammatory cascade by either cytokine (TNF, IL-1) or lipid mediator (PAF) antagonism or increasing host defense (G-CSF) may have a major impact on the treatment of sepsis in the most severely ill patients. However, at this moment, no phase III clinical trial provides positive results for the septic population as a whole (Table 1). Con-

Table 1. Summary of investigational anti-cytokine therapy of sepsis

Treatment		Company	Phase	Inclusion criteria	Number of PTS	Endpoint	Efficacy (trend)
Anti-TNF MoAB							
– Murine	CB0006	Celltech	II	Sepsis syndrome	80	Safety and pharmacokinetics	Survival + (subgroup)
	Bay x 1351	Miles & Bayer	III	Sepsis [no shock] Septic shock	400 994	28-day mortality 28-day mortality	Survival – Survival +
– Chimeric	cA2	Centocor	I–II	Sepsis	?	Safety and pharmacokinetics	?
	CDP571	Celltech	II	Septic shock	40	Safety and pharmacokinetics	?
– $F(ab)_2$	MAK195[F]	Knoll	II	Sepsis syndrome	122	Safety and pharmacokinetics	Survival + (subgroup)
sTNF-R1							
– r-p75-IgG		Immunex	II	Sepsis syndrome	120	Safety and pharmacokinetics	Survival – ($p<0.05$)
– r-p55-IgG	Ro 45-2051	Hoffmann-La Roche	II	Sepsis syndrome	200	Safety and pharmacokinetics	ongoing
IL-1ra	Antril	Synergen	II	Sepsis syndrome	99	Safety and pharmacokinetics	Survival + ($p<0.015$)
			III	Sepsis syndrome	901	28-day mortality	Survival + (subgroup)
Anti-PAF							
– natural	BN 52021	Ipsen-Beaufour	IIIa IIIb	Sepsis syndrome Gram-sepsis	262 600	28-day mortality 28-day mortality	Survival + (subgroup) ongoing
– analogue	BB-882	British Biotech	II	Sepsis syndrome	150	Safety and pharmacokinetics	ongoing
rhG-CSF	Neupogen	Amgen	II	Peritonitis	<50	Safety	ongoing

sequently, no recommendations can be made at present. We are waiting for the first positive results of large phase III clinical trials using such drugs to propose recommendations in the treatment strategy of severe infection.

Many questions remain unsolved [5]. First, is there an advantage in blocking TNF and IL-1, or one cytokine with a PAF antagonist at the same time? Although some animal studies suggest that blocking two cytokines is more effective than blocking each separately, there are no clinical studies at present to examine the effectiveness of combined therapy. Second, does blocking cytokine endanger host immune response? The clinical trial on soluble TNF receptors is a typical example. We have to be cautious in conducting clinical trials using such compounds, but at present, there are no rapid, predictive tests to determine which patients will benefit and which patients might worsen during cytokine blockade.

References

1. Bone RC (1992) Toward an epidemiology and natural history of SIRS. JAMA 101:1481–1483
2. Tracey KJ (1991) Tumor necrosis factor (cachectin) in the biology of septic shock syndrome. Circ Shock 35:123–128
3. Bone RC (1991) Physiopathology of sepsis. Ann Intern Med 115:457–469
4. Larrick JW (1989) Antibody inhibition of the immunoinflammatory cascade. J Crit Care 4:211–224
5. Dinarello CA, Gelfand JA, Wolff SM (1993) Anticytokine strategies in the treatment of the systemic inflammatory response syndrome. JAMA 269:1829–1835
6. Dhainaut JF, Mira JP, Fierobe L (1994) Platelet-activating factor: Pathophysiological changes and therapeutic implications in sepsis. In: Reinhart K, Eyrich K, Sprung C (eds) Sepsis. Springer-Verlag, Berlin, pp 397–413
7. Braquet P, Paubert-Braquet M, Bourgain RH, Bussolino F, Hosford D (1989) PAF/cytokines autoregulated feedback networks in microvascular injury: Consequences in shock, ischemia and graft rejection. J Lipid Med 1:75–112
8. Tracey KJ, Beutler B, Lowry SF, et al (1986) Shock and tissue injury induced by recombinant human cachectin. Science 234:470–474
9. Chang SW, Feddersen CO, Henson PM, Voelkel NF (1987) Platelet activating factor mediates hemodynamic changes and lung injury in endotoxin-treated rats. J Clin Invest 79:1498–1509
10. Hesse DG, Tracey KJ, Fong Y, et al (1988) Cytokine appearance in human endotoxemia and primate bacteremia. Surg Gynecol Obstet 166:147–153
11. Girardin E, Grau GE, Dayer JM, et al and the J5 Study Group (1988) Tumor necrosis factor and interleukin-1 in the serum of children with severe infectious purpura. N Engl J Med 319:397–400
12. Leaver HA, Qu JM, Smith G, Howie A, Ross WB, Yap PL (1990) Endotoxin releases platelet-activating factor from human monocytes in vitro. Immunopharmacology 20:105–113
13. Tracey KJ, Fong Y, Hesse DG, et al (1987) Anti-cachectin/TNF monoclonal antibodies prevent septic shock during lethal bacteraemia. Nature 330:662–664
14. Saunders RN, Handley DA (1987) PAF antagonists. Annu Rev Pharmacol Toxicol 27:237–255
15. Fisher CJ, Opal SM, Dhainaut JF, et al (1993) Influence of an anti-tumor necrosis factor monoclonal antibody on cytokine levels in patients with sepsis. Crit Care Med 21:318–327

16. Fast DJ, Schlievert PM, Nelson RD (1989) Toxic shock syndrome-associated staphylococcal and streptococcal pyogenic toxins are potent inducers of tumor necrosis factor production. Infect Immunol 57:291–294
17. Cabellos C, MacIntyre DE, Forrest M, Burroughs M, Prasad S, Tuomanen E (1992) Differing roles for platelet-activating factor during inflammation of the lung and subarachnoid space. The special case of streptococcus pneumoniae. J Clin Invest 90:612–618
18. Feuerstein G, Leader P, Siren AL, Braquet P (1987) Protective effect of a PAF-acether antagonist, BN 52021, in trichothecene toxicosis. Toxicology Letters 38:271–274
19. O'Reilly M, Silver GM, Greenhalgh DG, et al (1992) Treatment of intra-abdominal infection with G-CSF. J Trauma 33:679–682
20. Tracey KJ, Lowry SF, Fahey TJ III, et al (1987) Cachectin/tumor necrosis factor induces lethal shock and stress hormone responses in the dog. Surg Gynecol Obstet 164:415–422
21. Natanson C, Eichenholz PW, Danner RL, et al (1989) Endotoxin and tumor necrosis factor challenge in dogs simulate the cardiovascular profile of human septic shock. J Exp Med 169:823–832
22. Remick DG, Kunkel RG, Larrick JW, et al (1987) Acute in vivo effects of human recombinant tumor necrosis factor. Lab Invest 56:583–590
23. Pfeffer K, Matsuyama T, Kundig TM, et al (1993) Mice deficient for the 55-kd TNF receptor are resistant to endotoxin shock, yet succumb to L. monocytogenes infection. Cell 73:457–467
24. Beutler B, Milsark IW, Cerami AC (1985) Passive immunization against cachectin/tumor necrosis factor protects mice from lethal effect of endotoxin. Science 229:869–871
25. Fong Y, Tracey KJ, Moldawer LL, et al (1989) Antibodies to cachectin/TNF reduce interleukin-1β and interleukin-6 appearance during lethal bacteremia. J Exp Med 170:1627–1633
26. Ashkenazi A, Marsters SA, Capon DJ (1991) Protection against endotoxic shock by a tumor necrosis factor receptor immunoadhesin. Proc Natl Acad Sci USA 88:10535–10539
27. Hinshaw L, Olson P, Kuo G (1989) Efficacy of post-treatment with anti-TNF monoclonal antibody in preventing the pathophysiology and lethality of sepsis in the baboon. Circ Shock 27:362–369
28. Emerson TE, Lindsey DC, Jesmok GJ, et al (1992) Efficacy of monoclonal antibody against TNF-α in an endotoxemic baboon model. Circ Shock 38:75–84
29. Bagby GJ, Plessala KJ, Wilson LA, Thompson JJ, Nelson S (1991) Divergent efficacy of antibody to tumor necrosis factor-α in intravascular and peritonitis model of sepsis. J Infect Dis 163:83–88
30. Opal SM, Cross AS, Kelly NM, et al (1990) Efficacy of a monoclonal antibody directed against tumor necrosis factor in protecting neutropenic rats from lethal infection with *Pseudomonas aeruginosa*. J Infect Dis 161:1148–1152
31. Kindler V, Sappino AP, Grau GE, et al (1989) The inducing role of TNF in the development of bactericidal granulomas during BCG infection. Cell 56:731–740
32. Exley AR, Cohen J, Buurman W, et al (1990) Monoclonal antibody to TNF in severe septic shock. Lancet 335:1275–1277
33. Spooner C, Saravolatz L, Markowitz N, et al (1991) Safety and pharmacokinetics of murine antibody to human TNF. 31st Interscience Conference on Antimicrobial Agents and Chemotherapy, Chicago No 541 (Abst)
34. Wherry J, Abraham E, Wunderink R, et al (1994) Efficacy and safety of murine monoclonal antibody to human TNF (Bay x 1351). Intensive Care Med 20 (Suppl 1):S151 (Abst)
35. Zimmerman JL, Dillon K, Campbell W, Reinhart K (1994) Phase I/II trial of cA2, a chimeric anti-TNF antibody in patients with sepsis. Intensive Care Med 20 (Suppl 1):S151 (Abst)
36. Dhainaut JF, Vincent JL, Richard C (1994) CDP571, a CDR-grafted anti-human TNF antibody in septic shock: Safety, pharmacokinetics, and influence on cytokine levels. Am Rev Respir Dis (in press)

37. Reinhart K, Wiegand C, Kaul M (1994) Anti-TNF strategies with monoclonal antibody. Preliminary results with the specific monoclonal antibody MAK 195F. Intensive Care Med 20 (Suppl 1):S151 (Abst)
38. Kwiatkowski D, Molyneux ME, Stephens S, et al (1994) Response to monoclonal anti-TNF antibody in children with cerebral malaria. Q J Med (in press)
39. Beutler B, Milsark IW, Cerami A (1985) Cachectin/TNF: Production, distribution, and metabolic fate in vivo. J Immunol 135:3972–3977
40. Engelmann H, Novick D, Wallach D (1990) Two TNF-binding proteins purified from human urine: Evidence for immunological cross-reactivity with cell surface TNF receptors. J Biol Chem 265:1531–1536
41. van Zee KJ, Kohno T, Fischer E, et al (1992) TNF soluble receptors circulate during experimental and clinical inflammation and can protect against excessive TNF in vitro and in vivo. Proc Natl Acad Sci USA 89:4845–4849
42. Peppel K, Crawford D, Beutler B (1991) A TNF receptor-IgG heavy chain chimeric protein as a bivalent antagonist of TNF activity. J Exp Med 174:1483–1489
43. Sadoff J (1994) Phase II clinical trial on soluble TNF receptors (preliminary results) (personal communication)
44. Beutler B, Grau G (1993) TNF in the pathogenesis of infectious diseases. Crit Care Med 21:S423–S435
45. Eisenberg SP, Evans RJ, Arend WP, et al (1990) Primary structure and functional expression from complementary DNA of a human interleukin-1 receptor antagonist. Nature 343:341–346
46. Hannum CH, Wilcox CJ, Arend WP, et al (1990) Interleukin-1 receptor antagonist activity of a human interleukin-1 inhibitor. Nature 343:336–340
47. Arend WP, Welgus HG, Thompson RC, et al (1990) Biological properties of recombinant human monocyte-derived interleukin-1 receptor antagonist. J Clin Invest 85:1694–1697
48. Ohlsson K, Bjork P, Bergenfeld M, et al (1990) An interleukin-1 receptor antagonist reduces mortality from endotoxin shock. Nature 348:550–552
49. Fischer E, Marano MA, VanZee KJ, et al (1992) Interleukin-1 receptor blockade improves survival and hemodynamic performance in E. coli septic shock, but fails to alter host responses to sublethal endotoxemia. J Clin Invest 89:1551–1557
50. Wakabayashi G, Gelfand JA, Burke JF, et al (1991) A specific receptor antagonist for interleukin-1 prevents Escherichia coli-induced shock in rabbits. FASEB J 5:338–343
51. Aiura K, Gelfand JA, Burke JF, et al (1993) Interleukin-1 receptor antagonist prevents Staphylococcus epidermis-induced hypotension and reduces circulating levels of tumor necrosis factor and IL-1 in rabbits. Infect Immunol 61:3342–3350
52. Fischer E, VanZee KJ, Marano MA, et al (1992) Interleukin-1 receptor antagonist circulates in experimental inflammation and in human disease. Blood 79:2196–2199
53. Granowitz EV, Santos AA, Poutsiaica DD, et al (1991) Production of interleukin-1 receptor antagonist during experimental endotoxemia. Lancet 338:1423–1424
54. Fischer E, Marano MA, Barber A, et al (1991) A comparison between the effects of IL-1 alpha administration and sublethal endotoxemia in primates. Am J Physiol 261:442–452
55. Granowitz EV, Porat R, Mier JW, et al (1992) Pharmacokinetics safety, and immunomodulatory effects of human recombinant interleukin-1 receptor antagonist in healthy humans. Cytokine 4:353–360
56. Fisher CJ, Slotman GJ, Opal SM, et al (1994) Initial evaluation of human recombinant interleukin-1 receptor antagonist in the treatment of sepsis syndrome: A randomized, open-label, placebo-controlled multicenter trial. Crit Care Med 22:12–21
57. Fisher CJ, Dhainaut JF, Opal SM, et al (1994) Recombinant human interleukin-1 receptor antagonist reduces the mortality of patients with septic syndrome as a function of disease severity. JAMA (in press)
58. Knaus WA, Harrell F, Fisher CJ, et al (1993) The clinical evaluation of new drugs for sepsis: A prospective study design based on survival analysis. JAMA 270:1233–1241

59. Wallace JL, Whittle BJR (1986) Prevention of endotoxin-induced gastrointestinal damage by CV-3988, an antagonist of platelet-activating factor. Eur J Pharmacol 124:209–210
60. Terashita Z, Imura Y, Nishikawa K, Sumida S (1985) Is platelet activating factor (PAF) a mediator of endotoxin shock? Eur J Pharmacol 109:257–263
61. Toyofuku T, Kubo K, Kobayashi T, Kusama S (1986) Effects of ONO-6240, a platelet activating factor antagonist, on endotoxin shock in unanesthetized sheep. Prostaglandins 31:271–280
62. Adnot S, Lefort J, Lagente V, Braquet P, Vargaftig BB (1986) Interference of BN 52021, a PAF-acether antagonist, with endotoxin-induced hypotension in the guinea-pig. Pharmacol Res Commun 18:197–200
63. Etienne A, Hecquet F, Soulard C, Spinnewyn B, Clostre F, Braquet P (1985) In vivo inhibition of plasma protein leakage and Salmonella enteridis-induced mortality in the rat by a specific PAF-acether antagonist: BN 52021. Agents Actions 17:368–370
64. Braquet P, Touqui L, Shen T, Vargaftig B (1987) Perspectives in platelet-activating factor. Pharmacol Rev 39:97–145
65. Rabinovici R, Yue TL, Farhat M, et al (1990) PAF and TNF interactions in endotoxemic shock: Studies with BN 50739, a novel PAF antagonist. J Pharmacol Exp Ther 255:258–263
66. Graham RM, Stephens CJ, Silvester W, et al (1994) Plasma degradation of platelet-activating factor in severely ill patients with clinical sepsis. Crit Care Med 22:204–212
67. Dhainaut JF, Tenaillon A, Le Tulzo Y, et al (1994) PAF receptor antagonist, BN 52021, in the treatment of severe sepsis. Crit Care Med (in press)
68. Clark SC, Kamen R (1987) The human hematopoietic CSF. Science 236:1229–1237
69. Crawford J, Ozer H, Stoller R, et al (1991) Reduction by G-CSF of fever and neutropenia induced by chemotherapy in patients with small-cell lung cancer. N Engl J Med 325:164–170

Sepsis and Acute Lung Injury

G. R. Bernard, E. Holden, and J. W. Christman

Introduction

Sepsis syndrome is associated with diffuse microvascular injury (predominantly lung injury) which appears to be related to a wide variety of physiologically active and tissue destructive mediators. The exact cause and effect relationship between mediators and pathophysiology is becoming increasingly better understood but much remains to be elucidated. Even in those situations where biochemical mechanisms have been well worked out in animal models, it remains to be seen whether or not the findings can be transferred to humans with sepsis. The tremendous homogeneity of the sepsis syndrome population make clinical studies of this group difficult and meaning of clinical findings subject to interpretation. Increasingly, however, the availability of high quality assays and pharmacologic interventions has placed this type of research on more firm footing. In this chapter, the clinical implications of the release of bioactive lipids and free radicals of oxygen will be explored in the light of the available clinical data just now becoming available.

Role of Diffuse Membrane Damage in Sepsis and Acute Lung Injury (ALI)

The cellular damage produced by toxin and bacteriologic-induced activation of the immune system has been reviewed elsewhere [1]. Briefly, a major line of reasoning is that monocytes and macrophages recognize breaches in the immune barrier and react by producing a variety of second messengers designed to prepare the remainder of the immune system to deal with the invasion, bacteriologic or otherwise [2]. Phagocytosis is one of the fundamental mechanisms used by leukocytes, particularly macrophages and granulocytes, to destroy invading microorganisms. A principle feature of the phagocytic process involves the activation of NADPH oxidase (oxidative burst), a cell membrane associated enzyme system capable of converting molecular oxygen to superoxide anion (O_2-). Superoxide is rapidly converted to hydrogen peroxide (H_2O_2) either spontaneously or enzymatically with the participation of superoxide dismutase (SOD) with the spontaneous conversion almost as efficient as the enzymatic conversion. H_2O_2 is a powerful but relatively slow oxidant in biologic systems but it can damage DNA, react with sulfhydryl groups on structurally or enzymatically important proteins, and has other toxic effects. H_2O_2 is converted (detoxified) by catalase to water and oxygen or it enters in the multiple-step, iron catalyzed Fenton or Haber-Weiss reactions in which it is converted to hydroxyl radical. The hydroxyl radical is extremely reactive and in fact, is considered the most reactive free radical produced in biologic systems. Side products of this reactive species are lipid peroxides, hypochlorous acid and other highly reactive species.

The chronic infections seem in patients with chronic granulomatous disease of childhood, a genetic disorder in which the host lacks NADPH oxidase, attests to the importance of this enzyme in homeostasis and infectious disease prevention. As long as this potent oxidant activity is fairly well contained in the phagosome, little if any collateral tissue damage ensues. In the robust immune response of sepsis syndrome, it seems likely that the containment process is inadequate and that this results in damage to host tissues. The primary line of defense in the proper management of the process is a series of enzymes and free radical scavengers. SOD is important in first detoxification step of superoxide anion, conversion to hydrogen peroxide. SOD is found primarily as an intracellular enzyme although preliminary studies in patients with sepsis suggest that in this clinical condition, substantial quantities can be detected in plasma (personal communication, John Repine). Whether this is a result of cell damage, appropriate release triggered by the oxidant stress of sepsis or otherwise, the role of plasma and cellular SOD in sepsis remains to be elucidated.

Hydrogen peroxide is rapidly converted to water and oxygen by catalase, an enzyme with relatively low activity or by glutathione peroxidase, a more efficient enzyme. Glutathione peroxidase is different from catalase in other ways in that it is also active against lipid peroxides and it consumes glutathione in the catalytic process (i.e. converts glutathione (GSH) to oxidized glutathione (GSSG)) [3]. The difference in substrate specificity between catalase and GSH peroxidase is critically important. It is possible that much of the free radical attack on cell membranes results in the production of lipid peroxides rather than hydrogen peroxide. In order for the cell to recover from this injury, it must possess the ability to detoxify both types of peroxides.

Secondary defense against reactive oxygen metabolites is provided by vitamin E (α-tocopherol), β-carotene (a precursor of vitamin A), and thiols (sulfhydryl containing compounds such as methionine, cysteine and GSH). These easily oxidizable compounds provide a ready substrate for the reduction of free radicals. GSH is particularly attractive as a substrate because once oxidized to GSSG, it is easily regenerated (reduced) enzymatically through an energy consuming process by GSH reductase [3].

Oxidant Stress in Sepsis

Although the best known and possibly the most important oxidant stress in sepsis is oxidant burst, there are a variety of other potential sources of reactive oxygen species in this clinical syndrome. Supplemental oxygen, often required in therapy when ALI occurs, may place additional oxidant stress on the lung, drug metabolism may result in free radicals, and ischemia reperfusion injury may produce tissue injury through the production of free radicals. Free radical release may occur in the latter when hypoxanthine is converted to xanthine by xanthine oxidase. Xanthine oxidase is the form of the enzyme xanthine dehydrogenase present in ischemic tissues [4].

Relationship of Oxidant Stress to Free Radical Generation

Membrane phospholipids are the richest source of bioactive lipids in the body. During activation of inflammatory cells, phospholipases are activated resulting in the cleavage of arachidonic acid from cell membranes. Once free of the phospholipid bilayer, arachidonic acid is readily and rapidly converted to a very large variety of bioactive lipids. Through the action of 5-lipoxygenase, leukotriene B4, a potent chemoattractant, and leukotrienes C4, D4, and E4, potent bronchoconstrictors, vasoconstrictors which are also possibly important in the increased microvascular permeability associated with sepsis are released [5]. The other classic route of arachidonate metabolism is through the cyclooxygenase pathway. The major lipid mediators produced by this pathway include PGE, PGI_2, thromboxane-B_2 (TxB_2), and there are others [6]. There are still other very active lipids released as a result of cell membrane damage including platelet activation factor (PAF) [7].

The relative production of these different bioactive lipids from cell membranes is somewhat cell specific. Macrophages and platelets are the greatest source of thromboxane. There are some cell culture data suggesting that pulmonary macrophages produce more thromboxane than macrophages obtained from the peritoneum. Prostacyclin, on the other hand, is produced largely by systemic vascular bed endothelial cells. Systemic (peritoneal macrophages) are also a rich source. PAF and leukotrienes are produced by almost all cells tested to date.

Inhibition of leukotriene production in sepsis models has been of interest for several years [8]. Only recently have relatively non-toxic and potent 5-lipoxygenase inhibitors become available such that intensive testing could proceed. Such agents are currently in clinical testing for airway inflammatory changes of asthma but clinical trials in sepsis or ARDS have not been reported. Clinical studies of inhibition of the leukotriene pathway in sepsis seem rational given what we know about the adverse and long lasting effects of leukotrienes in animal models and in patients with ARDS. Recent data from patients with sepsis induced ARDS indicate very large and sustained increases in leukotriene metabolites (Fig. 1) [5].

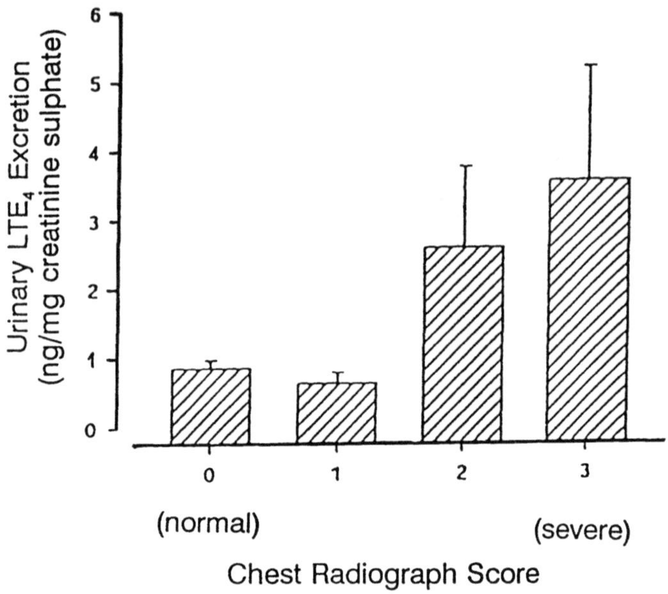

Fig. 1. Radiographic evidence of pulmonary edema and urinary LTE_4 excretion in patients with ARDS. Urinary LTE_4 excretion (ng/mg creatinine, mean ± SEM) values were compared to the chest radiograph scores obtained on the same days as the urine samples. There was a trend toward increased LTE_4 excretion on occasions where radiography revealed moderate (score = 2) and severe (score = 3) pulmonary edema. (From [5] with permission)

PGE is an anti-inflammatory prostaglandin and may be important in providing negative feedback to the inflammatory process [9]. Acting as an anti-inflammatory agent, excess quantities of this bioactive lipid are hypothesized to result in a relatively immunocompromised state in some critically ill patients and thus in these patients it may be harmful. On the other hand, the anti-inflammatory nature of the E-series prostaglandins have made them attractive in the clinical study of ARDS as potential therapy [10, 11]. It remains to be seen just how the balance between too much and too little PGE will finally settle out. This form of therapy is still under active study.

Thromboxane-B_2 is a potent bronchoconstrictor, a pulmonary vasoconstrictor, and this lipid activates platelets and causes them to aggregate. The concept of reducing the effect of thromboxane in sepsis has been tested through use of thromboxane synthetase inhibitors or by agents or by thromboxane-receptor antagonists [12].

Prostaglandin-I_2 (PGI_2) has anti-inflammatory actions as well as vaso- and bronchodilator effects which essentially oppose those of thromboxane. The balance between the two as well the relative number of receptors for each is probably important in determining the net physiologic effects of the release of these lipid mediators in sepsis. Compounding the problem is the fact that these metabolites have very short plasma and tissue half-lives making studies of the parent/active compounds impossible. Thromboxane, for example, has a plasma half-life of approximately 30 sec under normal conditions. It is conceivable that this time could be prolonged under conditions of rapid production such as sepsis, so that the usual pathways of metabolism are overwhelmed. But for made clinical as well as animal studies of these mediators very difficult. Still, these two lipids are the most studied the time being, animal and human studies must rely on the measurements of inactive metabolites. These issues have of the arachidonic acid metabolites.

Relationship between Free Radicals and the Arachidonic Acid Cascade

Any process by which the lipid membrane of cells is perturbed has the potential for activating phospholipases and for subsequent release of arachidonic acid. Free radicals of oxygen, easily capable of lipid peroxidation through the processes described above are major contenders for this role. It is possible that an early step in the process of development of the systemic inflammatory response is the disturbance of a critical mass of endothelial (microvascular) cell membrane lipids such that local reparative and/or containment processes are overwhelmed. As key mediators such as leukotrienes, thromboxane and prostacyclin enter the general circulation host, physiology begins to be altered in a variety of ways. The manner of host response is likely dictated by the relative preponderance of each mediator in each tissue bed as well as by the timing of the appearance of these substances. For example, if prostacyclin reaches the systemic vascular bed in large quantities and is relatively unopposed by thromboxane or other vasoconstrictors, low systemic vascular resistance and shock may result. If the final result is shock, which occurs in approximately 40–60% of sepsis syndrome patients at one time or another in their illness, and if shock is sustained, additional ischemia reperfusion occurs, more oxidants are produced and the cycle is not only repeated, but amplified. If, on the other hand, PGE or anti-inflammatory cytokines are released in sufficient quantities, then the cycle of inflammation with diffuse microvessel and organ damage could be broken and homeostasis could then be restored. Further complicating the complete understanding of these effects is that the local demographics of blood flow, receptor density and other factors may also impact the net physiologic response.

The complexity of the systemic inflammatory response is such that the details of the players and their interactions will probably be worked out only in controlled basic research models. On the other hand, considering the importance of timing and mediator and organ interaction on the process, no theory of the operation of the systemic inflammatory response can be taken as fact until there is adequate testing in humans. The heterogeneous nature of human diseases underlying this process clinically dictates that a major approach to the problem must be to employ inhibitors (or augmenters in cases where this is justified, i.e., PGE_1) of the purported mediators and observe the effect. The work to be described below with antioxidants and cyclooxygenase inhibitors is aimed directly at this process.

Relationship between Nuclear Factor kappa B, Cytokines and Inflammation

Reactive oxygen species may contribute to lung inflammation by modulating the production of inflammatory cytokines. Acute lung inflammation is distinguished by increased numbers of neutrophils within parenchyma. The exact mechanism responsible for the accumulation of neutrophils has not been fully characterized but a pervasive hypothesis is that neutrophils are recruited to the lung in response to chemotactic cytokines. Interleukin 8 (IL-8) belongs to a family of chemokines [13] and has been implemented in the pathogenesis of a wide variety of acute inflammatory conditions including ARDS [14], chronic bronchitis [15], cystic fibrosis [16], septic shock syndrome [17, 18], idiopathic pulmonary fibrosis [19], and empyema [20]. Experimental *in vitro* data, based on molecular techniques, indicate that reactive oxygen species (ROS) are involved in the regulation of the IL-8 gene. For example, exposure to hyperoxia induces IL-8 gene expression by blood monocytes [21] and oxygen scavengers block IL-8 gene expression in *ex vivo* stimulated whole blood [22].

IL-8 is produced by monocytic phagocytes and by a wide variety of nonleukocytic cells, including lymphocytes, fibroblasts, and epithelial and endothelial cells, when stimulated with endotoxin, IL-1, or tumor necrosis factor (TNF). There is little, if any, detectable constitutive production of IL-8 or expression of IL-8 mRNA by unstimulated cells. Within 1 h of stimulation, IL-8 mRNA is expressed, reaches maximal levels by 2–3 h and gradually declines thereafter. This transcriptional activation, at least in part, involves the binding of nuclear regulatory proteins, nuclear factor kappa B (NF-κB) and nuclear factor IL-6 (NF-IL-6), to specific promoter sequences present in the promoter region of the IL-8 gene [23, 24]. Gel mobility shift analysis has indicated that the NF-IL-6-like factor constitutively binds to the region between −94 and −81, whereas an inducible factor binds to the NF-κB binding element in the region between −80 and −71 of the IL-8 gene. The combination of the NF-IL-6 and NF-κB binding elements are both essential and sufficient for IL-8 promoter activity. The nuclear translocation and binding activity of NF-κB appears to be, at least in part, modulated by alteration in the redox state of the cell [25–30]. Agents which result in cellular oxidative stress are potential activators of NF-κB which could result in transcriptional activation of genes, like IL-8, which are dependent on NF-κB regulatory elements. This mechanism may provide a possible link which relates oxidative stress and acute inflammatory lung disease.

NF-κB exists in most cells as a non-DNA binding form in the cytoplasm composed of three subunits: a DNA-binding P-50 protein, a DNA-binding

P-65 protein, and an inhibitory subunit called IκB which is bound to the P-65. IκB inhibits DNA-binding of NF-κB and appears to be responsible for the cytoplasmic localization of the complex. The release of IκB appears to trigger the activation of the NF-κB transcription factor with translocation to the nucleus and binding to the NF-κB sequence in the IL-8 gene or other responsive genes. Several lines of evidence indicate that ROS can influence the binding affinity of NF-κB following stimulation. NF-κB is directly activated by H_2O_2 treatment of cells from an inactive cytoplasmic form to an active nuclear form [25, 26]. N-acetylcysteine (NAC) can block NF-κB induction by H_2O_2. As discussed, NAC is a thiol compound which is a direct ROS scavenger and restores intracellular glutathione levels. Since, NAC blocks NF-κB activation, it is reasoned that ROS mediate the activation of NF-κB. Various other stimuli including endotoxin, TNF, and phorbol 12-myristate 13-acetate (PMA) activate NF-κB and this activation can also be blocked by prior treatment with NAC and other antioxidants including the iron chelators pyrrolidine dithiocarbamate (PDTC) [27, 28]. Further evidence of the involvement of ROS in activation of NF-κB lies in the observation that treatment of cells with TNF and PMA can both deplete intracellular GSH stores and result in release of H_2O_2 and O_{2-} [26]. These data appear to indicate that many different agents induce the DNA-binding form of the cytoplasmic form of NF-κB by a mechanism which involves ROS.

Clinical Studies of the Antioxidant Approach with N-Acetylcysteine and Oxothiazolidine Carboxylate

As discussed above, GSH (glutamyl-cysteinyl-glycine) is particularly important in host defense against oxidative stress. Animal studies have shown that the lung is a net importer of reduced GSH [31]. Recent data have demonstrated a relative deficiency of pulmonary GSH, as estimated by bronchoalveolar lavage, in patients with ARDS [32]. Cysteine, though not generally considered an essential amino acid and therefore not included in routine parenteral nutrition, has been considered by some to conditionally essential in the critically ill in that its availability is dependent of the efficiency of conversion from other substrates such as methionine. NAC an antioxidant that also is rapidly converted to cysteine has been an attractive candidate for study in sepsis and ARDS. Extensive preclinical testing has continued to provide support for this hypothesis [33, 34].

Given the success in preventing tissue injury with NAC in a wide variety of cell and animal models and, given the relative safety of NAC in humans treated for acetaminophen overdose, a pilot study was performed in patients with established ARDS. The pilot was designed to answer several questions: 1) is circulating red blood cell GSH decreased in patients with established ARDS?; 2) can this very large reservoir for GSH be effectively augmented by NAC?; and 3) if circulating GSH can be augmented, what are the pathophysiological effects and safety of this intervention?

Thirty patients who had an illness known to be associated with ARDS and who met all the following criteria were eligible for randomization (double-blind, placebo-controlled): 1) arterial blood gases revealing a PaO_2 of ≤ 70 mm Hg while they were breathing at least 40% oxygen, or a PaO_2/PAO_2 (ratio of partial pressure of arterial oxygen to partial pressure of alveolar oxygen) of ≤ 0.3 (regardless of level of PEEP); 2) bilateral diffuse infiltrates on chest radiography compatible with pulmonary edema; and 3) a pulmonary artery wedge pressure ≤ 19 mm Hg. N-acetylcysteine (Zambon Laboratories, Cadempino, Switzerland) was delivered as an IV solution with a loading dose of 150 mg/kg delivered over 30 min followed by 16 maintenance doses of 24 mg NAC/kg repeated every 4 h for a total of 17 doses. All patients received the full course of placebo or active drug. Key physiologic variables were similar at entry in the NAC and placebo groups indicating a successful randomization. The mean amount of shunting, PEEP levels, and hemodynamic variables were similar to those previously reported for ARDS patients.

The results of these pilot studies indicate that GSH as measured by red cell GSH is substantially depleted in ARDS, possibly by as much as two-thirds [33]. The rationale for measuring red cell GSH is that the vast majority of circulating GSH is in the red cell, with very little in plasma. Given that serial tissue biopsies of lung or liver are difficult and probably not justifiable at this stage of understanding of GSH metabolism in ARDS, the only substantial tissue readily available for assay is the red cell. The loading dose of NAC was clearly effective in increasing plasma cysteine levels to roughly 10 fold over entry. Levels declined during the maintenance doses to only 2 fold over entry. There was no similar change in plasma cysteine from baseline noted over the 5 day treatment period in the placebo group. Erythrocyte GSH levels increased by over 50% from entry placing these levels near normal, but this did not occur until 72 h into the treatment period.

Physiologic effects were measured including PaO_2/PAO_2 ratio which improved rapidly in both treatment groups presumably due to use of mechanical ventilation, CPAP and other clinical support measures, but there was no significant difference in the rate of improvement between groups. Chest radiographs scored for presence of pulmonary edema (0 = normal, 1 = mild, 2 = moderate, 3 = severe) using the scoring method described in previous Vanderbilt studies revealed that our patients had moderate to severe pulmonary edema at entry. By 120 h post-study entry, there was a clear improvement in the NAC treated patients both as compared to entry levels and as compared to placebo controls with further improvement over placebo patients by 120 h.

Cardiac output tended to improve rapidly after the loading dose of NAC in the treated group by approximately 30% and the placebo group was unchanged but this difference did reach statistical significance. This increase in cardiac output translated into an increase in both oxygen delivery and oxygen consumption of similar magnitude in the NAC treated patients but not in the control group. There are now data from others suggesting a mechanism for this observation. Studies of cardiac function in models of ischemia/reperfusion indicate that oxidant injury is part of the reperfusion response which can be partially prevented or reversed by antioxidants [35].

Recently, additional pilot studies in patients with established ARDS have been conducted. Forty-six patients were randomized (double-blind, placebo-controlled) to receive either NAC (Fluimucil™, The Zambon Corporation, Cadempino, Switzerland) or oxothiazolidine carboxylate (OTC, Procysteine™, Free Radical Sciences, Cambridge, MA). The dosing regimen called for 70 mg/kg/day of NAC, 63 mg/kg/day OTC or an equal volume of placebo. The dosages for OTC and NAC are molar equivalents of each other, i.e. they provide for the same delivery of cysteine on a molar basis. Treatment was extended to 10 days total and the dosing regimen in this protocol did not provide for a loading dose. The study drugs were well tolerated and there were no adverse effects attributed to either agents. The preliminary analysis of this study confirms the presence and degree of cysteine and red cell GSH depletion in patients with ARDS. Of note is that although red cell GSH rose substantially with either treatment, some patients were still partially depleted at the end of the treatment period on day 10. This would suggest that dosing was either not maximized, that the machinery for production of red cell GSH was impaired, or that it takes more than 10 days of therapy to fully replete patients. Follow-up studies will be needed to address these issues. A large variety of physiologic responses were monitored during the total of 30 days from study entry. Favorable trends in reversal of PaO_2/FiO_2 criteria for ARDS, bilirubin levels, total white cell counts, and cardiac index were observed.

Two additional clinical studies of NAC have recently been reported. Suter el al. [36] reported a group of 61 patients with mild to moderate ALI randomized to receive NAC, 40 mg/kg/day, or placebo. The 1-month mortality was 22% in the NAC group versus 35% in the placebo group, p=NS. The percentage of patients requiring mechanical ventilation in the NAC group fell from 69 to 17% in three days versus a fall from 76 to 48% in the placebo group, p=0.01.

Jepsen et al. [37] studied a group of 66 ICU patients with ARDS randomizing to either NAC (150 mg/kg/load and 20 mg/kg/h for six days) or placebo. No differences were detected in PaO_2/FiO_2, chest radiograph, compliance or mortality over the 7 day study period. NAC did appear to impact the coagulation system as measured by serial platelet counts, fibrinogen and antithrombin III.

Clinical Studies of Cyclooxygenase Inhibition with Ibuprofen

Animals studies conducted over the past 25 years have supported the potential of cyclooxygenase inhibitors in the treatment of sepsis syndrome. In later years, the role of thromboxane and prostacyclin production has been elucidated in the acute alterations in pulmonary function seen following endotoxemia [38]. Snapper and colleagues [39], working with the chronically instrumented sheep model, demonstrated that pretreatment with the cyclooxygenase inhibitor meclofenamate blocked the early pulmonary hypertension and fall in dynamic compliance and lung volume seen after endotoxin infusion. Treatment with ibuprofen, even after established endotoxin-induced lung dysfunction in sheep, results in improved lung mechanics and pulmonary hemodynamics [40], suggesting that prostanoid production is persistent and continues to alter lung function.

Based on these and other data, a double-blind, randomized, placebo-controlled pilot study of the effect of ibuprofen (800 mg per rectum every 4 h for 12 h) in 30 patients with sepsis syndrome was undertaken [36]. Patients with

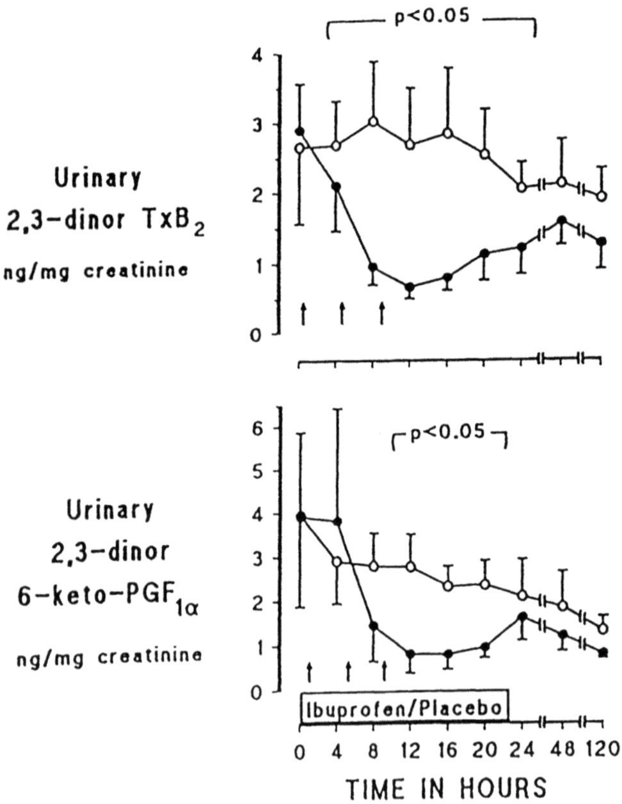

Fig. 2. Urinary concentrations of systemic eicosanoids in patients with sepsis syndrome. Urinary concentrations of 2,3-dinor-thromboxane-B_2 and 2,3-dinor-6-keto-$PGE_{1\alpha}$ normalized to urinary creatinine concentration. The arrows indicate the timing of the three doses of ibuprofen (800 mg) or placebo; p values refer to comparisons of ibuprofen group with placebo group for time-matched treatment periods. Open circles = placebo (n=8); closed circles = ibuprofen (n=9). (From [38] with permission)

abnormal vital signs including fever with at least one organ system failure secondary to sepsis were enrolled. Ibuprofen-treated patients experienced a significant decrease in heart rate, body temperature, peak airway pressure and minute ventilation. The ibuprofen-treated group experienced a significant decrease in urinary 2,3-dinor-6-keto-$PGF_{1\alpha}$ and 2,3-dinor-thromboxane B_2, whereas levels in the placebo-treated patients remained high for at least 120 h (Fig. 1). There was a positive correlation between the thromboxane metabolite and peak airway and pulmonary artery pressures, and an inverse correlation between the prostacyclin metabolite and mean systemic blood pressure. There also appeared to be a trend toward an increase in blood pressure especially for those patients in shock at study entry (Fig. 2) and more rapid resolution of pulmonary changes in ARDS blood gas criteria (Fig. 3). The findings in this study were consistent with the hypothesis that both constrictor and dilator prostaglandins contribute to the pathophysiology in septic patients.

The success of this pilot study using a limited course of ibuprofen in sepsis syndrome has led to the constitution of a multicenter working group supported by the Lung Division of the National Institutes of Health, National Heart Lung and Blood Institute. Seven clinical centers in North America are coordinating their efforts to determine if IV ibuprofen, 10 mg/kg (maximum 800 mg)/6 h for 8 doses, delivered early in the course of sepsis syndrome has an impact on the mortality and organ failure of this major clinical process (Fig. 4 and Table 1).

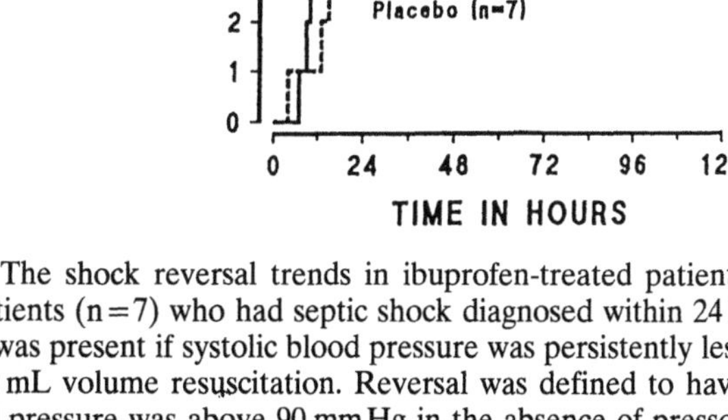

Fig. 3. Reversal trend in shock. The shock reversal trends in ibuprofen-treated patients (n=8) versus placebo-treated patients (n=7) who had septic shock diagnosed within 24 h of study entry are shown. Shock was present if systolic blood pressure was persistently less than 90 mmHg after at least 500 mL volume resuscitation. Reversal was defined to have occurred when the systolic blood pressure was above 90 mmHg in the absence of pressor therapy. The differences were not statistically significant ($p=0.12$). (From [38] with permission)

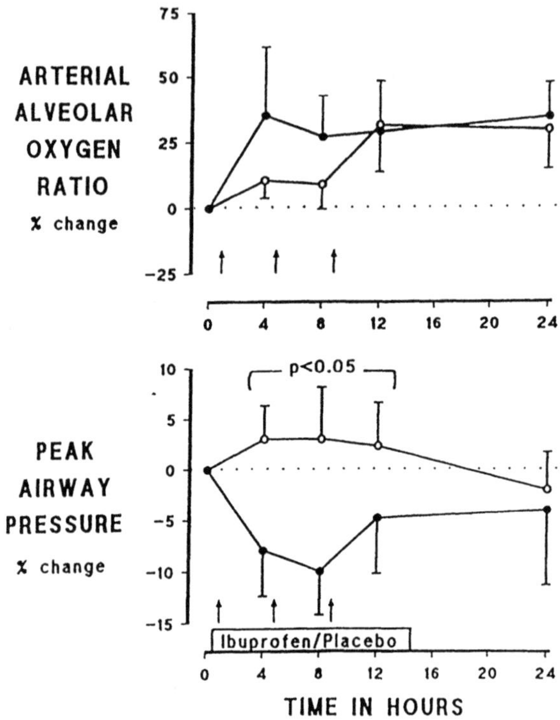

Fig. 4. Effect of cyclooxygenase inhibition on oxygenation and airway pressure. Effect of ibuprofen on arterial to alveolar PO_2 ratio (PaO_2/PAO_2) and peak airway pressure (for those patients requiring mechanical ventilation; PEEP has been subtracted) expressed as percent change from study entry. The arrows indicate the timing of the three doses of ibuprofen (800 mg) or placebo; p values refer to comparisons of ibuprofen group with placebo group for time-matched treatment periods. (Top) open circles = placebo (n=14); closed circles = ibuprofen (n=16). (Bottom) open circles = placebo (n=10); closed circles = ibuprofen (n=12)

Conclusion

Sepsis and ARDS, with their attendant high morbidity and mortality, remain difficult management problems and continue to constitute a major drain on health care resources. There is now a firm foundation to the understanding of the systemic inflammatory response which has markedly improved the climate for the conduct of clinical studies. The ability to accurately measure mediators or their metabolites and to block these mediators in a somewhat selective fashion (e.g. ibuprofen vs methylprednisolone) has also improved the outlook for progress in this area. Specifically, a large body of data derived from animal models suggest that therapies aimed at preventing unrestrained production of arachidonic acid metabolites and augmenting host antioxidant defenses are rational approaches for clinical trials in patients

Table 1. Entry data for patients entered into the study of ibuprofen in sepsis syndrome[a]. (From [38] with permission)

	Placebo (n=14)	Ibuprofen (n=16)
Age, yr	54.3±3.9	53.8±3.6
Vital signs		
Temperature, °F	100.5±0.5	100.5±0.5
Heart rate, beats/min	108±6	112±5
Respiratory measurements		
Respiratory rate, breaths/min	21±3	17±2
PaO_2/PAO_2	0.36±0.05	0.35±0.03
Mechanical ventilation, n (%)	11 (79)	13 (81)
FiO_2	0.60±0.07	0.60±0.05
Minute ventilation, L/min	13.4±1.6	13.9±1.1
Total thoracic compliance, mL/cm H_2O	52±7	47±7
Pulmonary edema score[b]	0.9±0.3	1.4±0.3
Cardiovascular function		
Patients with pulmonary artery catheter, n (%)	7 (50)	9 (56)
Cardiac output, L/min	6.49±0.67	6.13±0.89
Paw, mmHg	18±2	12±2[c]
Systemic blood pressure, mmHg	86±4	87±4
Ppa, mmHg	30±2	26±4
SVR, dyne·cm·s^{-5}	909±152	1084±195
PVR, dyne·cm·s^{-5}	152±27	245±107
Renal and hepatic function		
Serum creatinine, mg/dL	1.2±0.1	1.6±0.3
Patients with creatinine >4, n (%)	0 (0)	1 (6)
Creatinine clearance, mL/min	72±14	62±15
Bilirubin, mg/dL	2.8±0.8	2.0±0.6
Patients with bilirubin >4, n (%)	4 (29)	2 (13)
SGPT, IU/L	41±17	46±7
Other data		
WBC, thousands/mm^3	15±2	15±2
Platelet count, thousands/mm^3	219±47	301±55
Positive cultures, n (%)	12/14 (86)	14/16 (88)
Gramnegative, n	9	9
Positive blood cultures, n (%)	7/14 (50)	4/16 (25)
Gram-negative	3	1
Sepsis onset to treatment, h	7.2±0.7	7.6±0.6

[a] Data are shown as mean±SEM.
[b] 0=normal; 1=mild; 2=moderate; 3=severe.
[c] Indicates $p<0.05$ ibuprofen group versus placebo.

with either sepsis or ALI. Large scale clinical trials in these areas are ongoing and, if these interventions prove effective, patients with sepsis and ALI will have a better prognosis and Science will have gotten one step closer toward a better understanding of the basic biologic processes underlying these closely related syndromes.

Specific Conclusions

1. Though there is Level II data available for the use of antioxidants, specifically N-acetylcysteine, in acute lung injury, the studies have demonstrated conflicting results with one study showing benefit and a second study unable to demonstrate benefit. Routine therapy with N-acetylcysteine cannot be recommended at this time and remains experimental (Fig. 5).
2. Level II data exist supporting the use of ibuprofen in sepsis syndrome. The study was a pilot study and the number of patients too small to permit a recommendation regarding routine clinical use. This therapy should be considered experimental.

Acknowledgements: This work was supported in part by NIH NHLBI HL 19153 (SCOR in acute lung injury) and by NHLBI HL RO1 43167 (Cardiopulmonary effects of ibuprofen in sepsis).

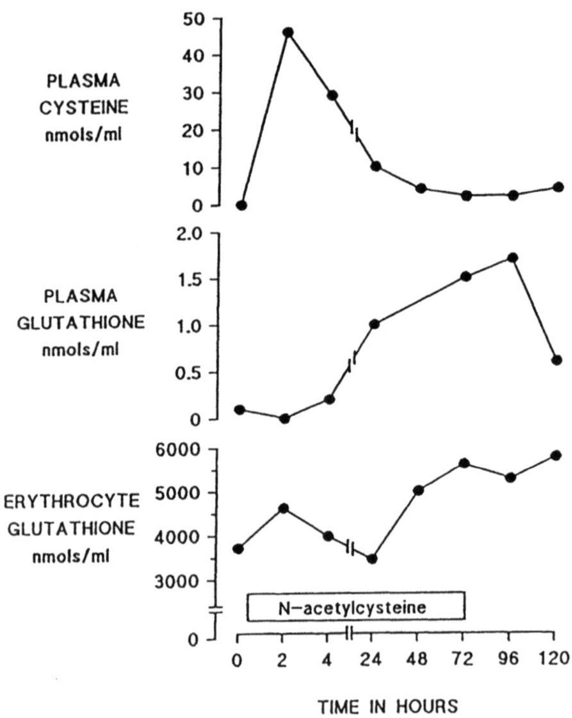

Fig. 5. Effect of N-acetylcysteine in a patient with ARDS. Therapy consisted of an IV loading dose of 150 mg/kg followed by 24 mg/kg every 4 h for 72 h. The loading dose had a profound and immediate effect on plasma cysteine while the plasma and red cell glutathione levels did not increase until approximately 24 h of therapy. (From [33] with permission)

References

1. Weiss SJ (1989) Tissue destruction by neutrophils. N Engl J Med 320:365–376
2. Bone RC, Balk RA, Cerra FB, et al (1992) Definitions for sepsis and organ failure and guidelines for the use of innovative therapies in sepsis. Chest 101:1644–1655
3. Grisham MB, McCord J (1986) Chemistry and cytotoxicity of reactive oxygen metabolites. In: Taylor AE, Matalon S, Ward PA (eds) Physiology of oxygen radicals. American Physiologic Society, Bethesda, MD, pp 1–18
4. Parks D, Granger DN (1986) Xanthine oxidase: Biochemistry, distribution and physiology. Acta Physiol Scand 548:87–99
5. Bernard GR, Korley V, Chee P, et al (1991) Persistent generation of peptido leukotriene in patients with the adult respiratory distress syndrome. Am Rev Respir Dis 144:262–267
6. Brigham KL, Meyrick B, Bernard GR (1986) Free radicals and arachidonic acid metabolites in endotoxin-induced pulmonary endothelial injury. In: Taylor AE, Matalon S, Ward PA (eds) Physiology of oxygen radicals. American Physiologic Society, Bethesda, MD, pp 1–18
7. Christman BW, Lefferts PL, King GA, Snapper JR (1988) Role of circulating platelets and granulocytes in PAF-induced pulmonary dysfunction in awake sheep. J Appl Physiol 64:2033–2041
8. Coggeshall JW, Christman BW, Lefferts PL, et al (1988) Effect of inhibition of 5-lipoxygenase metabolism of arachidonic acid on response to endotoxemia in sheep. J Appl Physiol 65:1351–1359
9. Brigham KL, Zadoff A, Serafin WE, Oates JA (1985) Prostaglandin E_2 (PGE_2) attenuates the pulmonary vascular response to endotoxemia in unanesthetized sheep. Clin Res 33:579 (Abst)
10. Holcroft JW, Vassar MJ, Weber CJ (1986) Prostaglandin E_1 and survival in patients with the adult respiratory distress syndrome: A prospective trial. Ann Surg 203:371–378
11. Bone RC, Slotman G, Maunder R, et al (1989) Randomized double-blind, multicenter study of prostaglandin E_1 in patients with the adult respiratory distress syndrome. Chest 96:114–119
12. Brigham KL (1985) Metabolites of arachidonic acid in experimental vascular lung injury. Federation Proc 44:43–45
13. Oppenheim JJ, Zachariae COC, Mukaida N, et al (1991) Properties of the novel proinflammatory supergene "intercrine" cytokine family. Annu Rev Immunol 9:617–648
14. Donnelly SC, Strieter RM, Kunkel SL, et al (1993) Interleukin-8 and development of adult respiratory distress syndrome in at-risk patient groups. Lancet 341:643–647
15. Richman-Eisenstat JB, Jorens PG, Hebert CA, et al (1993) Interleukin-8: An important chemoattractant in sputum of patients with chronic inflammatory airway diseases. Am J Physiol 264:L413–418
16. Dean TP, Dai Y, Shute JK, et al (1993) Interleukin 8 concentration are elevated in bronchoalveolar lavage, sputum, and sera of children with cystic fibrosis. Pediatric Res 34:162–166
17. Hack CE, Hart M, van Schijndel RJ, et al (1992) Interleukin-8 in sepsis: Relation to shock and inflammatory mediators. Infec Immun 60:2835–2842
18. Halstensen A, Ceska M, Brandtzaeg P, et al (1993) Interleukin-8 in serum and cerebrospinal fluid from patients with meningococcal disease. J Infect Dis 167:471–475
19. Carre PC, Mortenson RL, King TE, et al (1991) Increased expression of the interleukin 8 gene by alveolar macrophages in idiopathic pulmonary fibrosis. J Clin Invest 88:1802–1810
20. Broaddus VC, Hebert CA, Vitangcol RV, et al (1992) Interleukin-8 is a major neutrophil chemotactic factor in pleural liquid of patients with empyema. Am Rev Respir Dis 146:825–830
21. Metinko AP, Kunkel SL, Standiford TJ, Strieter RM (1992) Anoxia-hyperoxia induced monocyte-derived interleukin-8. J Clin Invest 90:791–798

22. DeForge LE, Fantone JC, Kenney JS, Remick DG (1992) Oxygen radical scavengers selectively inhibit interleukin 8 production in human whole blood. J Clin Invest 90:2123–2129
23. Mukaida N, Mahe Y, Matsushima K (1990) Cooperative interaction of nuclear factor-kappa B- and cis-regulatory enhancer binding protein-like factor binding elements in activating the interleukin-8 gene by pro-inflammatory cytokines. J Biolog Chem 265:21128–21133
24. Mukaida N, Shiroo M, Matsushima K (1989) Genomic structure of the human monocyte-derived neutrophil chemotactic factor IL-8. J Immunol 143:1366–1371
25. Schreck R, Albermann K, Baeuerle PA (1992) Nuclear factor kappa B: An oxidative stress-responsive transcription factor of eukaryotic cells (a review). Free Rad Res Comm 17:221–237
26. Schreck R, Rieber P, Baeuerle PA (1991) Reactive oxygen intermediates as apparently widely used messengers in the activation of the NF-κB transcription factor and HIV-1. EMBO J 10:2247–2258
27. Toledano MB, Leonard WJ (1991) Modulation of transcription factor NF-kappa B binding activity by oxidation-reduction in vitro. Proc Natl Acad Sci USA 88:4328–4332
28. Hayashi T, Ueno Y, Okamoto T (1993) Oxidoreductive regulation of nuclear factor kappa B. Involvement of a cellular reducing catalyst thioredoxin. J Biolog Chem 268:11380–11388
29. Schreck R, Grassmann R, Fleckenstein B, Baeuerle PA (1992) Antioxidants selectively suppress activation of NF-κB by human T-cell leukemia virus type I Tax protein. J Virol 66:6288–6293
30. Schreck R, Meier B, Mannel DN, Droge W, Baeuerle PA (1992) Dithiocarbamates as potent inhibitors of nuclear factor κB activation in intact cells. J Exper Med 175:1181–1194
31. Martensson J, Jain A, Frayer W, Meister A (1989) Glutathione metabolism in the lung: Inhibition of its synthesis leads to lamellar body and mitochondrial defects. Proc Natl Acad Sci USA 86:5296–5300
32. Pacht ER, Timerman AP, Lykens MG, Merola AJ (1991) Deficiency of alveolar fluid glutathione in patients with sepsis and the adult respiratory distress syndrome. Chest 100:1397–1403
33. Bernard GR (1991) N-acetylcysteine in experimental and clinical acute lung injury. Am J Med 91 (Suppl 3c):54–59
34. Bernard GR, Lucht WD, Niedermeyer ME, et al (1984) Effect of N-acetylcysteine on the pulmonary response to endotoxin in the awake sheep and upon in vitro granulocyte function. J Clin Invest 73:1772–1784
35. Forman MB, Puett DW, Cates CU, et al (1990) Glutathione redox pathway and reperfusion injury. Effect of N-acetylcysteine on infarct size. Circulation 78:202–213
36. Suter PM, Domenighetti G, Schaller MD, Laverriere MC, Ritz R, Perret C (1994) N-acetylcysteine enhances recovery from acute lung injury in man: A randomized, double-blind, placebo-controlled clinical study. Chest 105:190–194
37. Jepsen S, Herlevsen P, Knudsen P, Bud MI, Klausen MO (1992) Antioxidant treatment with N-acetylcysteine during adult respiratory distress syndrome: A prospective, randomized, placebo-controlled study. Crit Care Med 20:918–923
38. Bernard GR, Reines HD, Halushka PV, et al (1991) Prostacyclin and thromboxane A_2 formation is increased in human sepsis syndrome: Effects of cyclooxygenase inhibition. Am Rev Respir Dis 144:1095–1101
39. Snapper JR, Hutchison AA, Ogletree ML, Brigham KL (1983) Effects of cyclooxygenase inhibitors on the alterations in lung mechanics caused by endotoxemia in the unanesthetized sheep. J Clin Invest 72:63–76
40. Wright PW, Bernard GR (1989) Mechanisms of the late hemodynamic and airway mechanics response to endotoxin in the awake sheep. Am Rev Respir Dis 140:672–678

Increasing Oxygen Delivery in Sepsis

L. Gattinoni, L. Brazzi, and P. Pelosi,

Introduction

The concept of increasing oxygen delivery (DO_2) has been applied in various diseases and syndromes, including sepsis, in order to correct impaired oxygen transport to tissues, possible mismatch between regional blood flow and regional oxygen demand, or altered tissue capability for oxygen extraction. Whatever method used to increase oxygen delivery (volume load, cardioactive drug, etc.) the rationale for increasing oxygen delivery is based on the following hypothesis:

1) global or regional impairment of DO_2 to the cell creates an oxygen debt;
2) oxygen debt may induce anaerobic metabolism and/or impair cell function without inducing anaerobic metabolism;
3) oxygen debt is disclosed by an increased oxygen consumption (VO_2) when DO_2 is increased; and
4) increasing DO_2 corrects the oxygen debt, consequently VO_2 increases and, possibly, outcome improves.

In this chapter, we will discuss the rationale of increasing DO_2 and the preliminary data obtained in a group of septic patients in which the effects of DO_2 increase on survival was tested in a randomized, prospective trial.

The Oxygen Debt

Oxygen Debt involving Anaerobic Metabolism

The oxygen debt may be defined as the amount of energy demand, which must be satisfied by anaerobic metabolism. The oxygen debt was first identified in sport medicine and occurs when the oxygen demand exceeds the oxygen availability [1]. Acidosis develops and no further work can be performed. There is no doubt that oxygen debt may occur in diseases as advanced shock, and it has been clearly demonstrated both in animals and in humans [2, 3]. However, this is a preterminal state in which acidosis develops, VO_2 sharply decreases, and, in the absence of correction of the underlying cause, death occurs shortly.

This condition is classically described by the DO_2/VO_2 curve. At a critical point of DO_2 (300 ml/min/m^2 in man, 7–8 ml/kg/min in animals) [4], when VO_2 begins to decrease, lactic acidosis develops and the "dying process" begins, if delivery is not restored.

It is more questionable if the oxygen debt, as previously defined, may be payed by the anaerobic metabolism over an extended period of time, i.e. 24 h or more. Let's consider a patient with a VO_2 of 250 ml/min. This corresponds, for a caloric equivalent of oxygen equal to 5 cal (i.e. 1 mL O_2=5 cal), to an energy demand of 1800 Kcal/24 h. If, in this particular patient, an oxygen debt of 10% of the energy demand occurs, the anaerobic metabolism must provide 125 cal/min, i.e. 180 Kcal/24 h. As each mole of ATP generates 7.3–7.5 Kcal, the number of moles of ATP required will be 24.3 (i.e. 180 Kcal/24 h divided by 7.4 Kcal derived by each mole of ATP=24.3 mole ATP/24 h). ATP is derived from the anaerobic metabolism of glucose. Each mole of glucose produces anaerobically 2 moles of ATP, and 2 moles of lactate. The anaerobic production of the required 24.3 moles ATP/24 h is then associated to the production of 24.3 moles of lactate, i.e. 24300 mmol/24 h. This impressive amount largely exceeds the possibility of metabolism of lactate by the liver and kidney. Moreover, the complete oxidation of 1 mole of lactate produces 3 moles of CO_2. This is equivalent to the oxydation of 24.3 moles of lactate/24 h which produces 1134 mL CO_2/min!

This example clearly indicates that the oxygen debt requiring an energy supply from anaerobic metabolism cannot be maintained for an extended period of time.

Oxygen Debt without Anaerobic Metabolism

There is another possibility to explain an oxygen debt which not necessarily implies a shift to anaerobic metabolism. It is in fact possible that in the presence of impaired DO_2, the cell decreases, at least in part, its metabolic functions. As an example, the cells with high turnover may decrease the multiplication rate, the gut cells may decrease the absorption rate, the wound repair may decrease, etc. This condition could be equivalent to a starving organism which decreases its metabolic rate. This "starving-like state" could explain an oxygen debt in the absence of clear signs of anaerobic metabolism and would result in a cellular-organ dysfunction without immediate risk of death. Unfortunately, this hypothesis, to our knowledge, has never been investigated in critically ill patients.

Oxygen Supply Dependency

In normal physiology, the independent variable for the DO_2/VO_2 relationship is VO_2, i.e. the energy demand. Increasing energy demand, as during muscle exercise, causes an increase in DO_2, mainly through an increase in cardiac index (CI). In heavy exercise, CI increase is associated with an increase in oxygen extraction. However, a series of reports (see below) pointed out that, in various diseases or syndromes, the increase in DO_2, obtained with different methods (volume load, cardioactive drugs, decrease of positive end-expiratory pressure, and physical methods as leg elevations or chest physiotherapy) was associated with an increase in VO_2 at levels of DO_2 higher than its critical value (300 ml/min/m^2). This phenomenon, usually called oxygen supply dependency, was described both with and without concurrent acidosis. The oxygen supply dependency is generally interpreted as the presence of a masked oxygen debt, which is payed when DO_2 is increased. While this interpretation is widely accepted in the presence of acidosis (unmasked oxygen debt), where oxygen debt is associated with anaerobic metabolism, it appears more questionable in the absence of acidosis. In this case, the oxygen debt should be only associated with impaired cell/organ functions, without need of energy from anaerobic metabolism, i.e. "starving-like" state.

To further complicate the issue, a great debate arose about the methodology used to study the oxygen supply dependency phenomena. Most of the studies (see below) used the reverse Fick method to measure VO_2 instead of a direct measurement of expired gases. As with the reverse Fick method, most of the variables used to compute DO_2 are also used to compute VO_2, the association DO_2/VO_2 could be artefactual (mathematical coupling of the shared variables) [5]. This originated a great debate over the years, splitting the investigators in "believers" and "non-believers" in oxygen supply dependency.

The real existence of the oxygen supply dependency in the absence of acidosis is not only of pathophysiological or academic interest, but may deeply affect the therapeutical approach in critically ill patients. The use of "supranormal" hemodynamic values, advocated by Shoemaker et al. [6], finds its rationale in the presence of oxygen supply dependency phenomena, i.e. oxygen supply dependency discloses a masked oxygen debt, increasing DO_2 to supranormal values, pays the debt, and outcome improves.

Literature Review

We reviewed 80 studies [7–86] dealing with increasing DO_2 and/or oxygen supply dependency in various diseases and syndromes. Although in this chapter we will, specifically, deal with sepsis or septic shock, it was interesting to consider the problem of oxygen supply dependency more widely. Most of the studies were performed in sepsis (26 studies – 555 patients), ARDS (15 studies – 479 patients), and surgical setting (17 studies – 2262 patients) (Table 1); 4 studies were performed including patients with mixed pathology [80–83] while 3 studies included specifical group of patients as cancer patients [84], obese with obstructive sleep-apnea patients [86], and patients with hepatic failure [86]. Only 6 studies, to our knowledge, were randomized for increasing DO_2, 4 in surgical patients [23, 26, 27, 33], one in septic pa-

Table 1. Diagnostic categories in which oxygen supply dependency was investigated

Etiology	Ref.	No. of studies	No. of prospective	No. of retrospective	No. of randomized	No. of patients
ARDS	[7–21]	15	14	1	0	479
Surgical	[22–38]	17	16	1	4	2262
COPD	[39–41]	3	3	0	0	57
Heart failure	[42–50]	9	9	0	0	394
Sepsis	[51–76]	26	26	0	1	555
Trauma	[77–79]	3	3	0	0	217
Mixed etiologies	[80–83]	4	4	0	1	195
Others	[84–86]	3	3	0	0	42
Total		80	78	2	6	4201

tients [67] and one in heterogeneous critically ill patients [83]. As shown in Table 2, out of 80 studies which look for increasing DO_2 and/or oxygen supply dependency, 57 studies (72%, 3537 patients) found, at least in some of the patients, oxygen supply dependency, while 22 studies (28%, 575 patients) did not. It is interesting to note that in quite all the categories of patients, there was a prevalence of authors who found an oxygen supply dependency; however it should be remembered that in the majority of these studies, VO_2 was determined by indirect method, thus influencing DO_2/VO_2 relationship, as shown below. One study, where DO_2 was increased to a specific endpoint ($CI > 2.5$ l/min/m^2) did not evaluate oxygen supply dependency [27].

Table 3 summarizes the various methods used to change DO_2: volume load and cardiocirculatory drugs, alone or in combination, were used more frequently (14 volume load alone, 23 vasoactive drugs alone, and 14 fluids and drugs in combination), while 16 studies were only observational and DO_2 was not deliberately increased.

Table 2. Presence or absence of oxygen supply dependency in different diagnostic categories

Etiology	Ref.	DO_2/VO_2 dependency (No. of patients)	DO_2/VO_2 independency (No. of patients)	Total (No. of patients)
ARDS	[7–21]	10 (366)	5 (113)	15 (479)
Surgical*	[22–38]	12 (2029)	4 (144)	16 (2173)
COPD	[39–41]	2 (51)	1 (6)	3 (57)
Heart failure	[42–50]	7 (339)	2 (55)	9 (394)
Sepsis	[51–76]	19 (397)	7 (158)	26 (555)
Trauma	[77–79]	2 (150)	1 (67)	3 (217)
Mixed etiologies	[80–83]	3 (172)	1 (23)	4 (195)
Others	[84–86]	2 (33)	1 (9)	3 (42)

* One study [27] did not evaluate oxygen supply dependency

Table 3. Methods used to change oxygen delivery

	Ref.	DO_2/VO_2 dependency (No. of patients)	DO_2/VO_2 independency (No. of patients)	Total (No. of patients)
Drugs	[17, 39, 41, 44, 46–49, 51, 57–61, 63–65, 68, 73–76, 86]	16 (379)	7 (183)	23 (562)
PEEP	[7–9, 13, 16, 20, 21]	5 (116)	2 (33)	7 (149)
Fluids	[11, 12, 14, 15, 18, 43, 45, 52, 53, 55, 56, 66, 70, 84]	10 (251)	4 (84)	14 (335)
Fluids + Drugs*	[23, 24, 26, 27, 29, 31, 33, 34, 54, 67, 69, 72, 78, 80, 83]	9 (1153)	5 (226)	14 (1379)
Legs elevation	[40, 85]	1 (30)	1 (11)	2 (41)
Chest physiotherapy	[30, 37, 38]	3 (63)	–	3 (63)
None	[10, 19, 22, 25, 28, 32, 35, 36, 42, 50, 62, 71, 77, 79, 81, 82]	13 (1543)	3 (40)	16 (1583)
Total		57 (3535)	22 (577)	79 (4112)

* One study [27] did not evaluate oxygen supply dependency

As shown in Table 4, among the 29 studies which evaluated the effect of increasing DO_2 on mortality, 24 (83%) reported an improved outcome with an increased DO_2, and a DO_2/VO_2 dependency was found in the great majority of them (21 studies, 88%). However, it is important to notice that most of the studies (50 studies, 63%) evaluating DO_2/VO_2 dependency did not deal with survival.

Lactic acidosis does not seems to influence the presence of oxygen supply dependency. Table 5 shows that even if only 26 studies out of the 79 considered the lactate levels, a similar frequency of DO_2/VO_2 dependency was observed in the presence of lactic acidosis (12 studies out of 15, 80%) or in the absence of lactic acidosis (8 studies out of 11, 73%).

The possible importance of the methodology to evaluate the DO_2/VO_2 dependency is shown in Table 6 in which the studies were classified according to the method used to determine VO_2. For a given method, the studies were then classified as showing "presence" or "absence" of DO_2/VO_2 dependency according to the conclusions of the author itself. As an example, when in a given study, part of the patients showed DO_2/VO_2 dependency while some others did not, that study was classified as showing "presence" or "absence" of DO_2/VO_2 dependency according to the final statement of the author, as "... in summary, in a group of patients with ARDS ... we found a direct relationship between DO_2 and VO_2 ..." [8] or "... our study suggest the hypothesis that inadequate VO_2 relative to demand is characteristic of

Table 4. Improved or not improved outcome increasing DO_2 as a function of presence or absence of oxygen supply dependency

	Ref.	DO_2/VO_2 dependency (No. of patients)	DO_2/VO_2 independency (No. of patients)	Total (No. of patients)
Survival improvement*	[9, 13, 17, 22–24, 26, 29, 31, 33, 35, 42, 43, 53, 57, 58, 61, 65, 67, 68, 73, 78, 79, 83]	21 (2492)	3 (229)	24 (2721)
No survival improvement	[10, 28, 45, 63, 82]	2 (104)	3 (100)	5 (204)
No evaluation	[7, 8, 11, 12, 14–16, 18–21, 25, 30, 32, 34, 36–41, 44, 46–52, 54–56, 59, 60, 62, 64, 66, 69–72, 74–76, 77, 80, 81, 84–86]	34 (939)	16 (248)	50 (1187)
Total		57 (3535)	22 (577)	79 (4112)

* One study [27] did not evaluate oxygen supply dependency

many patients ..." [12]. As a result, DO_2/VO_2 was found in 49 out of 63 studies (78%), where the VO_2 was determined from reverse Fick method, and only 8 out of 16 studies (50%), where VO_2 was independently determined.

Table 5. Presence or absence of oxygen supply dependency as a function of acid base status

	Ref.	DO_2/VO_2 dependency (No. of patients)	DO_2/VO_2 independency (No. of patients)	Total (No. of patients)
High lactic acid	[9, 12, 14, 43, 45, 46, 52–55, 61, 63, 66, 68, 84]	12 (385)	3 (105)	15 (490)
Normal lactic acid	[7, 11, 42, 48, 49, 70, 71, 73–75, 80]	8 (199)	3 (54)	11 (253)
No measurement*	[8, 10, 13, 15–21, 23–26, 28–32, 35–41, 44, 47, 50, 51, 56–60, 62, 64, 65, 67, 72, 76–79, 81–86]	37 (2951)	16 (418)	53 (3369)
Total		57 (3535)	22 (577)	79 (4112)

* One study [27] did not evaluate oxygen supply dependency

Table 6. Presence or absence of oxygen supply dependency as function of the method used to measure O_2 consumption

	Ref.	DO_2/VO_2 dependency (No. of patients)	DO_2/VO_2 independency (No. of patients)	Total (No. of patients)
Reverse Fick	[7–10, 12–16, 19–24, 26, 29, 31–36, 42–48, 50–69, 72–74, 76, 77–84, 86]	49 (3377)	14 (428)	63 (3805)
Oxygen uptake	[11, 17, 18, 25, 28, 30, 37–41, 49, 70, 71, 75, 85]	8 (158)	8 (149)	16 (307)
Total		57 (3535)	22 (577)	79 (4112)

* One study [27] did not evaluate oxygen supply dependency

We do not want to achieve any definitive conclusion from this brief review, but a few points deserve some comments. It is worth noting that among the studies supporting the hypothesis of a reduction in mortality rate and morbidity when cardiac output and DO_2 were deliberately increased, relatively few are randomized even if many authors suggest an extensive application of this kind of therapeutical approach. Moreover, many of the randomized studies quoted above were performed in relatively small groups of young patients; groups were not always well matched; and the treatment regimen was often unclear. Consequently, considerable doubts could be cast on the efficacy of this type of treatment both in surgical and in critically ill patients. Moreover, other questions regarding the safety of this kind of therapeutical approach remain unsolved since the increase of cardiac output and DO_2 requires the use of invasive procedures and inotropes, and the frequency of adverse reaction is reported only in a limited number of studies. Another important observation was that increased lactic acidosis did not seem to be well correlated with the presence of DO_2/VO_2 dependency. Clinicians often state that in patients with severe sepsis, blood lactate levels are elevated (>2 mmol/L), supporting the hypothesis that hypermetabolism results in a metabolic state wherein substrate availability and metabolic rate exceed regional DO_2, such that anaerobic metabolism occurs. Since anaerobic metabolism is quite inefficient to produce adequate energy, it induces the formation of lactic acid. However, the lactic acid levels reflect the balance of many biochemical processes including normal aerobic and anaerobic metabolism, wash-out of lactic acid from the tissues, and metabolism of lactic acid in the liver, gut, kidneys, heart and brain. The presence of these various processes causes an extreme difficulty to consider blood lactate levels as a reliable marker of anaerobic metabolism in clinical practice, as suggested by our data. In our brief review, the presence of lactic acidosis was not related to the presence of a DO_2/VO_2 dependency, as expected. In conclusion, the DO_2/VO_2 dependency phenomenon does not seem clearly related either to any particular etiology or to methods used to change DO_2. Furthermore, the method used for VO_2 measurement (expired gas analysis versus reverse Fick method) must be carefully considered when interpreting the DO_2/VO_2 dependency studies.

Pathophysiology and Hemodynamic Treatment in Septic Shock

Although gram-negative bacteremias have been reported to occur frequently, the proportion of these cases which are associated with sepsis or septic shock are difficult to estimate. However the mortality rate associated with septic shock is 30 to 60%, unaltered by recent advances in antibiotic therapy and improvements in hemodynamic monitoring. Sepsis is defined as an infection associated with systemic manifestations. In this condition, the patient is defined "toxic", although more specific criteria are positive blood cultures or a presumed site of infection associated with several symptoms and signs as tachycardia, tachypnea, fever or hypothermia, leukocytosis and delirium. The hemodynamics in septic patients is characterized by an hyperdynamic status with a high cardiac output and low peripheral vascular resistances. Furthermore, endocrine alterations as hyperglycemia, hypertriglyceridemia and hypocalcemia may occur during sepsis.

During sepsis in the early stages, the homeostasis of the whole body is sufficiently maintained. However in the late stages, these regulatory mechanisms fail and the evidence of cardiocirculatory shock ensues. Septic shock is characterized by an hyperdynamic stage and, sometimes, by a preterminal hypodynamic stage. During the hyperdynamic stage, the presence of high cardiac output, low pulmonary artery occlusion pressure and low peripheral vascular resistances is typical.

The hemodynamics during septic shock has been extensively investigated [87–90] and a global myocardial dysfunction has been shown. As mentioned above, during septic shock, cardiac output was high but this effects was due to tachycardia since stroke volume was generally low.

When the left ventricular stroke work was measured, it clearly revealed a typical left ventricular failure. Moreover, the relative importance in myocardial depression during septic shock significantly correlated with survival [91]. Some authors have suggested the possible presence of a circulatory myocardial depressant factor as probably responsible for this cardiac dysfunction [91]. Septic shock patients are characterized by an abnormal oxygen extraction resulting in low extraction ratios with normal to high mixed venous hemoglobin saturations and lactic acidosis. Several potential mechanisms have been proposed to explain this defect looking at peripheral oxygen utilization: 1) peripheral arterial-venous shunting of blood due to maldistribution of blood flow resulting from microthrombosis and disturbed autoregulation in the microvasculature; 2) histotoxic injury caused by endotoxin release which produces cellular damage; and 3) diffuse capillary leak syndrome that would decrease the effective capillary density. Whatever the mechanism, peripheral defects in oxygen utilization may be overcome by increasing perfusion and DO_2. Consequently, if the hypothesis of oxygen debt is correct, an improvement in survival should be expected if cardiac output and DO_2 are therapeutically increased. Few randomized studies have evaluated the beneficial effects of augmenting cardiac output and DO_2 on mortality in patients with septic shock. Tuchschmidt et al. [67] in a recent randomized study, evaluated the therapeutic benefit of augmenting DO_2 in a group of patients with septic shock. The authors did not find any significant difference in survival between the normal treatment (NT) and optimal treatment group (OT) (28 in OT vs 50% in NT, $p=0.14$). However, since some patients of the NT group were spontaneously hyperdynamic and some of the OT group did not achieve their desired endpoint, patients were arbitrarily subset using a midpoint cardiac index of 4.5 $L/min/m^2$. With this kind of analysis, the authors found that patients with cardiac index >4.5 $L/min/m^2$ both in OT and NT had a better survival than patients with cardiac index <4.5 $L/min/m^2$. They concluded that outcome in patients with septic shock appears to be related to the level of systemic DO_2, therefore the titration of therapy to increase levels of cardiac index and DO_2 might be associated with improval survival from septic shock. However Tuchschmidt et al. [67] simply demonstrated that healthier patients die less often than less healthy ones, despite therapy. Based on these data, it is not clear that global increases in DO_2 will benefit patients with sepsis or septic shock.

Another problem is to evaluate if augmenting DO_2 is associated with increased risks for the patients. In fact volume replacement may precipitate pulmonary edema and induce acute left and right ventricular failure. The use of inotropes, such as dopamine or dobutamine, may increase the myocardial oxygen demand, and favor cardiac arrhythmias with an increase in global tissue oxygen demand. On the other side, vasopressors may worsen regional ischemia. Thus aggressive resuscitative therapies which aim to augment cardiac index and DO_2 levels above "normal" levels are no of proven value and may be, indeed, detrimental.

The $S\bar{v}O_2$ Study

We report data of a subgroup of 182 patients classified as septic or in septic shock and enrolled in a large multicenter randomized trial where three different hemodynamic goals were compared: in group I treatment was adapted to reach and maintain a normal cardiac index (2.5–3.5 $L/min/m^2$); in group II treatment was adapted to reach and maintain a supranormal cardiac index (>4.5 $L/min/m^2$); in group III treatment was adapted to reach and maintain a normal $S\bar{v}O_2$, i.e. $\geq 70\%$. All patients had a modified SAPS score >11 and underwent 5 days of active hemodynamic treatment: volume load, dobutamine-dopamine vasodilators. At baseline, VO_2 was not related to the final outcome. However, CI, DO_2 and extraction ratio were all predictors of the final outcome (Table 7). The hemodynamic status before active treatment was

Table 7. VO_2, CI, DO_2 and extraction ratio in septic patients (n = 182)

	No. of patients	No. of deaths	Mortality rate, %
VO_2 (mL/min/m^2)			
<120	52	31	60
120–160	51	36	71
>160	69	32	46
CI (L/min/m^2)*			
<2.5	29	22	76
2.5–4.5	103	62	60
>4.5	47	18	38
DO_2 (mL/min/m^2)*			
<400	50	34	68
400–600	70	45	64
>600	59	23	39
ER (%)*			
<30	101	50	50
30–60	63	42	67
>60	8	7	88

* $p < 0.01$

well balanced within the three groups, i.e. there was no significant differences in CI, DO_2 and extraction ratio between the three groups at baseline. From the basal hemodynamic data of these 182 septic patients, the rationale of increasing DO_2 seems reasonable. In fact, lower cardiac index and DO_2 were associated with significantly higher mortality, supporting the basic observations of Shoemaker et al. [26, 31, 35, 78] and others [13, 22, 25, 58, 59, 61, 67, 73]. In other words, the severity of the pathophysiological status at admission in ICU markedly negatively influences outcome, despite any kind of following treatment (i.e. more severe disease, more probability to die). Furthermore, as shown in Figure 1, in this patients population, increasing DO_2 over time did not increase VO_2; consequently, we did not find any DO_2/VO_2 dependency in our patients with septic shock.

The possible presence of oxygen supply dependency in septic shock is currently largely debated. Tuchschmidt et al. [92] found an DO_2/VO_2 dependency in a group of patients with septic shock below a critical DO_2 of 15 mL/kg/min, with survivors tending to have higher deliveries. Haupt et al. [53] showed that septic patients with increased arterial lactate levels had increases in VO_2 when DO_2 was increased to levels >8 mL/kg/min. Likewise, Kaufman et al. [52] found that VO_2 increased in septic shock patients by increasing DO_2 with fluid resuscitation. In our study, the mortality rate of the three randomized groups was not significantly different (Table 8). This means that in these septic patients, increasing DO_2 to supranormal values failed to increase VO_2 and did not change the mortality rate compared to maintain DO_2 to physiological levels or to maintain $S\bar{v}O_2$ within physiological values.

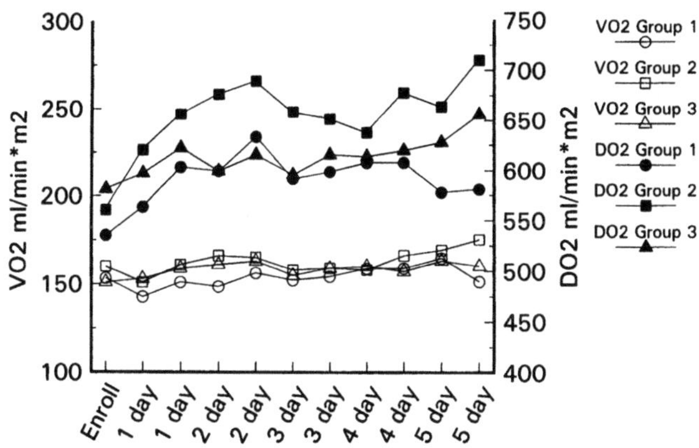

Fig. 1. Oxygen delivery (DO_2, black symbols) and oxygen consumption (VO_2, white symbols) in a group I, II, III as a function of the days of treatment

Conclusion

Increasing DO_2 finds its rationale in the presence of an unmasked (acidosis presence) or masked (acidosis not detectable) oxygen debt.

In the presence of acidosis, there is no doubt that an impaired delivery must be restored, otherwise death occurs in a relatively short time. The issue is far more complicated when we deal with a masked oxygen debt. The questions are: 1) does masked oxygen debt exist?; 2) how much DO_2 must be increased?

The proof of a masked oxygen debt is indirect, i.e. it is inferred from the presence of oxygen supply dependency above the critical level of DO_2. There is some evidence that most of the studies which found oxygen supply dependency had a methodologic problem (reverse Fick method), so that the existence of the oxygen supply dependency is then doubtful. However, even assuming that a masked oxygen debt exists, how much must DO_2 be increased? Data from the $S\bar{v}O_2$ study do not support the use of supranormal hemodynamic treatment as mortality rate was similar in patients with normal or supranormal hemodynamic treatment. Moreover, $S\bar{v}O_2$ study does not support the presence of a masked oxygen debt in an average population of septic patients, as we did not find, despite the use of reverse Fick method, any evidence of increasing VO_2 when increasing DO_2.

Table 8. Mortality rate in septic patients (n = 182) in the $S\bar{v}O_2$ study

	Group 1	Group 2	Group 3
No. of patients	57	66	59
No. of deaths	29	35	41
Mortality rate, %	51	53	69

References

1. Margaria R, De Caro L (1956) Il lavoro muscolare. In: Vallardi F (ed) Principi di fisiologia umana, Milano, pp 1834–1856
2. Holtzman S, Schuler JJ, Earnest W, et al (1974) Carbohydrate metabolism in endotoxemia. Circ Shock 1:181–193
3. Cain SM (1977) Oxygen delivery and uptake in dogs during anemic and hypoxic hypoxia. J Appl Physiol 42:228–234
4. Edwards JD (1993) Clinical controversies concerning oxygen transport principles: More apparent than real? In: Vincent JL (ed) Yearbook of intensive care and emergency medicine 1993. Springer Verlag, Berlin, Heidelberg, New York, pp 385–405
5. Hanique G, Dugernier T, Laterre PF, et al (1994) Evaluation of oxygen uptake and delivery in critically ill patients: A statistical reappraisal. Intensive Care Med 20:19–26
6. Shoemaker CW (1989) Pathophysiologic and fluid management of postoperative and posttraumatic ARDS. In: The Society of Critical Care Medicine. WB Saunders Company, Philadelphia, pp 615–636
7. Danek SJ, Lynch JP, Weg JG, et al (1980) The dependence of oxygen uptake on oxygen delivery in the adult respiratory distress syndrome. Am Rev Respir Dis 122:387–395
8. Mohsenifar Z, Goldbach P, Tashkin DP, et al (1983) Relationship between O_2 delivery and O_2 consumption in the adult respiratory distress syndrome. Chest 84:267–271
9. Rashkin MC, Bosken C, Baughman RP (1985) Oxygen delivery in critically ill patients. Relationship to blood lactate and survival. Chest 87:580–584
10. Karisman K, Burns SR (1985) Regulation of tissue oxygen extraction is disturbed in adult respiratory distress syndrome. Am Rev Respir Dis 132:109–114
11. Annat G, Viale JP, Percival C, et al (1986) Oxygen delivery and uptake in the adult respiratory distress syndrome. Am Rev Respir Dis 133:999–1001
12. Kruse JA, Haupt MT, Puri VK, et al (1990) Lactate levels as predictors of the relationship between oxygen delivery and consumption in ARDS. Chest 98:959–962
13. Russell JA, Ronco JJ, Lockhat D, et al (1990) Oxygen delivery and consumption and ventricular preload are greater in survivors than in non-survivors of the adult respiratory distress syndrome. Am Rev Respir Dis 141:659–665
14. Fenwick JC, Dodek PM, Ronco JJ, et al (1990) Increased concentrations of plasma lactate predict pathologic dependence of oxygen consumption on oxygen delivery in patients with adult respiratory distress syndrome. J Crit Care 5:81–86
15. Clarke C, Edwards JD, Nightingale P, et al (1991) Persistence of supply dependency of oxygen uptake at high levels of delivery in adult respiratory distress syndrome. Crit Care Med 19:497–502
16. Lorente JA, Renes E, Gomez-Aguinaga MA, et al (1991) Oxygen delivery-dependent oxygen consumption in acute respiratory failure. Crit Care Med 19:770–775
17. Hankeln KB, Gronemeyer R, Held A, et al (1991) Use of continuous non-invasive measurement of oxygen consumption in patients with adult respiratory distress syndrome following shock of various etiologies. Crit Care Med 19:642–649
18. Ronco JJ, Phong PT, Walley KR, et al (1991) Oxygen consumption is independent of changes in oxygen delivery in severe adult respiratory distress syndrome. Am Rev Respir Dis 143:1267–1273
19. Appel PL, Shoemaker WC (1992) Relationship of oxygen consumption and oxygen delivery in surgical patients with ARDS. Chest 102:906–911
20. Ranieri VM, Giuliani R, Eissa NT, et al (1992) Oxygen delivery-consumption relationship in septic adult respiratory distress syndrome patients: The effects of positive end-expiratory pressure. J Crit Care 7:150–157
21. Spec Marn A, Tos L, Kremzar B, et al (1993) Oxygen delivery consumption relationship in adult respiratory distress syndrome patients: The effects of sepsis. J Crit Care 8:43–50

22. Bland RD, Shoemaker WC, Abraham E, et al (1985) Hemodynamic and oxygen transport patterns in surviving and non-surviving postoperative patients. Crit Care Med 13:85–90
23. Shoemaker WC, Appel PL, Kram HB, et al (1988) Prospective trial of supranormal values of survivors as therapeutic goals in high-risk surgical patients. Chest 94:1176–1186
24. Shoemaker WC, Appel PL, Kram HB (1988) Tissue oxygenation debt as a determinant of lethal and non-lethal postoperative organ failure. Crit Care Med 16:117–120
25. Vermeij CG, Feenstra BWA, Bruining HA (1990) Oxygen delivery in postoperative and septic patients. Chest 98:415–420
26. Shoemaker WC, Kram HB, Appel PL, et al (1990) The efficacy of central venous and pulmonary artery catheters and therapy based upon them in reducing mortality and morbidity. Arch Surg 125:1332–1338
27. Beraluk JF, Abrahams JH, Gilmour I, et al (1991) Preoperative optimization of cardiovascular hemodynamics improves outcome in peripheral vascular surgery: A prospective, randomized clinical trial. Ann Surg 214:289–297
28. Vermeij CG, Feenstra BWA, Adrichem WJ, et al (1991) Independent oxygen uptake and oxygen delivery in septic and postoperative patients. Chest 99:1438–1443
29. Shoemaker WC, Appel PL, Kram HB (1991) Oxygen transport measurements to evaluate tissue perfusion and titrate therapy: Dobutamine and dopamine effects. Crit Care Med 19:672–688
30. Weissman C, Kemper M (1991) The oxygen uptake-oxygen delivery relationship during ICU intervention. Chest 99:430–435
31. Shoemaker WC, Appel PL, Kram HB (1992) Role of oxygen debt in the development of organ failure, sepsis and death in high risk surgical patients. Chest 102:208–215
32. Boyd O, Ground RM, Bennett ED (1992) The dependency of oxygen consumption on oxygen delivery in critically ill postoperative patients is mimicked by variations in sedation. Chest 101:1619–1624
33. Boyd O, Ground RM, Bennett ED (1993) A randomized clinical trial of the effect of deliberate perioperative increase of oxygen delivery on mortality in high risk surgical patients. JAMA 270:2699–2707
34. Boyd O, Ground RM, Bennett ED (1993) The use of dopexamine hydrochloride to increase oxygen delivery perioperatively. Anesth Analg 76:372–376
35. Shoemaker WC, Appel PL, Kram HB (1993) Hemodynamic and oxygen transport response in survivors and non-survivors of high risk surgery. Crit Care Med 21:977–990
36. Lugo G, Arizbe D, Dominguez G, et al (1993) Relationship between oxygen consumption and delivery during anesthesia in high risk surgical patients. Crit Care Med 21:64–69
37. Harding J, Kemper M, Weissman C (1993) Alfentanil attenuates the cardiopulmonary response of critically ill patients to an acute increase in oxygen demand induced by chest physiotherapy. Anesth Analg 77:1122–1129
38. Weissman C, Kemper M (1993) Stressing the critically ill patient: The cardiopulmonary and metabolic responses to an acute increase in oxygen consumption. J Crit Care 8:100–108
39. Brent BN, Matthay RA, Mahler DA, et al (1984) Relationship between oxygen uptake and oxygen transport in stable patients with chronic obstructive disease. Am Rev Respir Dis 129:682–686
40. Albert RK, Schrijen F, Poincelot F (1986) Oxygen consumption and transport in stable patients with chronic obstructive pulmonary disease. Am Rev Respir Dis 134:678–682
41. Mohsenifar Z, Jasper AC, Koerner SK (1988) Relationship between oxygen uptake and oxygen delivery in patients with pulmonary hypertension. Am Rev Respir Dis 138:69–73
42. Shibutani K, Komatsu T, Kubal K, et al (1983) Critical level of oxygen delivery in anesthetized man. Crit Care Med 11:640–643

43. Komatsu T, Shibutani K, Okamoto K, et al (1987) Critical level of oxygen delivery after cardiopulmonary bypass. Crit Care Med 15:194–197
44. Creamer JE, Edwards JD, Nightingale P (1990) Hemodynamic and oxygen transport variables in cardiogenic shock secondary to acute myocardial infarction and response to treatment. Am J Cardiol 65:1297–1300
45. Dietrich KA, Conrad SA, Hebert CA, et al (1990) Cardiovascular and metabolic response to red blood cell transfusion in critically ill volume-resuscitated non-surgical patients. Crit Care Med 18:940–944
46. Vincent JL, Roman A, De Backer D, et al (1990) Oxygen uptake/supply dependency. Ann Rev Respir Dis 142:2–7
47. Pittet JF, Lacroix JS, Gunning K, et al (1992) Different effects of prostacyclin and phentolamine on delivery dependent O_2 consumption and skin microcirculation after cardiac surgery. Can J Anesth 39:1023–1029
48. Teboul JL, Annane D, Thuillex C, et al (1992) Effects of cardiovascular drugs on oxygen consumption-oxygen delivery relationship in patients with congestive heart failure. Chest 101:1582–1587
49. Ruokonen E, Takala J, Kari A (1992) Regional blood flow and oxygen transport in patients with low cardiac output syndrome after cardiac surgery. Crit Care Med 21:1304–1311
50. Routsi C, Vincent JL, Bakker J, et al (1993) Relation between oxygen consumption and oxygen delivery in patients after cardiac surgery. Anesth Analg 77:1104–1110
51. Jardin F, Sportiche M, Bazin M, et al (1981) Dobutamine: A hemodynamic evaluation in human septic shock. Crit Care Med 9:329–332
52. Kaufman BS, Rackow EC, Falck JL (1984) The relationship between oxygen delivery and consumption during fluid resuscitation of hypovolemic and septic shock. Chest 85:336–340
53. Haupt MT, Gilbert EM, Carlson RW (1985) Fluid loading increases oxygen consumption in septic patients with lactic acidosis. Am Rev Respir Dis 131:912–916
54. Gilbert EM, Haupt MT, Mandanas RY, et al (1986) The effect of fluid loading, blood transfusion and catecholamine infusion on oxygen delivery and consumption in patients with sepsis. Am Rev Respir Dis 134:873–878
55. Astiz ME, Rackow EC, Falck JL, et al (1987) Oxygen delivery and consumption in patients with hyperdynamic septic shock. Crit Care Med 15:26–28
56. Wolf YG, Cotev S, Perel A, et al (1987) Dependence of oxygen consumption on cardiac output in sepsis. Crit Care Med 15:198–205
57. Bihari D, Smithies M, Gimson A, et al (1987) The effects of vasodilation with prostacyclin on oxygen delivery and uptake in critically ill patients. N Engl J Med 317:397–403
58. Edwards JD, Brown GCS, Nightingale P, et al (1989) Use of survivors' cardiorespiratory values as therapeutic goals in septic shock. Crit Care Med 17:1098–1103
59. Vincent JL, Roman A, Kahn RJ (1990) Dobutamine administration in septic shock: Addition to a standard protocol. Crit Care Med 18:689–693
60. Martin C, Saux P, Eon B, et al (1990) Septic shock: A goal-directed therapy using volume loading, dobutamine and/or norepinephrine. Acta Anaesthesiol Scand 34:413–417
61. Palazzo MG, Suter PM (1991) Delivery dependent oxygen consumption in patients with septic shock: Daily variations, relationship with outcome and the sick-euthyroid syndrome. Intensive Care Med 17:325–332
62. Reinhart K, Bloos F, Konig F, et al (1991) Reversible decrease of oxygen consumption by hyperoxia. Chest 99:690–694
63. Bakker J, Coffernils M, Leon M, et al (1991) Blood lactate levels are superior to oxygen derived variables in predicting outcome in human septic shock. Chest 99:956–962
64. Mackenzie SJ, Kapadia F, Nimmo GR, et al (1991) Adrenaline in treatment of septic shock: Effects on haemodynamics and oxygen transport. Intensive Care Med 17:36–39

65. Edwards JD (1991) Oxygen transport in cardiogenic and septic shock. Crit Care Med 19:658–663
66. Steffes CP, Bender JS, Levison MA (1991) Blood transfusion and oxygen consumption in surgical sepsis. Crit Care Med 19:512–517
67. Tuchschmidt J, Fried J, Astiz M, et al (1992) Elevation of cardiac output and oxygen delivery improves outcome in septic shock. Chest 102:216–220
68. Wysocki M, Besbes M, Roupie E, et al (1992) Modification of oxygen extraction ratio by change in oxygen transport in septic shock. Chest 102:221–226
69. Silverman HJ, Tuma P (1992) Gastric tonometry in patients with sepsis. Effects of dobutamine infusions and packed red blood cell transfusions. Chest 102:184–188
70. Marik PE, Sibbald JW (1993) Effect of stored blood transfusion on oxygen delivery in patients with sepsis. JAMA 269:3024–3029
71. Ronco JJ, Fenwich JC, Tweeddale MG, et al (1993) Identification of the critical oxygen delivery for an anaerobic metabolism in critically ill septic and non-septic humans. JAMA 270:1724–1730
72. Moran JL, O'Fathartaigh MS, Peisach AR, et al (1993) Epinephrine as an inotropic agent in septic shock: A dose profile analysis. Crit Care Med 21:70–77
73. Vallet B, Chopin C, Curtis SE, et al (1993) Prognostic value of the dobutamine test in patient with sepsis syndrome and normal lactate values: A prospective multicenter study. Crit Care Med 21:1868–1875
74. De Backer D, Berré J, Zhang H, et al (1993) Relationship between oxygen uptake and oxygen delivery in septic patient: Effects of prostacyclin versus dobutamine. Crit Care Med 21:1658–1664
75. Ruokonen E, Takala J, Kari A, et al (1993) Regional blood flow and oxygen transport in septic shock. Crit Care Med 21:1296–1303
76. Lorente JA, Landin L, De Pablo R, et al (1993) Effects of blood transfusion on oxygen transport variables in severe sepsis. Crit Care Med 21:1312–1318
77. Feustel PJ, Fortune JB, Stratton H, et al (1990) Oxygen delivery and consumption in head-injured and multiple trauma patients. J Trauma 30:1259–1266
78. Fleming A, Bishop M, Shoemaker W, et al (1992) Prospective trial of supranormal values as goals of resuscitation in severe trauma. Arch Surg 127:1175–1181
79. Bishop MH, Shoemaker WC, Appel PL, et al (1993) Relationship between supranormal circulatory values, time delay and outcome in severely traumatized patients. Crit Care Med 21:56–63
80. Nimmo GR, MacKenzie SJ, Walker SW, et al (1992) The relationship of blood lactate concentration, oxygen delivery and oxygen consumption in septic shock and the adult respiratory distress syndrome. Anesthesia 47:1023–1028
81. Gutierrez G, Bismar H, Dantzker DR, et al (1992) Comparison of gastric intramucosal pH with measures of oxygen transport and consumption in critically ill patients. Crit Care Med 20:451–457
82. Maynard N, Bihari D, Beale L, et al (1993) Assessment of splanchnic oxygenation by gastric tonometry in patients with acute circulatory failure. JAMA 270:1203–1210
83. Yu M, Levy MM, Smith P, et al (1993) Effect of maximizing oxygen delivery on morbidity and mortality rates in critically ill patients: A prospective, randomized controlled study. Crit Care Med 21:830–838
84. Silverman HJ, Abrams J, Rubin LJ (1988) Effects of interleukin-2 on oxygen delivery and consumption in patients with advanced malignancy. Chest 94:816–821
85. Williams AJ, Mohsenifar Z (1989) Oxygen supply dependency in patients with obstructive sleep apnea and its reversal after therapy with nasal continuous positive airway pressure. Am Rev Respir Dis 140:1308–1311
86. Wendon JA, Harrison PM, Keays R, et al (1991) Arterial-venous pH differences and tissue hypoxia in patients with fulminant hepatic failure. Crit Care Med 19:1362–1364
87. Siegel J, Greenspan M, Del Guercio LRM (1967) Abnormal vascular tone, defective oxygen transport and myocardial failure in human septic shock. Ann Surg 165:504–508

88. Parrillo JE, Brach C, Shelhamer JH, et al (1985) A circulating myocardial depressant substance in humans with septic shock. J Clin Invest 76:1539–1545
89. Weil MH, Nishijima H (1978) Cardiac output in bacterial shock. Am J Med 64:920–927
90. Tuchschmidt J, Oblitas D, Fried J (1991) Oxygen consumption in sepsis and septic shock. Crit Care Med 19:664–671
91. Parker MH, Suffredini AF, Natanson C, et al (1989) Responses of left ventricular function in survivors and non-survivors of septic shock. J Crit Care 4:19–23
92. Tuchschmidt J, Fried J, Swinney R, et al (1989) Early hemodynamic correlates of survival in patients with septic shock. Crit Care Med 17:719–723

Designing the Optimum Clinical Trial for the Treatment of Sepsis

Critical Evaluation of the Design and Conduct of Previous Clinical Trials in Sepsis

C. J. Fisher and D. J. Cook

Introduction

Sepsis is the clinical manifestation of the host-derived systemic inflammatory response resulting from invasive infection. Sepsis begins with a nidus of infection, frequently gram-negative or gram-positive organisms, which proliferate and either invade the bloodstream (bacteremia) or release various substances into the bloodstream. Microbial cellular components such as endotoxin, peptidoglycan, teichoic acid antigen, or various exotoxins released by microorganisms are thought to initiate the host systemic inflammatory response by stimulating monocytes or macrophages, endothelial cells or neutrophils to release the endogenous mediators of sepsis. The most important of these mediators are the proinflammatory cytokines, tumor necrosis factor-α (TNF), IL-1, and IL-8. These proinflammatory mediators in turn initiate a cascade of events resulting in the Systemic Inflammatory Response Syndrome (SIRS). Sepsis syndrome may be viewed as a dysregulation syndrome of these messenger molecules. Once initiated, this clinical syndrome can become self-perpetuating and independent of the original infection. A variety of approaches have been attempted to modulate this cascade of events.

In this chapter, we critically appraise the clinical trials of therapy directed against the mediators of sepsis, and provide levels of evidence to aid in the interpretation of these studies according to their methodologic rigor. These trials are summarized in Table 1; a representative group of them is discussed in considerable detail in this chapter. Recommendations regarding future investigations in this field are also presented.

Steroids

In 1976, Schumer reported results using steroids in septic patients [1]. This study was conducted in a single center, was randomized and blinded, and reported data collected both retrospectively and prospectively. Both decadron and methylprednisolone were used as active study drugs. Although the study reported positive results, a combination of its poor study design, two different steroids and variable doses of steroids made it very difficult to

Table 1. Summary of clinical trials in sepsis: Levels of evidence

Intervention	Level of evidence	Recommendation
Steroids	1 meta-analysis of 9 RCTs (Level I)	Grade B Recommendation steroids are not recommended for routine clinical use in sepsis or septic shock
Monoclonal antibodies	2 RCTs 2 unpublished RCTs (Level I)	Grade A Recommendation Monoclonal antibodies are contraindicated in sepsis and septic shock
Polyclonal immunoglobulins	2 RCTs (Level II)	Grade B Recommendation Polyclonal immunoglobulins are not recommended for sepsis or septic shock
TNF antibodies	1 RCT 1 unpublished RCT Case Series (Level II)	Grade A Recommendation Anti-TNF is contraindicated for routine clinical use in sepsis or septic shock
Soluble TNF receptors	1 unpublished RCT Case Series (Level V)	Grade A Recommendation Soluble TNF receptor is contraindicated for routine clinical use in sepsis or septic shock
PAF receptor antagonists	1 RCT 1 unpublished RCT Case Series (Level II, V)	Grade B Recommendation PAF-antagonists are not recommended for routine clinical use in sepsis or septic shock
Antiserum	2 RCTs (Level II)	Grade B Recommendation J5Antisera is not recommended for routine clinical use in sepsis or septic shock
IL-1ra	2 RCTs (Level II)	Grade B Recommendation IL-1ra is not recommended for sepsis or septic shock

RCT – randomized clinical trial; Level I Evidence – published randomized clinical trials with adequate power or meta-analysis with homogeneity of individual trial results; Level II Evidence – published randomized clinical trials with possibility of type I or type II errors; Level V – published Case Series data

interpret. Subsequently, Sprung and colleagues [2] reported results from a single center demonstrating a transient benefit using steroids with no overall increase in survival. Based on this suggestive, albeit anecdotal, clinical data, as well as a large number of animal studies reporting very positive results using steroids (primarily methylprednisolone), two other large, well designed, clinical trials (out of eight conducted) will be described herein.

The Methylprednisolone in Severe Sepsis and Septic Shock Study Group evaluated the role of high-dose methylprednisolone sodium succinate in 382 patients [3]. This study, supported by Upjohn, was the first study in sepsis to use an optimal study design. The trial was prospective, multicenter, randomized, double-blinded, and placebo-controlled. High-dose methylprednisolone (30 mg/kg) was administered within two hours of the diagnosis of sepsis syndrome and repeated every 6 h for a total of 4 doses. Block randomization was used and a small dose of mannitol plus 5% dextrose in water (D5W) was used as the placebo. The study endpoints were 14-day mortality and reversal of shock. Overall, the study results were negative. However, in patients with creatinine greater than 2.0 mg/dL, mortality doubled and reversal of shock fell by 50% in the methylprednisolone treated group. Retrospective analysis of the effect of methylprednisolone in ARDS demonstrated that steroids were deleterious. Some controversy remains regarding the interpretation of the elevated creatinine in one group and the apparent increase in the incidence of shock and mortality in the steroid group.

The VA Cooperative Clinical Trial of Steroids in Sepsis [4], also supported by Upjohn, reported their trial at the same time. The entry criteria differed slightly, most notably by the inability to admit patients with an altered mental status who were not able to give their own informed consent. The result of this difference is seen in the lower placebo mortality found in the VA Cooperative trial. This trial also reported no benefit with steroids (give dose regimen) but did not show a statistically significant deleterious effect on 14-day mortality. Similar to the Methylprednisolone Sepsis Study, the VA Cooperative Trial was prospective, multicenter, randomized, double-blinded, and placebo-controlled (small dose of mannitol plus D5W, as above). Unfortunately, the VA Cooperative Trial was stopped prematurely, and therefore, did not enroll the total number of patients defined in its original analytical plan. Even if full patient accrual had occurred, the study would have been negative, based on the results reported.

Although there is a scientific rationale for the potential role for steroids in sepsis and septic shock, two well conducted clinical trials to date have failed to demonstrate any benefit. Meta-analysis of all 9 clinical trials using steroids (see Chapter by J. Carlet et al.) remains unconvincing (Level I Evidence).

Anti-endotoxin Approaches

Endotoxin is the lipopolysaccharide (LPS) component of gram-negative cell walls; lipid A is to biologically active component of endotoxin which is highly conserved among different gram-negative species. Approximately two-thirds of all cases of sepsis syndrome are associated with gram-negative bacteria and it has been demonstrated that endotoxin stimulates release of TNF-α, IL-1, IL-6, IL-8 and platelet activating factor (PAF), resulting in many of the severe systemic manifestations of gram-negative sepsis. Therefore, endotoxin, and in particular, lipid A, are attractive targets for immunotherapy.

Antiserum

In 1982, Ziegler et al. reported the results of a polyclonal, human antiserum obtained from volunteers vaccinated with a mutant (J5) strain of *Escherichia coli* [4]. The volunteers were firemen who were phlebotomized for control preimmune serum and then were vaccinated with the mutant J5 *E. coli.* Three hundred four patients were carefully screened over a 7 year period by investigators from each study site for evidence of gram-negative infection associated with a systemic response, and 212 patients were enrolled into the trial. Entry into the trial, which was sponsored by NIH, was largely based on the clinical impression of gram-negative sepsis by the investigators rather than a specific menu of clinical entry criteria. The trial design was prospective, multicenter, randomized, double-blinded, and placebo-controlled (using preimmune serum). One hundred three patients received one unit of J5 antiserum with an observed mortality of 22% while 109 patients received one unit of placebo (preimmune serum) with an observed mortality of 39%, for a reduction in 14-day mortality of 44% ($p=0.01$). One hundred ninety-one (90%) of the 212 patients enrolled into the trial had gram-negative bacteremia.

Subsequently, Baumgartner et al. [6] evaluated J5 antiserum in surgical patients at high risk of developing septic shock. Overall, these authors found the incidence of shock to be 2.3 times higher in the 136 patients who received placebo (preimmune serum) compared to the 126 patients who receive J5 antiserum. When further analyzing the subgroup who underwent abdominal surgery, the incidence of shock was 5.6 times higher in the placebo treated group.

It would appear from these clinical trials that J5 antiserum is active and beneficial in patients with gram-negative infection. Unfortunately, J5 antiserum is difficult to standardize into reproducible doses and suffers from the potential infectious complications of using human blood products. Further, it is very important to note that in the trial of Ziegler et al. [5], only patients with gram-negative infections were enrolled and 90% of patients enrolled had gram-negative bacteremia. Clearly, therefore, the opportunity to demonstrate and effect against endotoxin was present. These facts alone totally differentiate this trial from any other clinical trial in sepsis.

At present, based on the above, antiserum is not recommended for the routine clinical use in sepsis (Level II Evidence).

Immune Globulin

An alternative approach to administering antiserum to patients with sepsis is to administer immune globulins. Unfortunately, despite a great deal of research, the data available to interpret the effectiveness of immunoglobulin supplemental therapy in patients with sepsis is, at best, meager. Most studies are small, and almost all fail significantly in clinical trial design, most notably through lack of randomization, lack of double-blind, or lack of concurrent placebo control. In 1988, Calandra and colleagues [7] reported the results of a randomized, double-blind clinical trial evaluating the effectiveness of IgG antibody purified from pooled plasma from *E. coli*-immunized volunteers. These authors reported no difference in mortality between patients given IgG antibody (30 patients) and those given standard IgG (41 patients). In 1991, Dominioni et al. [8] showed a reduction in mortality from 67 to 38% in 62 surgical patients (primarily abdominal) using supplemental IgG (Sandoglobulin) in patients with a sepsis score greater than 20. Recently, these authors have updated their observations with 100 patients total (1986 to 1994), with sepsis scores 17 or greater (L. Dominioni, personal communication). They report 37% mortality in the IgG treated group versus 61% in the placebo treated group ($p=0.05$).

Schedel [9] reported his results from a single center using a polyclonal immunoglobulin preparation IgGMA (Pentaglobin). Patients were enrolled in the trial over a 3-year period, only if they had a measurable endotoxin level >12.5 pg/mL and met sepsis syndrome criteria. Fifty-five patients were studied, and the mortality rate was 9 of 28 patients (32%) in the placebo group (no immunoglobin preparation) compared to 1 of 27 in the IgGMA (4%) treated group. It is interesting to note that survivors had lower endotoxin levels after 24 h and higher anti-lipid A IgG titers. Although this study is small and unblinded, it demonstrates the potential power of using endotoxin assays as a screening tool for study entry.

The results of other clinical studies using immunoglobulins are inconclusive regarding their effectiveness in reducing mortality in sepsis syndrome. These trials have enrolled between 24 and 329 patients with dosage ranging from 0.6 to 1.6 g IgG/kg body weight. Failure to detect significant reduction in mortality is, at least in large part, due to poor study design and inadequate sample size.

Immunoglobulins are not currently recommended for routine use in sepsis (Level II Evidence).

Monoclonal Antibodies To Endotoxin

Monoclonal antibodies to endotoxin have been developed using the heat-inactivated mutant J5 *E. coli* and two have been tested in humans. One is predominately human IgM (HA-1A, Centocor), produced by a heteromyeloma, and the other is murine in origin (E5, Xoma), developed in murine splenocytes and produced in mouse ascites.

Ziegler et al. [10] enrolled 543 patients over 18 months in a prospective, randomized, double-blind, placebo-controlled (albumin) clinical trial evaluating the effectiveness of a single dose of 100 mg of HA-1A in reducing 28-day all cause mortality in patients with gram-negative sepsis. Randomization generally resulted in balanced groups, although there were slight, statistically insignificant, imbalances in the organ failure subgroups, as well as the group infected with *Pseudomonas,* which favored the HA-1A treated group.

On an intention-to-treat analysis, HA-1A did not reduce mortality. The placebo mortality was 43% compared to 39% in the HA-1A treated group. However, in the subgroup with gram-negative bacteremia (200 patients), mortality was reduced by 39% ($p=0.014$). Mortality was reduced by 42% in patients with gram-negative bacteremia and shock ($p=0.017$).

Although these results with HA-1A appeared quite promising and led to licensing in most of Europe, the FDA requested a confirmatory trial. This trial was called the CHESS Trial (Centocor HA-1A Efficacy in Septic Shock) and was undertaken at 513 community hospitals (R. Mc Closky, personal communication). The entry criteria were suspected gram-negative infection with recent onset (within 24 h) of shock at study entry. The primary endpoint was 14-day all cause mortality in the predefined subgroup of patients with gram-negative bacteremia with shock present within 24 h of study entry. The study design called for 5000 patients to be enrolled with 1000 patients meeting the primary endpoint of gram-negative bacteremia and shock. Two thousand one hundred ninety-nine patients were enrolled in the trial. A prespecified interim analysis occurred when 500 patients with gram-negative bacteremia were enrolled. This interim analysis revealed that the mortality in patients without gram-negative bacteremia who received HA-1A, exceeded the placebo mortality ($p=0.1$). On this predetermined stopping rule, the trial was stopped. By the time the trial was finally stopped, 621 patients with gram-negative bacteremia were enrolled and the difference between the HA-1A treated group without gram-negative bacteremia and placebo was not significant ($p=0.13$, which would not have stopped the trial). Based on this interim analysis, HA-1A was voluntarily withdrawn from the European market and withdrawn by Centocor from the FDA evaluation process. Unfortunately, due to the poor study design and the lack of data collected, we will never know if there were imbalances between the study groups or if there was a true detrimental effect of HA-1A to explain these results.

Greenman et al. [11] enrolled 486 patients with 468 evaluable patients over a 17 month period in a prospective, randomized, double-blind, placebo-controlled clinical trial evaluating the effect of two doses of the murine IgM monoclonal antibody E5 (2 mg/kg at study entry and 2 mg/kg at 24 h) on reducing the 30-day all cause mortality in patients with gram-negative sepsis. Randomization was generally well matched with the exception of the age distribution (64 years in the placebo group which was higher than the treated group at 60 years, $p=0.05$).

E5 did not reduce mortality in the intention-to-treat analysis. On retrospective analysis, E5 reduced mortality in the subgroup (137 patients) with gram-negative infection without shock from 43% in the placebo to 30% in the E5 treated group. In patients with refractory shock, mortality was 45% in E5-treated patients compared to 40% in the placebo treated patients. Refractory shock in this trial was defined as shock that did not respond to either fluid resuscitation or vasopressor therapy.

Based on the results of the first trial, a second randomized, double-blind, placebo-controlled (human serum albumin) was performed with the primary endpoint being 30-day mortality in patients with gram-negative infection without shock at study entry. Eight hundred forty-seven patients were randomized and 530 had documented gram-negative infection. Mortality was 70% in the E5 group and 74% in the placebo group ($p=0.21$). E5 improved the resolution of organ dysfunction present at study entry in the first trial, but failed to reproduce this result in the second trial. Currently, a third trial with E5 is under way.

At present, the evidence to support monoclonal antibody therapy directed against endotoxin is non-conclusive and at present this therapy should still be considered experimental (Level II Evidence). Further details on this important subject may be found in the chapter by T. Calandra and J. D. Baumgartner.

Anti-tumor Necrosis Factor Approaches

TNF-α is thought to play a major role in shock and organ failure associated with sepsis. Considerable experimental evidence exists to suggest that blocking TNF-α may prevent the sequelae and reduce mortality of septic shock. In 1990, Exley and Cohen [12] first reported administering a murine IgG monoclonal antibody directed against human TNF-α (CB0006, Celltech) to 14 patients with septic shock. No untoward reactions were observed. Recently, Fisher and colleagues [13] reported the first prospective, randomized clinical trial using a murine monoclonal anti-TNF antibody (CB0006). This trial was open-label with escalating doses of CB0006. Eighty patients were enrolled and no survival benefit was found for the total study population, but 35 patients with increased circulating TNF concentrations (>50 pg/mL) present at study entry appeared to benefit by the high dose anti-TNF antibody treatment (86% 28-day survival).

The North America Septic Shock Trial 1 (NORASEPT-1) using a murine IgG anti-TNF monoclonal antibody (Bayer-Miles) was stopped in July 1992 following an interim analysis which demonstrated futility for an overall positive outcome but suggested the possibility of a treatment effect in the patients with septic shock (J. Wherry, personal communication). A follow-up NORASEPT-2 clinical trial in patients with septic shock was initiated in January, 1994. The results of NORASEPT-1 have not been published at this time. Centocor recently conducted a Phase I–II trial using their chimeric anti-TNF antibody (cA2) alone and in combination with HA-1A. This is the first time combination immunotherapy has been administered to humans with sepsis (J. Zimmerman, personal communication). The trial was not designed to determine efficacy. At the time of this writing, two Phase II clinical trials using a Fab′2 murine anti-TNF antibody (Knoll) which is highly human specific have been completed (C. J. Fisher and K. Reinhart, personal communications).

At the present time, insufficient clinical data exist to support the use of anti-TNF monoclonal antibodies in the routine management of sepsis (Level II Evidence).

Soluble TNF Receptors

An alternate approach to anti-TNF monoclonal antibodies is soluble TNF receptors. These receptors are shed from the cell surface and bind circulating TNF before it can signal the target cell. These receptors have been cloned and fused in a variety of fashions with IgG. The preliminary results of the soluble TNF receptor (rhu TNFR:Fc) from Immunex unfortunately revealed a negative dose-response result which is alarming (C. J. Fisher, personal communication). The results of this clinical trial will require careful review because of the potential ramifications of a deleterious response to an anti-TNF approach. A clinical trial with another soluble TNF receptor (Roche) has just been started.

Anti-Interleukin-1 Approaches

Interleukin-1 (IL-1) is a major endogenous mediator in the sepsis cascade. The administration of TNF-α or IL-1β either alone or in combination has been shown to reproduce many of the physiologic and laboratory changes observed in animal models and patients with sepsis syndrome. Several possible approaches to IL-1 blockade exist, including soluble IL-1 receptors, antibodies directed against IL-1 receptor, inhibition of IL-1 converting enzyme, and IL-1 receptor antagonist (IL-1ra). Only IL-1ra has been tested in clinical trials.

IL-1 Receptor Antagonist

IL-1ra is a naturally occurring human protein, produced by macrophages and other cells in response to IL-1, endotoxin, and other microbial products, which recognizes and binds to both Type I and Type II IL-1 receptor, yet possesses no IL-1 agonist activity.

Fisher et al. [14] recently published the results of a Phase II randomized, open-label, placebo-controlled clinical trial evaluating the dose-response efficacy of IL-1ra (Synergen). Ninety-nine patients were randomized into placebo or one of three treatment groups with IL-1ra given at 17, 67, or 133 mg/h. Mean APACHE II score at study entry was 22.3. At study entry, 65% of the patients were in shock and 30% were bacteremic. Intention-to-treat analysis revealed a dose-dependent survival advantage with IL-1ra treatment ($p=0.015$). Twenty-eight day all cause mortality rates were: 11 (44%) deaths among 25 placebo patients; 8 (32%) deaths among 25 patients receiving

IL-1ra 17 mg/h; 6 (25%) deaths among 24 patients receiving IL-1ra 67 mg/h; and 4 (16%) among 25 patients receiving IL-1ra 133 mg/h. A dose-related survival benefit was observed with infusion of IL-1ra in patients with septic shock at study entry (n=65; p=0.002) and in patients with gram-negative infection (n=45; p=0.04). A significant dose-related reduction in the APACHE II score was achieved by the end of infusion (p=0.038). Patients with an increased circulating IL-6 concentration of >100 pg/mL at study entry demonstrated a dose-related survival benefit with IL-1ra treatment (p=0.009).

Based on the promising results of the Phase II trial, a Phase III trial was conducted and recently reported by Fisher and colleagues [15]. This trial was a prospective, randomized, double-blind, placebo-controlled trial evaluating the efficacy of IL-1ra in the treatment of patients with sepsis syndrome. The trial consisted of three arms: placebo; 1.0 mg/kg/h of IL-1ra; and 2.0 mg/kg/h of IL-1ra. Patients received an initial loading dose of 100 mg of IL-1ra or placebo infused over 60 sec followed by study drug infused intravenously for 72 h. Eight-hundred ninety-three patients were enrolled at 63 centers. A significant increase in survival time was not observed with IL-1ra treatment compared to placebo in all patients studied (n=893, generalized Wilcoxon statistic, p=0.22) or in patients with shock at study entry (n=713, generalized Wilcoxon statistic, p=0.23), the two primary efficacy analysis specified *a priori* for this trial. This corresponds to a 15 and a 14% reduction in 28-day all cause mortality, respectively. Results from secondary analysis using endpoints specified *a priori* suggest an increase in survival time with IL-1ra treatment in patients with one or more organ dysfunction (ARDS, DIC, renal dysfunction, and/or hepatobiliary dysfunction) present at study entry (n=563, linear dose-response, p=0.009). In patients with a predicted risk of mortality >24%, a retrospective analysis demonstrated an increase in survival time with IL-1ra treatment (n=580, linear dose-response, p=0.005). This corresponds to a 22% reduction in 28-day all cause mortality. Further, retrospective analysis combining patients with both > one organ dysfunction and a predicted risk of mortality >24% (n=411, linear dose-response, p=0.002) also demonstrated an increase in survival time.

Although the intention-to-treat results of the Phase III IL-1ra trial were not significant, they were within the 95% confidence limits of the Phase II trial. Further, and perhaps of greater interest, are the results of the prespecified organ failures. These criteria can be readily applied at the bedside to identify patients who may benefit from this therapy. Of equal note, is the use of risk assessment as a tool to stratify patients regarding potential benefit for immunotherapy. Future trials may well benefit from using these tools in their trial design. A follow-up Phase III trial of IL-1ra using this approach is currently under way.

At present, IL-1ra is a promising experimental agent for the treatment of sepsis, currently not recommended for routine clinical use (Level II Evidence). Future studies will define the role of this therapy in the treatment of patients with sepsis syndrome.

Anti-Platelet Activating Factor Approaches

In addition to the major proinflammatory cytokines TNF and IL-1, bioactive lipids, especially platelet activating factor (PAF), play a significant role in mediating the endogenous response to sepsis. Platelet activating factor is produced by a variety of cells, including endothelial cells, platelets, leukocytes, monocytes and lymphocytes and is a potent phospholipid, autocoid mediator involved in sepsis. Because PAF is stimulated by endotoxin, and potentially by gram-positive bacterial products, it is an attractive target for immunotherapy.

PAF Receptor Antagonist

A variety of structurally different PAF antagonists have been tested in gram-negative sepsis in animals and been proven beneficial. Dhainaut and colleagues [16] have recently reported the results of the first clinical trial using a PAF-antagonist (BN 52021, Beaufour-Ipsen) in clinical sepsis. This was a prospective, randomized, double-blind, placebo-controlled trial. Two-hundred sixty-two patients were enrolled and received either a 120 mg dose of BN 52021 intravenously every 12 h over a 4-day period, or placebo. The intent-to-treat 28-day all cause mortality was 51% for the placebo and 42 % for the BN 52021 group (p=0.17). However, in patients with gram-negative sepsis, there were 30 deaths (57%) among the 53 placebo patients compared to 22 deaths (33%) among the 67 BN 52021 treated patients (p=0.01). Further, in the subgroup of patients with gram-negative sepsis who were in shock at study entry mortality was 65% for the placebo compared to 37% for the BN 52021 treated patients (p=0.01). Although this was a negative study on a intent-to-treat basis, once again, the subgroup with gram-negative infection with or without shock demonstrates efficacy on subgroup analysis. Currently, a Phase III trial with BN 52021 is nearing completion (J.F. Dhainaut, personal communication).

The currently available evidence is insufficient to recommend routine clinical use of anti-PAF treatment in the management of sepsis (Level II Evidence).

What Have We Learned?

Although no Phase III clinical trial has demonstrated a positive result on an intent-to-treat analysis yet, much can be learned from these studies. There appears to be a consistent theme that the subgroup of patients with gram-negative infection (with or without bacteremia) is a population which demonstrates responsiveness to immunotherapy. This is true with a variety of immunotherapeutic approaches as has been demonstrated. Although targeting this population may appear difficult, we believe this is a solvable problem. Further, it appears that patients with one or more organ failures present at study entry are discriminating in terms of demonstrating efficacy. In addition, shock also appears to be a marker of septic patients who may be responsive to immunotherapy, although one must be careful with the definition. Finally, the evolving field of risk assessment appears very promising in terms of stratifying patients and perhaps using risk assessment in combination with organ failure to identify patients at greatest risk with maximal opportunity to benefit from these novel therapies.

Recommendations for Future Research

1. Large multicenter, double-blind, placebo-controlled randomized trials of sufficient power are necessary to maximize internal validity, minimize random error, avoid type II error and enhance the generalizability of trial results.
2. Definitions for the target population must be explicit, reproducible, and include illness severity scores.
3. Protocols for the investigational treatment, as well as cointerventions (antibiotics, etc.) should be standardized.
4. Outcomes should be clinically relevant, reproducible, specified *a priori*, and should include both measures of benefit and harm.
5. Analyses should be planned *a priori*, and include, at a minimum, an intention-to-treat analysis and a power calculation.
6. All patient outcomes (withdrawals, drop-outs, cross-overs, success and failures) should be reported.
7. Full and rapid reporting of all clinical trials in sepsis, regardless of their results, is mandatory, to avoid publication bias and to inform the ICU community about this rapidly growing literature.

References

1. Schumer W (1976) Steroids in the treatment of clinical septic shock. Ann Surg 184:333–341
2. Sprung CL, Caralis PV, Marcial EH, et al (1984) The effect of high-dose corticosteroids in patients with septic shock. N Engl Med 311:1137–1143
3. Bone R, Fisher CJ, Clemmer T, et al (1987) A controlled clinical trial of high dose methylprednisolone in the treatment of severe sepsis and septic shock. N Engl J Med 317:653–658
4. The Veterans Administration Systemic Sepsis Cooperative Study Group (1967) Effect of high-dose glucocorticosteroid therapy on mortality in patients with clinical signs of systemic sepsis. N Engl J Med 317:659–665
5. Ziegler EJ, McCutchan JA, Fierer J, et al (1982) Treatment of gram-negative bacteremia and shock with human antiserum to a mutant Escherichia coli. N Engl J Med 307:1225–1230

6. Baumgartner JD, Glauser MP, McCutchan JA, et al (1985) Prevention of gram-negative shock and death in surgical patients by antibody to endotoxin core glycolipid. Lancet 2:59–63
7. Calandra T, Glauser MP, Schellekens J, Verhoef J (1988) Treatment of gram negative septic shock with human IgG antibody to Escherichia coli J5: A prospective, double-blind, randomized trial. J Infect Dis 158:312–319
8. Dominioni L, Dionigi R, Zanello M, et al (1991) Effects of high dose IgG on survival of surgical patients with sepsis scores of 20 or greater. Arch Surg 126:236–240
9. Schedel I, Driekhausen U, Nentwig B, et al (1991) Treatment of gram-negative septic shock with an immunoglobin preparation: A prospective, randomized clinical trial. Crit Care Med 19:1104–1113
10. Ziegler EJ, Fisher CJ, Sprung CL, et al (1991) Treatment of gram negative bacteremia and septic shock with HA-1A human monoclonal antibody against endotoxin. N Engl J Med 324:429–436
11. Greenman RL, Schein RMH, Martin MA, et al (1991) A controlled clinical trial of E5 murine monoclonal IgM antibody to endotoxin in the treatment of gram-negative sepsis. JAMA 256:1097–1102
12. Exley AR, Cohen J, Buurman W, et al (1990) Murine monoclonal antibody to recombinant human tumor necrosis factor in the treatment of severe septic shock. Lancet 335:1275–1276
13. Fisher CJ, Opal SM, Dhainaut JF, et al (1993) Influence of an anti-tumor necrosis factor monoclonal antibody on cytokine levels in patients with sepsis. Crit Care Med 21:318–327
14. Fisher CJ, Slotman GJ, Opal SM, et al (1994) Initial evaluation of human recombinant interleukin-1 receptor antagonist in the treatment of sepsis syndrome: A randomized, open-label, placebo-controlled multicenter trial. Crit Care Med 22:12–21
15. Fisher CJ, Dhainaut JF, Opal SM, et al (1994) Recombinant human interleukin-1 receptor antagonist in the treatment of patients with the sepsis syndrome: Results from a randomized, double-blind, placebo-controlled trial. JAMA (in press)
16. Dhainaut JF, Tenaillon A, Le Tulzo Y, et al (1994) Platelet activating factor receptor antagonist BN 52021 in the treatment of severe sepsis: A randomized, double-blind, placebo-controlled multicenter trial. Crit Care Med (in press)

Evaluation of the Adequacy of Source Control

J. C. Marshall and S. F. Lowry

Introduction

The management of life-threatening infection rests on three principles:

1. optimal physiologic resuscitation and support;
2. debridement of devitalized tissue, drainage of abscesses, and definitive surgical management of ongoing sources of contamination; and
3. administration of systemic antimicrobial therapy to which the infecting organism is sensitive.

The advent of mediator-directed therapy has introduced the prospect of a fourth principle: that of selective modulation of the injurious sequelae of the host response. However, although the systemic inflammatory mediator response may contribute to morbidity in critical illness, it also plays a critical role in the early localization and elimination of an infectious challenge [1–3]. Animal studies demonstrate that mediator manipulation can have diametrically opposite effects depending on the adequacy of the control of infection [4], raising the distinct possibility that benefit or harm in the clinical arena may depend on the adequacy of the control of a focus of infection.

The term *source control*, as it is used here, can be defined as those physical measures undertaken to eradicate a focus of infection, to eliminate ongoing microbial contamination, and to render the local environment inhospitable to microbial growth and tissue invasion. Source control is the mainstay of the treatment of life-threatening infection, while antimicrobial therapy as appropriately viewed as adjunctive therapy. But while the principles of optimal supportive care and antimicrobial therapy can be assessed on the basis of data from a number of controlled clinical and laboratory studies, source control as a concept has been established more on the basis of surgical dictum, and there are few data that permit the evaluation of specific approaches.

The objectives of this chapter will be to review the biologic principles of source control as they apply to the study of novel mediator-directed therapy, to summarize available approaches to the evaluation of the adequacy of source control, and to propose a generic approach to the evaluation of source control in the context of clinical trials of mediator-directed therapy in sepsis.

Source Control: The Biologic Rationale

Outcome following an infectious challenge can be conceptualized as a function of three factors: the inoculum of the infecting organism and its intrinsic virulence, the adequacy of the innate host response, and the nature of the environment in which the infection evolves [5]. It is intuitively evident that measures that will reduce the size of the infecting inoculum or alter the local environment to favor local host defenses over microbial proliferation will lead to an improved clinical outcome.

Animal studies demonstrate that the size of the bacterial inoculum is an important factor in determining whether an experimental challenge will be successfully cleared by the host [6–8]; epidemiologic studies of wound infection support this hypothesis [9]. Conversely, a critical objective of source control techniques is a reduction of the microbial load.

For a given inoculum of microorganisms, outcome is significantly dependent on systemic factors reflecting the status of antigen-specific and non-specific host immunity [7, 10, 11] as well as on local environmental factors that can be potentially modified by the particular technique of source control. Normal host defenses can be impaired, and microbial infectivity increased, by the local presence of such adjuvants as foreign bodies including suture materials [12], devitalized tissue [13], barium sulfate [14], hemoglobin [8], and fibrin [15]. Even the presence of significant volumes of sterile saline in the peritoneal cavity will impair local host defenses [16]. It follows from this that the surgical management of an infectious focus should strive to remove devitalized tissue and foreign debris, and to secure careful hemostasis [17].

Finally, early studies demonstrated that a delay in the treatment of experimental infection resulted in impairment of local host defense mechanisms, and a reduced susceptibility to antimicrobial agents [6]; clinical studies of peritonitis [18, 19] and necrotizing soft tissue infections [20] confirm that delay in therapy is associated with increased mortality.

A large number of experimental models have been developed to study the biology of overwhelming infection and endotoxemia and the effects on outcome of various interventions [21]. It is striking that surgical therapy has not been evaluated systematically in these models, and that few, if any, include a maneuver directed towards control of the source of infection in their design. Not only is the biologic rationale for source control poorly defined, but its impact on outcome has not been adequately factored into experimental models.

Divergent Effects of Response Manipulation in Models of Controlled and Uncontrolled Infection

The biologic rationale for mediator-directed therapy in sepsis is a large body of experimental evidence that activation of the endogenous host systemic inflammatory response is responsible for much of the morbidity and mortality associated with systemic infection [1, 22, 23]. Teleologically, however, it is apparent that a phenomenon as well-conserved as the systemic inflammatory response must have evolved to subserve a role that has survival benefit for the host: experimental studies support the hypothesis that the septic response is an important component of the early, non-specific response to infection and of the pathways that effect microbial killing. The corollary of this hypothesis is that the effects of mediator antagonism will differ depending on whether the experimental challenge is live bacteria or bacterial products, and on whether or not an infectious challenge has been satisfactorily contained.

The experimental literature is replete with reports that demonstrate that modulation of endogenous host defenses can have contradictory consequences, depending on the nature of the challenge. Tumor necrosis factor (TNF) has been shown to be a critical early mediator of the physiologic sequelae of endotoxin [24], and administration of a blocking antibody to TNF protects mice against endotoxin challenge [25], and primates against gram-negative bacteremia [26]. However administration of TNF itself is protective in a rodent model of disseminated infection [27], and interruption of the normal interactions between TNF and host cells compromises the normal biologic response against *Listeria monocytogenes* [28, 29]. Competitive blockade of interleukin 1 (IL-1) with the IL-1 receptor antagonist (IL-1ra) provides protection in models of endotoxemia [30] and bacteremia [31], while the administration of IL-1 is protective in a model of gram-negative peritonitis [32] or in neonatal gram-negative bacteremia [33]. A similar dichotomy is seen with the anti-inflammatory cytokine, IL-10, whose administration is beneficial in endotoxemia [34], but whose blockade is protective in systemic *Candidiasis* [35].

The contradictory results of cytokine manipulation in animal models argue for caution in the use of these strategies in the clinical situation. It is unknown which, if any, of the numerous animal models of invasive infection best models the process as it arises in the complex setting of human critical illness [21]; descriptive clinical studies suggest that the usual clinical entry criteria for such trials define an heterogeneous group of patients whose outcome is independently influenced by factors reflecting the presence and control of infection, the severity of the clinical septic response, and the degree of organ dysfunction that develops [36].

It must be acknowledged that we are not currently able to stratify patients with clinical evidence of sepsis into groups that are homogeneous with respect to their underlying disease or their predicted response to mediator manipulation, and this inability to differentiate patients who might benefit from such interventions from those who might be made worse is likely a factor in the inconsistent or contradictory results obtained from early clinical trials involving antagonism of IL-1 or TNF. Careful evaluation of source control in patients entered into clinical trials becomes a critical part of the *post hoc* evaluation of these experimental therapies.

Evaluation of Source Control

There is currently no standardized approach to the evaluation of the adequacy of source control for clinical trials in sepsis; such evaluations are generally performed by a clinical evaluation committee on a case by case basis. In the absence of consensus on the critical components of such an evaluation and in the face of limited data upon which to base consensus, this model remains the optimal available approach. It is obviously important that the individuals performing these evaluations be experienced in the clinical management of these complex disease processes, and in the advantages and weaknesses of differing approaches.

Our objective here is to outline what we see as the important issues to be addressed in assessing the adequacy of source control. The development of a formalized approach to such a process will not only standardize practices, but will permit *post hoc* analyses of the impact of the adequacy of source control on the response to therapy.

Components of the Evaluation of Source Control

Evaluation of the adequacy of source control techniques requires consideration of a number of factors.

Was Culture-proven Bacterial or Fungal Infection Present? A recurring problem in clinical trials of mediator-directed therapy has been an *a priori* failure to identify at least one infecting organism in as many as one quarter or one third of patients studied. Although such therapies may have efficacy in the treatment of non-infectious causes of the systemic inflammatory response syndrome, both the biologic rationale of mediator manipulation and the need for homogeneity in the patient groups studied demand that a concerted effort be made to document the presence of an infectious process prior to patient enrollment. Moreover, it is incumbent on the principle investigator to make this determination: the complexity of the patient population studied is such that it is inappropriate to leave patient selection to the study nurse or junior house staff.

The need to document the presence of infection at the outset of the study places a greater emphasis on the type of source control techniques employed, for it carries an implicit obligation to define and treat a discrete process, rather than simply to place faith in the dubious efficacy of broad spectrum empiric antimicrobial therapy.

Was the Infection One for Which Measures beyond Supportive Care and Antimicrobial Therapy are Indicated? Most viral and some non-viral infectious diseases (meningitis, spontaneous bacterial peritonitis, and disseminated *Candidiasis,* for example) are treated exclusively by supportive measures and antimicrobial therapy. For most bacterial infections, however, additional source control measures are indicated. Pneumonia, for example, is managed by suctioning and chest physiotherapy to drain secretions, while the therapy of secondary bacterial peritonitis is directed towards correction of the underlying problem responsible for peritoneal contamination (often involving surgical resection and diversion of gastrointestinal contents), debridement of injured tissue, and drainage of discrete foci of infection. Source control measures applicable to specific infections are summarized in Table 1; they include the removal of contaminated foreign bodies, relief of obstruction and anatomic correction of sites of ongoing bacterial contamination, debridement of devitalized tissue, and drainage of discrete abscesses or collections of infected material.

If a process amenable to source control techniques is identified, then the adequacy of the measures employed must be assessed.

Were Adequate Measures Undertaken to Control the Identified Source of Infection? Definitive management of a focus of infection entails such measures as the surgical or percutaneous drainage of an abscess, debridement of necrotic tissue, and removal of colonized foreign bodies. The optimal therapy for a given clinical situation will be influenced by a number of factors, making generalizations about specific interventions difficult. In the management of intraabdominal infections, for example, appropriate management

Table 1. Source control methods for common ICU infections

Site of infection	Source control techniques
Sinusitis	Drainage of sinuses
Pneumonia	Physiotherapy, suctioning
Empyema	Drainage, decortication
Mediastinitis	Drainage and debridement Diversion
Peritonitis	Resection, repair, or diversion of ongoing sources of contamination Drainage of abscesses Debridement of necrotic tissue
Cholangitis	Bile duct decompression
Pancreatic infection	Drainage or debridement
Urinary Tract	Drainage of abscesses Relief of obstruction Change catheter
Line-related bacteremia	Remove catheter, change site
Endocarditis	Valve replacement
Septic arthritis	Joint drainage and debridement
Soft tissue infection	Debridement of necrotic tissue Drainage of discrete abscesses
Prosthetic device infection	Device removal

options range from percutaneous drainage under ultrasound or CT guidance [37] to strategies involving planned relaparotomy or an open abdomen approach [38]; benefits for one approach over another have not been established. Removal of a colonized central venous line or Foley catheter is a simple and effective means of source control for catheter-related bacteremia and cystitis respectively. The decision to remove an infected foreign device may be very difficult, however, if the device is an infected vascular graft or a heart valve [39].

Were Sources of Ongoing Microbial Contamination Adequately Controlled? Definitive source control of a focus of invasive infection requires not only adequate debridement and drainage, but also measures taken to eliminate ongoing contamination. In the case of perforated sigmoid diverticulitis, for example, standard therapy entails not only drainage of local infection, but also resection of the diseased colon and proximal fecal diversion by means of a colostomy, the so-called Hartmann procedure [40]. In other locations, where surgical resection is not feasible, control of ongoing contamination may be achieved by ensuring that a well-controlled fistula has been created.

Was the Implementation of Adequate Source Control Measures Undertaken in a Timely Fashion? Beyond the steps taken to treat a local focus of infection, evaluation of the adequacy of source control measures must also consider the timeliness of such intervention; delay in the institution of adequate surgical therapy appears to be a significant risk factor for the development of the multiple organ dysfunction syndrome (MODS) [41, 42].

Approaches to the Evaluation of Source Control

The disease processes responsible for life-threatening infection in the critically ill are complex, and consequently, the evaluation of the adequacy of source control is difficult. Because formal models for the assessment of source control have not been developed, there is a need for retrospective studies to develop and test such models. Ideally these would be performed using existing databases of patients enrolled in clinical trials of biologic response modification, testing the hypothesis that the adequacy of source control has a differential impact on survival in the control and experimental arms of such trials.

The adequacy of source control can be expressed as a binary categorical variable -adequate or inadequate-, however conversion to an ordinal or a continuous variable reflecting the extent to which source control is optimal could facilitate the process of developing and testing such an evaluative tool. Several complementary approaches are available to evaluate source control in individual cases; each has its advantages and limitations.

Expert Consensus on the Approach Employed: The adequacy of a particular source control technique can be evaluated prospectively, before the clinical outcome is known, by consideration of the specific therapy instituted. Such an approach necessitates the establishment of an expert panel, blinded not only to the treatment group but also to the outcome of the particular case. Decisions regarding the adequacy of therapy are made with reference to optimal standards of practice at the time the therapeutic decision was made, without consideration of whether the approach led to survival of the patient. For example, in considering a patient with perforated sigmoid diverticulitis and a localized left lower quadrant abscess, an expert panel might consider percutaneous CT-guided abscess drainage or a Hartmann resection as adequate therapy, drainage and proximal diversion as suboptimal therapy, and proximal diversion alone as inadequate therapy. Such a decision would be dependent not on the subsequent course of the patient, but on the evaluation of the panel regarding the optimal approach at the time the attending surgeon was faced with the clinical decision.

Evaluation of source control by a consensus panel permits the optimal evaluation of a novel agent under real life clinical conditions when the therapeutic decision must be made, and provides for the incorporation of the intangible element of clinical judgment into the evaluation of therapy. At the same time, however, it introduces an inescapable element of subjectivity, and makes it difficult to develop objective criteria to aid in deciding which patients might benefit from therapy.

Radiographic Evidence of Adequate Response to Therapy: The adequacy of many source control measures can be evaluated radiographically by documenting the resolution or persistence of the focus of infection. Follow-up evaluation by CT-scan or ultrasonography can define whether a persistent undrained collection is present, while sinograms can ascertain whether adequate drainage of a breach of the GI tract has been achieved.

Although it is possible to establish *a priori* radiographic criteria for the evaluation of the adequacy of source control measured against a gold standard of retrospective clinical judgment, these criteria will of necessity be inadequate. A residual fluid collection on an abdominal CT-scan may reflect undrained infection or loculated sterile fluid; a therapeutic decision is generally made by interpreting the radiographic findings in light of the clinical state of the patient. Moreover certain processes that clearly need source control intervention (intestinal infarction as an example) are not well-diagnosed radiographically.

Microbiologic Evidence of the Adequacy of Source Control: The persistence of an infecting organism despite systemic antimicrobial therapy suggests that the source of the infection has not been adequately controlled. For example, recurrent bacteremia is an indication for valve replacement in patients with endocarditis [43], and may suggest suppurative thrombophlebitis requiring vein excision [44]. Similarly, microbial persistence in the dialysate of patients on chronic ambulatory peritoneal dialysis suggests either colonization of the catheter requiring its removal, or a perforation of the GI tract [45].

The use of microbiologic criteria for the evaluation of the adequacy of source control has limitations. Cultures may be rendered negative in a patient with ongoing contamination by the concomitant use of antibiotics, moreover persistent culture positivity from a drain situated in an intraabdominal abscess or empyema cavity may reflect adequate, rather than inadequate source control. For many common infectious processes the correlation between microbial cultures and the presence of infection is weak. It has been suggested, for example, that the absence of bacteremia is a sign of intraabdominal infection in the patient manifesting a fever following laparotomy [46].

Attenuation of the Clinical Manifestations of SIRS as a Measure of the Adequacy of Source Control: In clinical practice, the resolution of clinical manifestations of a systemic inflammatory response (SIRS) is most commonly used to evaluate the overall response to therapy. Stone et al. [47] evaluated more than 2500 patients enrolled in 11 prospective trials of antibiotic therapy and found that no patient developed recurrent infection when the temperature and white counts were normal, and the differential smear showed fewer than 73% granulocytes, at the time of discontinuation of antibiotic therapy; in contrast recurrent infection developed in 19% of patients who only had a normal temperature, and in 3% of patients who had a normal temperature and white count, but an abnormal differential. Although the persistence of SIRS is generally held to be an indication for further investigation or more definitive source control intervention, there are few data available to evaluate the accuracy of this belief.

While the resolution of signs of systemic inflammation is common following appropriate therapy for patients outside the ICU, clinical manifestations do not correlate well with the presence of infection, or the adequacy of its therapy in the critically ill patient [23]. Non-infectious causes of SIRS including tissue trauma and drug reactions are relatively common in the ICU; conversely, systemic manifestations may be blunted by coexistent immunosuppressive disorders or the use of corticosteroids. While resolution of SIRS may suggest that source control is adequate, persistent SIRS is by no means specific for inadequate source control.

Persistence or Resolution of Organ Dysfunction as a Measure of the Adequacy of Source Control: The development of MODS has been classically associated with uncontrolled, often occult, infection [48, 49], an association that stimulated enthusiasm for the surgical technique of blind laparotomy-abdominal exploration undertaken to control an occult infectious focus in the absence of radiographic evidence of abdominal infection [50]. Uncontrolled infection is a common cause of MODS, and evidence of remote organ dysfunction in the critically ill patient should trigger an aggressive search for an unidentified focus of infection [5, 48], particularly when MODS evolves rapidly, or arises in the setting of a complicated disease process. However, like SIRS, organ dysfunction in the critically ill patient is not specific for uncontrolled infection, moreover adequate control of infection does not necessarily lead to the reversal of organ dysfunction [51]. In the absence of a systematic method of describing the severity of MODS, the association of organ dysfunction with infection is primarily conceptual and qualitative, and organ dysfunction lacks utility as a quantitative measure of the adequacy of source control.

Autopsy Evidence of the Adequacy of Source Control: The gold standard for the evaluation of the adequacy of source control is *post mortem* examination. A careful *post mortem* examination should be undertaken in every non-survivor enrolled in clinical trials in sepsis, and consent for such examinations must be vigorously sought.

In summary, the adequacy of source control may be evaluated by a number of complementary methods including expert consensus on the approach employed, objective radiographic or microbiologic findings, and evidence of the persistence or resolution of the acute and chronic manifestations of the systemic inflammatory response. Its failure may often be determined at the time of autopsy. None of these methods is by itself definitive, moreover there is a striking paucity of published data to permit their evaluation.

When Should the Adequacy of Source Control be Determined?

The adequacy of source control requires evaluation at two separate times within the context of a clinical trial of a novel therapeutic agent for sepsis: at the time that therapy is instituted, and retrospectively, after the patient has recovered or died. These evaluations address, respectively, the *effectiveness* and the *efficacy* of the experimental intervention.

An effectiveness study evaluates an intervention as it might be used in clinical practice. In the therapy of sepsis, much is unknown at the time that therapy is instituted. The use of immunotherapy for gram-negative infection, for example, was complicated by the fact that bacterial culture results were generally unavailable at the time the therapeutic decision was made [52]. Similarly, the logistical complexities involved in the care of the critically ill septic patient, and the inaccuracies inherent in clinical judgment result in inevitable delays or errors in management. Such problems are an inescapable reality of practice, and an effective therapy is one that can confer benefit even in the imperfect context of the real world.

The evaluation of source control as part of an effectiveness study requires that the evaluation be made on the basis of information that was available (or could have been available) to the attending physicians. Such an evaluation must rely heavily on expert consensus on the approach employed in the face of the available radiographic, bacteriologic, and clinical data.

An efficacy study evaluates the performance of an intervention under ideal circumstances. Efficacy analyses of mediator-directed therapy in sepsis are important for several reasons. They shed light on the *in vivo* biologic action of the agent, by assessing its action independent of the confounding effects of suboptimal therapy. Moreover, as the systemic inflammatory response becomes better characterized, and as new diagnostic approaches are developed, the basis for therapeutic decision-making may change, and studies based on older approaches may become obsolete.

The evaluation of source control as part of an efficacy study is by definition retrospective: the objective is to determine not whether the therapy selected was the optimal one, but whether the approach used, whether ideal or not, actually worked. Evaluation therefore depends on such factors as radiographic and bacteriologic improvement, clinical improvement, and, where available, autopsy results.

A Model for the Evaluation of Source Control

The adequacy of source control is a critical, but largely overlooked element of the evaluation of mediator-directed therapy in sepsis. Formal evaluation of the adequacy of source control must be a component of such clinical trials. Such evaluation must address both effectiveness and efficacy, and both should be reported when the study results are published. The approaches used for each of these evaluations differ (Tables 2 and 3), and ideally two separate evaluation committees should be established.

Effectiveness Evaluation

An effectiveness evaluation assesses therapy as it might be used in actual clinical practice. Since clinical decisions are categorical in nature (to treat or not to treat), an effectiveness evaluation should also be categorical (adequate or inadequate). This determination should be made through the process of a review of the data available at the time the patient was enrolled in the study, and by an expert panel including at least one intensivist and one

Table 2. Source control evaluation: effectiveness analysis

Objective	To determine whether the particular method of source control chosen at the time therapy was instituted was adequate or inadequate.
Approach	Expert panel, blinded to subsequent clinical course of patient, reviews clinical materials available at the time therapy was instituted.
Result of Evaluation	A categorical decision that the technique of source control was or was not adequate.

Table 3. Source control evaluation: efficacy analysis

Objective	To determine the adequacy of the method of source control in retrospect, judged against a gold standard of ideal therapy.
Approach	Review by committee of all materials available at the end of the study period to determine the adequacy of the technique of source control used, considering both the adequacy of the technique, and the timeliness of its use. Committee blinded to study arm.
Result of Evaluation	Grading of the adequacy and timeliness of intervention on a pre-established scale, for example: 1. optimal 2. minor concerns identified, unlikely to significantly affect outcome 3. moderate concerns with probability of significant effect on outcome 4. major concerns, highly likely to affect outcome.

surgeon. Under certain circumstances it may be appropriate for this panel to seek an independent assessment from a clinical expert in the specific area of the disease process being treated. This panel must remain blinded to the subsequent clinical course of the patient.

The mandate of the effectiveness evaluation committee is to determine whether the therapy instituted was the optimal approach, based on the data available at the time. Since both the clinical condition of the patient and the available data change over time, the committee should continue to review events over the first 48 or 72 h of therapy, to determine whether the clinical response to changing circumstances was adequate. Specific issues of interest to this process are summarized in Table 2.

Efficacy Evaluation

An efficacy evaluation assesses the performance of an intervention under ideal circumstances. Within the context of a clinical trial of mediator-directed therapy in sepsis, an efficacy evaluation can shed important light on the biology of the septic response, and on the identification of subgroups of patients who may benefit from the therapy. The evaluation is, of necessity, retrospective.

Source control evaluation as part of an efficacy analysis should evaluate two distinct aspects: the adequacy of control of the primary infectious process and of ongoing sources of contamination, and the timeliness of the source control intervention. Since this evaluation is retrospective, the efficacy evaluation committee can base its assessment on multiple factors including the appropriateness of the original intervention, bacteriologic and radiologic evidence of control of the source of infection, the resolution of clinical manifestations of SIRS, findings at the time of subsequent operative interventions, and, in the case of deaths, the results of *post mortem* examination. To facilitate *post hoc* data analysis, decisions regarding the success of drainage should be separated from those involving the timeliness of intervention. Moreover, the use of a scale to evaluate the adequacy of source control more accurately reflects the clinical reality that the management of a given case is a continuum of varying degree of success. It may be appropriate to evaluate efficacy at more than one time point, for example, at the time that therapy is initiated, at the conclusion of the experimental intervention, and at fixed time points subsequently.

Conclusions

Formal evaluation of the adequacy of source control is a critical component of any study to evaluate new strategies for the treatment of sepsis. Because modulation of the systemic inflammatory response may impair a critical component of local host defenses, it is biologically reasonable to expect that the net benefit of such a therapeutic strategy will depend on the adequacy of control of a focus of infection.

A formal template for the evaluation of source control has not yet been developed; indeed given the paucity of data available, the development of model approaches must await the availability of data from trials that have already been conducted. Nonetheless, the broad outlines of an evaluative process can be developed, as we have suggested here. Evaluation of source control should be performed from the perspective of both an effectiveness evaluation and an efficacy evaluation; differing approaches are required for these assessments.

The disappointing and often contradictory results of the initial forays into the field of therapeutic manipulation of the host inflammatory response [53, 54] suggest that we do not yet know which patients should receive these interventions. This underlines the need to develop models that evaluate differences in disease process and therapeutic adequacy, rather than simply generic illness severity [55]. The development of strategies for the formal evaluation of the adequacy of source control is an essential element of this process.

Recommendations

1. The adequacy and timeliness of source control is an important determinant of outcome in severe infection, but an under-emphasized component of the design and evaluation of clinical trials in sepsis.
2. A formal evaluative process to assess source control should be a component of the design of every trial of novel therapies in sepsis; this evaluation should include separate effectiveness and efficacy analyses.

3. An effectiveness analysis evaluates the adequacy of therapy at the time the therapeutic decision was made. Such an analysis should be performed by a committee with adequate representation from practising intensivists and surgeons; the committee is mandated to review the source control procedures instituted based on a review of clinical data available at the time of study entry. The committee must be blinded to the subsequent clinical course of the patient, and the decision of the committee is a categorical one, that source control was or was not adequate.
4. An efficacy analysis evaluates the performance of the experimental therapy under ideal conditions of source control. The efficacy analysis should be performed by a separate committee, also comprising practising intensivists and surgeons and blinded to the study arm, but not to the clinical outcome of the patient. The committee should have access to all clinical and laboratory data describing the course of the patient over the duration of the trial, and its conclusions should grade the adequacy of source control on a scale.
5. The evaluation of the adequacy of source control should take into account:
   - documentation of the presence of infection at the time of diagnosis of the septic process and the institution of therapy
   - timing relative to onset of the disease process
   - appropriateness of the actual technique of drainage or source control
   - persistence or resolution of the primary process based on clinical, bacteriologic, and radiographic parameters
   - the adjuvant measures undertaken to ensure optimal control (e.g. proximal diversion, debridement, resection)
   - complications directly a result of the method of source control (for example, bleeding or organ injury)
6. The development of methods for the formal evaluation of source control is a priority in future studies of the epidemiology of sepsis.
7. It is highly desirable that existing databases from completed trials in sepsis be available for study to assist in the development of appropriate evaluative models.

References

1. Lowry SF, VanZee KJ, Moldawer LL (1992) Strategies for modulation of systemic and tissue cytokine responses to sepsis. In: Lamy M, Thijs LG (eds) Update in Intensive Care and Emergency Medicine. Volume 16: Mediators of Sepsis. Springer-Verlag, Berlin, pp 345–361
2. Giroir BP (1993) Mediators of septic shock: New approaches for interrupting the endogenous inflammatory cascade. Crit Care Med 21:780–789
3. Natanson C, Hoffman WD, Suffredini AF, Eichaker PQ, Danner RL (1994) Selected treatment strategies for septic shock based on proposed mechanisms of pathogenesis. Ann Intern Med 120:771–783

4. Marshall JC (1994) Infection and the host septic response contribute independently to adverse outcome in critical illness: Implications for clinical trials of mediator antagonism. In: Vincent JL (ed) Yearbook of Intensive Care and Emergency Medicine 1994. Springer-Verlag, Berlin, pp 1–13
5. Meakins JL, Wicklund B, Forse RA, McLean APH (1980) The surgical intensive care unit: Current concepts in infection. Surg Clin N Am 60:117–132
6. Miles AA, Miles EM, Burke J (1957) The value and duration of defence reactions of the skin to the primary lodgement of bacteria. Br J Exp Pathol 38:79–96
7. Pennington JE (1979) Lipopolysaccharide Pseudomonas vaccine: Efficacy against pulmonary infection with Pseudomonas aeruginosa. J Infect Dis 140:73–80
8. Dunn DL, Nelson RD, Condie RM, Simmons RL (1993) Mechanisms of the adjuvant effect of hemoglobin in experimental peritonitis. VI. Effects of stroma-free hemoglobin and red blood cell stroma on mortality and neutrophil function. Surgery 93:653–659
9. Cruse PJ, Foord R (1973) A five-year prospective study of 23649 surgical wounds. Arch Surg 107:206–210
10. Cenci E, Romani L, Vecchiarelli A, Pucchetti P, Bistoni F (1989) Role of L3T4+ lymphocytes in protective immunity to systemic *Candida albicans* infection in mice. Infect Immun 57:3581–3587
11. Collins HH, Cross AS, Dobek A, Opal SM, McClain JB, Sadoff JC (1989) Oral ciprofloxacin and a monoclonal antibody to lipopolysaccharide protect leukopenic rats from lethal infection with *Pseudomonas aeruginosa*. J Infect Dis 159:1073–1082
12. James RC, McLeod CJ (1961) Induction of staphylococcal infection in mice with small inocula introduced on sutures. Br J Exp Pathol 42:266–277
13. Howe CW, Marston AT (1962) A study on sources of postoperative staphylococcal infection. Surg Gynecol Obstet 115:266–275
14. Bohnen JMA, Christou NV, Meakins JL (1987) Suppression of delayed cutaneous hypersensitivity and inflammatory cell delivery by sterile barium peritonitis. J Surg Res 43:430–435
15. Rotstein OD, Pruett TL, Simmons RL (1986) Fibrin in peritonitis. V. Fibrin inhibits phagocytic killing of *Escherichia coli* by human polymorphonuclear leukocytes. Ann Surg 203:413–419
16. Dunn DL, Barke RA, Ahrenholz DH, Humphrey EW, Simmons RL (1984) The adjuvant effect of peritoneal fluid in experimental peritonitis. Ann Surg 199:37–43
17. Meakins JL (1991) Surgeons, surgery, and immunomodulation. Arch Surg 126:494–498
18. Bohnen JMA, Boulanger M, Meakins JL, McLean APH (1993) Prognosis in generalized peritonitis. Relation to cause and risk factors. Arch Surg 118:285–290
19. Svanes C, Salveson H, Espehaug B (1989) A multifactorial analysis of factors related to lethality after treatment of perforated gastroduodenal ulcer 1935–1985. Ann Surg 209:418–423
20. Stamenkovic I, Lew PD (1984) Early recognition of potentially fatal necrotizing fasciitis. N Engl J Med 310:1689–1693
21. Fink MP, Heard SO (1990) Laboratory models of sepsis and septic shock. J Surg Res 49:186–196
22. Michalek SM, Moore RN, McGhee JR, Rosenstreich DL, Mergenhagen SE (1980) The primary role of lymphoreticular cells in the mediation of host responses to bacterial endotoxin. J Infect Dis 141:55–63
23. Marshall JC, Sweeney D (1990) Microbial infection and the septic response in critical surgical illness. Sepsis, not infection, determines outcome. Arch Surg 125:17–25
24. Tracey KJ, Beutler JB, Lowry SF, et al (1986) Shock and tissue injury induced by recombinant human cachectin. Science 234:470–474
25. Beutler B, Milsark IW, Cerami AC (1985) Passive immunization against cachectin/tumor necrosis factor protects mice from lethal effect of endotoxin. Science 228:869–871
26. Tracey KJ, Fong Y, Hesse DG, et al (1987) Anti-cachectin/TNF monoclonal antibodies prevent septic shock during lethal bacteremia. Nature 330:662–664

27. Alexander HR, Sheppard BC, Jensen JC, et al (1991) Treatment with recombinant human tumor necrosis factor-alpha protects rats against the lethality, hypotension and hypothermia of gram-negative sepsis. J Clin Invest 88:34–39
28. Nakane A, Minagawa T, Kato K (1988) Endogenous tumor necrosis factor (cachectin) is essential to host resistance against *Listeria monocytogenes* infection. Infect Immun 56:2563–2569
29. Pfeffer K, Matsuyama T, Kundig TM, et al (1993) Mice deficient for the 55 kd tumor necrosis factor receptor are resistant to endotoxic shock, yet succumb to *L. monocytogenes* infection. Cell 73:457–467
30. Ohlsson K, Bjork P, Bergenfeldt M, Hageman R, Thompson RC (1990) Interleukin-1 receptor antagonist reduces mortality from endotoxin shock. Nature 348:550–552
31. Wakabayashi G, Gelfand JA, Burke JF, Thompson RC, Dinarello CA (1991) A specific receptor antagonist for IL-1 prevents *E. coli*-induced shock in rabbits. FASEB J 5:338–343
32. Lange JR, Alexander HR, Merino MJ, Doherty GM, Norton JA (1992) Interleukin-1α prevention of the lethality of *Escherichia coli* peritonitis. J Surg Res 52:555–559
33. Mancilla J, Garcia P, Dinarello CA (1993) IL-1 receptor antagonist can either protect or enhance the lethality of *Klebsiella pneumoniae* sepsis in newborn rats. Infect Immun 61:926–932
34. Gerard C, Bruyns C, Marchant A, et al (1993) Interleukin 10 reduces the release of tumor necrosis factor and prevents lethality in experimental endotoxemia. J Exp Med 177:547–550
35. Romani L, Puccetti P, Mencacci A, et al (1994) Neutralization of IL-10 up-regulates nitric oxide production and protects susceptible mice from challenge with *Candida albicans.* J Immunol 152:3514–3521
36. Marshall JC, Shields J (1994) Infection, host response, and organ dysfunction contribute independently to outcome in sepsis syndrome: Towards a staging system for clinical sepsis. Presented at the 14th annual meeting of the Surgical Infection Society, Toronto, Ontario
37. Olak J, Christou NV, Stein LA, Meakins JL (1986) Operative vs percutaneous drainage of intraabdominal abscesses: Comparison of morbidity and mortality. Arch Surg 121:141–146
38. Christou NV, Barie PS, Dellinger EP, Waymack JP, Stone HH (1993) Surgical Infection Society intra-abdominal infection study. Prospective evaluation of management techniques and outcome. Arch Surg 128:193–199
39. Bandyk DF, Esses GE (1994) Prosthetic graft infection. Surg Clin N Am 74:571–590
40. Corder AP, Williams JD (1990) Optimal operative treatment in acute septic complications of diverticular disease. Ann Royal Coll Surg Engl 72:82–86
41. Fry DE, Pearlstein L, Fulton RL, Polk HC (1980) Multiple system organ failure. The role of uncontrolled infection. Arch Surg 115:136–140
42. Henao FJ, Daes JE, Dennis RJ (1991) Risk factors for multiorgan failure: A case-control study. J Trauma 31:74–80
43. Amoury RA (1988) Infections of the Heart. In: Howard RJ, Simmons RL (eds) Surgical Infectious Diseases. 2nd Ed. Appleton & Lange, Norwalk CT USA, Chapter 27
44. Hauser CJ, Bosco P, Davenport M (1989) Surgical management of fungal peripheral thrombophlebitis. Surgery 105:510–514
45. Spence PA, Mathews RE, Khanna R (1985) Indications for operation where peritonitis occurs in patients on chronic ambulatory peritoneal dialysis. Surg Gynecol Obstet 161:450–452
46. Le Gall JR, Fagniez PL, Meakins J, Brun-Buisson C, Trunet P, Carlet J (1982) Diagnostic features of early high post-laparotomy fever: A prospective study of 100 patients. Br J Surg 69:452–455
47. Stone HH, Bourneuf AA, Stinson LD (1985) Reliability of criteria for predicting persistent or recurrent sepsis. Arch Surg 120:17–20
48. Polk HC, Shields CL (1977) Remote organ failure: A valid sign of occult intra-abdominal infection. Surgery 81:310–313

49. Bell RC, Coalson JJ, Smith JD, Johanson WG (1983) Multiple organ system failure and infection in adult respiratory distress syndrome. Ann Intern Med 99:293–298
50. Hinsdale JG, Jaffe BM (1984) Re-operation for intra-abdominal sepsis: Indications and results in a modern critical care setting. Ann Surg 199:31–36
51. Norton LW (1985) Does drainage of intra-abdominal pus reverse multiple organ failure? Am J Surg 149:347–350
52. Ziegler EJ, Fisher CJ, Sprung CL, et al (1991) Treatment of gram-negative bacteremia and septic shock with HA-1A human monoclonal antibody against endotoxin. N Engl J Med 324:429–436
53. Siegel JP (1994) Clinical development of biological response modifiers. Can J Infect Dis 5 (Suppl A):S5A–S8A
54. Fisher CJ, Dhainaut J-F, Opal S, et al for the Phase III rhIL-1ra Sepsis Syndrome Study Group (1994) Recombinant human interleukin-1 receptor antagonist in the treatment of patients with sepsis syndrome. Results from a randomized, double-blind, placebo-controlled trial. JAMA 271:1836–1843
55. Knaus WA, Harrell FE, Fisher CJ, et al (1993) The clinical evaluation of new drugs for sepsis. A prospective study design based on survival analysis. JAMA 270:1233–1241

Statistical Considerations for the Design of the Optimal Clinical Trial

G. S. Doig and J. Rochon

Introduction

Although the general approach to the analysis of trials in sepsis therapy should be similar to the approach used for other intervention studies, there are several differences that make the field of sepsis research unique. Sepsis trials present a unique challenge because the patient population is heterogeneous, sepsis often presents with various comorbid disease states, and septic patients often receive different treatments for these comorbid states that are dependent on study center preferences.

Due to the slow rates of accrual at each study center, the typical sepsis randomized clinical trial is characterized by a large number of participating study centers each enrolling a few patients. Unfortunately these large multicenter trials have some not so obvious disadvantages with respect to costs, coordination and analysis. Many authors have previously dealt with comparisons of the design and conduct of single versus multicenter clinical trials, and these considerations are particularly relevant to the study of new therapies for sepsis [1, 2]. The purpose and focus of this chapter is to deal with statistical considerations particularly relevant to the conduct of the optimal multicenter randomized trial in sepsis therapy.

Trial Size in Sepsis Randomized Clinical Trials

A computerized search of the National Library of Medicine's Medline and the Institute for Scientific Information's Current Contents (Clinical Medicine) was performed using BRS On-line search services. Searching from 1966 to December 1993, using the key descriptors (MeSH headings) "sepsis" or "septic" and cross referenced with the text descriptor "random", a total of 120 abstracts were downloaded. Further investigation showed that 75 of these papers dealt with human subjects and of those 75, approximately 8 papers would qualify as Level I evidence (see chapter by Cook). All of the 8 Level I trials found by this search failed to show a significant treatment effect based on their primary intention-to-treat analysis.

The remaining trials all involve less than 100 patients and suffer from the problems inherent to all under-powered trials. Results from small trials can lead to two obvious types of errors: 1) the small trial is, by definition, underpowered and tends towards type II errors (declaring a difference to be nonsignificant when a true difference actually exists); and 2) due to the large confidence intervals generated by small numbers, positive results from small trials often tend to overestimate true treatment effects. The positive underpowered trial can thus lead to a third less obvious error: in using an optimistic overestimate of treatment effect, it is possible for subsequent trials to underestimate the sample size required to achieve the desired power and confidence.

The sepsis investigator has two primary methods with which to increase sample size: 1) conduct a long duration study in a single center; or 2) decrease the duration of the study by involving multiple centers. Of the 8 previously mentioned Level I sepsis trials, all have enrolled over 100 patients and all achieved this level of enrollment through the use of multiple study centers.

Multicenter Clinical Trials

The principle advantages of the multicenter trial are the faster rate of patient accrual and increased generalizability due to the increased number and diversity of participating centers. Since multicenter trials require the collaboration of the medical and research staff at each center, the trial often benefits from the input of many diverse talents. Unfortunately, this collaboration also often causes the trial to become sidetracked due to the lack of vision and direction from a single leading principal investigator.

An excellent example of the loss of direction that a multicenter design can suffer from is illustrated by a pair of articles from California. In the initial paper, Vasser et al. [3] investigated the use of a hypertonic saline/dextran solution for the resuscitation of trauma patients. Using an extremely well conceived single-center double-blind design, the investigators enrolled 166 trauma victims into initial resuscitation with either 250 mL 7.5% saline/6% dextran 70 or 250 mL lactated Ringer's solution. Analysis showed that treatment conferred a *trend* ($p=0.068$) towards survival in a clinically important subgroup: those with severe head trauma. The next logical step would have been to investigate this finding through either a refinement of study design or an increase in sample size.

The Multicenter Group for the Study of Hypertonic Saline in Trauma Patients, which was composed of some of the primary researchers involved in the previously mentioned study plus representatives of other contributing study centers, elected to investigate the problem further by increasing sample size through the design of a multicenter trial. The study design and blinding techniques of Vasser et al. [3] were adapted to include 6 trauma service systems and 4 fluid treatment groups (lactated Ringer's, 7.5% saline/6% dextran 70, 7.5% saline/12% dextran 70, and 7.5% saline) [4]. Enrollment of 386 patients resulted in approximately 80 patients per treatment group, which was extremely similar to the group size of the first study. Since the treatment groups were essentially the same size between the first single-center study and the subsequent multicenter study, the investigators lacked the statistical power to answer any of the questions raised by the first study. Had the investigators decided to maintain only 2 treatment groups (control and a single version of hypertonic saline), they probably could have contributed significantly to the dilemma of the use of hypertonic saline in the severe head trauma patient.

In addition to the problem of "research by committee", the multicenter trial can be very difficult to administrate and conduct. Most researchers have found that as the number of study centers increases, so do the problems associated with quality control, application of admission criteria, problems associated with enrollment, and number of protocol violations (Table 1). Addressing the problems associated with multicenter clinical trials can consume a large portion of the research budget, and an investigation of the cost relationships of various study combinations reveals that the most desirable design incorporates a large number of patients from a few study centers as opposed to a fewer number of patients from a large number of study centers.

Statistical Analysis

As a general principle, the primary analysis of any randomized control trial *must* be performed on an *intention-to-treat* basis. This means that as soon as the patient is randomized to a treatment arm, the patient is considered to have entered the study and must be included in the primary analysis whether or not the treatment is successfully completed.

Primary Outcomes

To date, all the major Level I sepsis studies have used all cause mortality as the primary study outcome, but have varied as to the follow-up period [5–8].

Table 1. Advantages of single versus multicenter studies

Single center
– improved quality control
– homogeneous patient population
– more cost effective
– can achieve large sample sizes over time
– simpler to analyze and interpret
Multicenter
– faster patient accrual
– increased generalizability of results
– collaboration improves quality

Total mortality as the primary outcome has the undeniable, highly desirable characteristics of being *unambiguous, easily measured,* and *important* [9].

The follow-up period of any clinical study should be sufficiently long such that the risk of outcome (mortality) due to the entry criteria (sepsis) is essentially zero at the conclusion of the study. Whatever the selected follow-up period, care must be taken to follow *all* patients for the complete duration of the trial in order to eliminate the possibility of selective dropouts.

The mortality rates reported in the control arms of the Level I ranges from 25 [5] to 43% (Table 2) [8]. Perhaps the best estimate of the mortality rate experienced by septic patients is provided by Knaus et al. [10], who used Bone et al.'s [5] definition of sepsis syndrome to classify patients. From the total collection of 58737 patients, 1195 met the criteria for sepsis syndrome and experienced a 28-day all cause mortality rate of 36%. Since mortality in sepsis is not a rare event, it does not limit effective study design and should therefore serve as the primary outcome for future studies.

Some interest has been expressed in using survival analysis [10], which would use a time to event (mortality) approach as the primary statistical outcome for sepsis trials. Time to event analysis is extremely important to consider when a therapy, such as AZT treatment for HIV infection, does not alter mortality rates, but may actually *delay* the onset of mortality and improve the quality of life experienced.

The primary advantage of the use of survival analysis is a small increase in statistical power, as compared to the direct comparison of mortality rates. Since most sepsis trials use 28-day mortality as the primary outcome, then survival analysis could only detect a significant improvement in patient' survival times over this study period. If this is the case, then given a therapy with a statistically significant survival time benefit, without evidence for a statistically significant mortality effect, the questions that must then be answered before survival time is adopted as the primary outcome are: Is a delay in mortality from day 3 to day 15 clinically important and does the patient benefit from having mortality delayed given that the extra time will most likely be spent in the ICU?

Recently, discussion has centered around using the joint distribution of a trend towards decreased mortality along with a significant benefit in organ

Table 2. Mortality experienced in control arms of sepsis studies

Trial	Ref.	Publication date	Mortality rate, %	95% CI, %	Patients No
Bone et al.	[5]	1987	25	19–31	191
Calandra et al.	[6]	1988	50	32–68	30
Ziegler et al.	[8]	1991	43	37–49	281
Knaus et al.	[10]	1993	36	33–39	1195
Fisher et al.	[14]	1994	44	25–64	25

function as the statistical outcome for future sepsis trials. Provided that the benefit to a specific organ system (e.g. renal, respiratory) has been explicitly demonstrated in previous studies, and that *unambiguous, easily measured* and *important* functional definitions of organ failure are applied (such as requirement for dialysis or mechanical ventilation), this approach could indeed result in fewer patients being required for definitive licensing studies. It should be noted however, that deviations from predicted mortality using scoring systems such as APACHE, MPM, SAPS or combined organ failure scores are not sufficiently accurate or precise to warrant their use as a surrogate mortality outcome in a well designed randomized clinical trial.

Controlling for Differences in Baseline Variables

Effective randomization and blinding are employed to remove potential sources of bias. Many definitions of bias exist in the statistical literature, but here we will use a working definition that includes *anything besides our treatment or random chance that can modify the strength and/or direction of the association between treatment and outcome.* Most randomized trials will employ a formal statistical test of baseline characteristics to determine if randomization "worked".

While statisticians will argue over the interpretation of P-values produced by comparison of randomized groups, most will agree that an imbalance in baseline characteristics should be explored for a potential effect on study outcome. In order for a baseline characteristic to have the potential to bias study results, it must be statistically associated with the study outcome *and* in a state of imbalance. If a baseline characteristic satisfies these two criteria, then it should be offered to a multivariate model to assess its impact on the treatment effect [11]. A multivariate model, when applied to large randomized trials, is much more desirable than stratification since more than one confounder can be investigated at a time. When a baseline measure is associated with both the treatment and the outcome, then it satisfies the classical definition of a confounding variable. These authors recommend that a P-value of less than 0.25 between randomized baseline groups should be used to indicate the potential for imbalance, and any groups displaying this level of imbalance should be assessed in a multivariate model to determine the magnitude and direction of their impact on treatment effect.

Since the addition of covariates to a multivariate model consumes degrees of freedom and further reduces the power of the investigation, additions to the model should be made judiciously and according to a previously determined methodology [11]. One approach would be to select a few, well researched, prognostic factors *a priori*, and adjust for only these factors if they satisfy the above outlined requirements of potential confounders. A list of possible prognostic factors is provided by Knaus in the chapter on Prognosis in Sepsis.

If all baseline characteristics are in balance, then the analysis of a single center trial resolves down to the application of a simple chi-square test, *t*-test or non-parametric test, depending on the study outcome.

Statistical control of confounders should be viewed as distinctly different from subgroup analysis. The intention of subgroup analysis is to investigate qualitatively different effects of treatment in clinically important subpopulations. When using additive multivariate models (least squares linear regression, logistic regression, survival regression), these qualitatively different effects are investigated by introducing treatment × factor interaction terms. Subgroup analysis based on prognostic factors can be performed if the factors are in balance after randomization (and hence do not qualify as confounders). Subgroup analysis is used for hypothesis generation, not hypothesis testing, and should never be used to alter overall trial conclusions.

Pooling Results Across Study Centers

As mentioned earlier, the decision to undertake a multicenter trial should not be taken lightly. Unfortunately, given the accrual rates for septic patients, the multicenter trial provides the only method for obtaining effective sample sizes within a realistic period of time. Multicenter trials should be designed such that: 1) the power is sufficient to show significance with the pooled treatment results; 2) there should be consistency over large centers in producing nominally significant results; and 3) there should be consistency over all centers with respect to direction of results. In order to meet all three criteria, there must be sufficient numbers of patients enrolled at each study center such that the effect estimators at each center are stable.

The basis for pooling treatment results across study centers depends on the satisfaction of 4 criteria: 1) the use of a common treatment protocol; 2) the uniform application of eligibility criteria; 3) equal motivation to enroll patients; and 4) randomization within study center [2]. As the number of centers involved in a study increases, so does the potential for the violation of one of these assumptions.

One of the major challenges to the sepsis researcher is the lack of homogeneity in the presentation of sepsis itself. Sepsis can present in a young healthy adult or in a geriatric trauma victim. The primary ICU admitting reason can be sepsis, or sepsis can be a complication in a patient receiving intensive care for a host of underlying disorders. Since study centers can range from large tertiary care teaching hospitals to smaller non-teaching community hospitals, these concurrent diseases (comorbidities) have the potential to be treated with vastly different approaches.

These differences in presentation, comorbidities and level of care can be controlled by randomization, but unfortunately patients are randomized *within* study centers, and not randomly assigned *between* study centers. This can result in significantly different patient populations and comorbidities at each center receiving different treatment regimes. Thus, with the combination of a lack of randomization between study centers, which can result in different patient populations at each center, and the presence of different treatment regimes for comorbidities at each center, we have the potential for a significant bias to enter into the analysis. This potential for bias is not new to most statisticians, especially those who have performed a meta-analysis, but this particular form of bias has been dealt with very poorly by previous sepsis multicenter randomized clinical trials.

Meta-Analysis and Study-Level Bias

In the field of meta-analysis, this potential for "study" bias is readily recognized and addressed. Since each study that contributes to a meta-analysis is conducted independently of the others, the study entry criteria, measurement of outcome and general study design all differ slightly. To control for these study differences, the overall estimate of treatment effect is obtained by using a model that considers the "contributions" of each study. The two most common models used are the fixed effects method of Mantel and Haenszel [12] and the random effects method of DerSimonian and Laird [13]. Individual studies can exhibit rather large effects in a meta-analysis, and although the potential exists for study centers to exhibit similar effects in sepsis trials, the magnitude of these effects will undoubtedly be much smaller [14].

Controlling for Study-Center Bias

The direction of the bias introduced by the possibility of study center effects could be either positive or negative on the overall outcome. Investigating and controlling for this potential bias will produce a more valid and unbiased estimate of treatment effect, but in order to effectively assess the impact of this bias, sufficient numbers of patients must be present in each study center. A rough estimate of the absolute minimum number of patients required at each study center to assess this "operator-dependent-variability" is 20 (10 treatment and 10 control patients).

The level of impact of the study center effect can be assessed statistically, and should the effect prove to be not statistically significant, then the data can be safely pooled and an analysis similar to the analysis conducted on a single center study can be conducted. If the study center effect is significant, then a pooling approach similar to that used in meta-analysis can be adopted to produce an unbiased estimate of overall treatment effect.

In the worst case scenario, as in meta-analysis, if a treatment × study center interaction exists, a valid overall treatment effect estimator cannot be obtained. In such a situation, the investigators must examine the clinical differences between study centers in detail to determine if a valid biological reason exists to explain the different treatment effects at each study center. Although it is not uncommon to have a significant interaction chi-square in meta-analysis, the institution of a common protocol at each study center of a multicenter trial makes this possibility less remote.

Conclusion

In order to accrue sufficient numbers of patients in a reasonable amount of time, a multicenter study design should be used to investigate novel sepsis therapies. The optimal design, from an analytical point of view, would include a few large study centers each accruing large numbers of patients as opposed to a large number of study centers each accruing a few patients.

To aid interpretation, reporting of future studies should include a breakdown of the number of patients accrued at, and mortality rate experienced by, each individual center. Reporting of each center's patient characteristics should also be included.

Accrual at each center should be of sufficient size so as to allow the interpretation of the direction and marginal significance of the results at individual centers. Prior to pooling the data, the assumptions supporting the ability to pool should be investigated by testing the significance of the study center effect and the homogeneity of individual center outcomes.

The estimators of overall treatment effect should be controlled for baseline prognostic factors that qualify as potential confounders and subgroup analysis should only be used for hypothesis generation, and not to modify the overall conclusion of the trial.

All of the above measures are required to ensure that the final estimator of treatment effect is valid and free from bias. If previous studies into potential therapies for sepsis had been more rigorously designed (from a statistical standpoint), perhaps we would have found useful some treatments that have been discarded, or at least perhaps we could have avoided costly, subsequent trials that proved futile and fruitless.

References

1. Meinart CL (1986) Single-center versus multicenter trials. In: Meinart CL (ed) Clinical trials: Design, conduct and analysis. Oxford University Press, New York, pp 23–30
2. Pocock SJ (1983) The size of a clinical trial: Multicentre trials. In: Pocock SJ (ed) Clinical trials: A practical approach. John Wiley & Sons, Chichester, pp 123–142
3. Vassar MJ, Perry CA, Gannaway WL, Holcroft JW (1991) 7.5% sodium chloride/dextran for resuscitation of trauma patients undergoing helicopter transport. Arch Surg 126:1065–1072
4. Vassar MJ, Fischer RP, O'Brien PE, et al and the Multicenter Group for the Study of Hypertonic Saline in Trauma Patients (1993) A multicenter trial for resuscitation of injured patients with 7.5% sodium chloride. The effect of added dextran-70. Arch Surg 128:1003–1011

5. Bone RC, Fisher CJ Jr, Clemmer TP, Slotman GJ, Metz CA, Balk RA (1987) A controlled clinical trial of high-dose methylprednisolone in the treatment of severe sepsis and septic shock. N Engl J Med 317:653–658
6. Calandra T, Glauser MP, Schellekens J, Verhoef J (1988) Treatment of gram-negative septic shock with human IgG antibody to Escherichia coli J5: A prospective, double-blind, randomized trial. J Infect Dis 158:312–319
7. Greenman RL, Schein RM, Martin MA, et al and The XOMA Sepsis Study Group (1991) A controlled clinical trial of E5 murine monoclonal IgM antibody to endotoxin in the treatment of gram-negative sepsis. JAMA 266:1097–1102
8. Ziegler EJ, Fisher CJ Jr, Sprung CL, et al and The HA-1A Sepsis Study Group (1991) Treatment of gram-negative bacteremia and septic shock with HA-1A human monoclonal antibody against endotoxin. A randomized, double-blind, placebo-controlled trial. N Engl J Med 324:429–436
9. Friedman LM, Schron EB (1992) Statistical problems in the design of antiarrhythmic drug trials. J Cardiovas Pharm 20 (Suppl 2):S114–S118
10. Knaus WA, Harrel FE, Fisher CJ, et al (1993) The clinical evaluation of new drugs for sepsis. A prospective study design based on survival analysis. JAMA 270:1233–1241
11. Beam TR, Gilbert DN, Kunin CM (1992) General guidelines for the clinical evaluation of anti-infective drug products. Clin Infec Dis 15 (Suppl 1):S5–S32
12. Mantel N, Haenszel W (1959) Statistical aspects of the analysis of data from retrospective studies of disease. J Natl Cancer Inst 22:719–728
13. DerSimonian R, Laird N (1986) Meta-analysis in clinical trials. Controlled Clin Trials 7:177–188
14. Fisher CJ, Slotman GJ, Opal SM, et al (1994) Initial evaluation of human recombinant interleukin-1 receptor antagonist in the treatment of sepsis syndrome: A randomized, open-label, placebo-controlled multicenter trial. Crit Care Med 22:12–21

The Monitoring and Reporting of Clinical Trials

R. J. Sylvester and F. Meunier

Introduction

A clinical trial may be defined as a carefully designed, prospective medical study which attempts to answer a precisely defined set of questions with respect to the effects of a particular treatment or treatments [1]. The first step in any clinical trial is to write a detailed protocol describing the trial's rationale and objectives, the treatments to be evaluated, and its conduct and logistics. If the results of a trial are to have an influence on the day-to-day practice of clinicians, the trial must be able to provide a *convincing reproducible* answer to an important question. It goes without saying that a poorly written protocol with insufficient attention being paid to the trial's methodology may not allow one to draw definitive, unbiased conclusions with respect to the question under study.

Scientifically rigorous clinical trials are essential to evaluate new therapeutic modalities or strategies, particularly in life threatening conditions such as sepsis. Norrby in particular has stressed the deficiencies which are often found in clinical trials of antibiotics and the need to carry out scientifically valid investigations [2–4]. The EORTC (European Organization for Research and Treatment of Cancer) Antimicrobial Therapy Cooperative Group reviewed the problems experienced and the lessons learned from four of their trials in febrile granulocytopenic cancer patients and set standards for the definition of infection and the criteria of response [5].

Controversy on the conduct of trials in sepsis still exists however with respect to such basic issues as the assessment of the outcome of therapy, both with respect to the definition of response and failure and also concerning whether or not modifications of the treatment regimen are permitted [6–8]. Clinical trials in sepsis have also become more complex over the past several years as new controversial therapeutic approaches are evaluated, including the use of glucocorticosteroids, pentoxifylline, naloxone, IL-1 receptor agonists, and anti-TNF and anti-LPS (endotoxin) monoclonal antibodies [9–10].

In an attempt to improve the design and conduct of clinical trials with anti-infective drugs and to update the 1977 US Food and Drug Administration (FDA) guidelines for the clinical evaluation of anti-infective drugs, the past several years have seen the publication of guidelines by a number of different authors and groups [11–16]. Of particular importance are the "guidelines for the evaluation of anti-infective drug products" [15] which were published in 1992 by the Infectious Diseases Society of America in cooperation with the FDA. These guidelines were subsequently adapted in 1993 by a European working party of the European Society of Clinical Microbiology and Infectious Diseases [16].

Over the past several years, the methodology of clinical trials has also become more and more complex with it becoming almost impossible for an isolated scientist to carry out a clinical trial by himself. Support for the conduct of clinical trials comes from various sources, such as the pharmaceutical industry, contract research organizations, various national groups, and international non-profit research organizations such as the EORTC. The EORTC, for example, provides the necessary infrastructure to aid its investigators in carrying out such trials. For non-pharmaceutical industry sponsored trials, the EORTC is the legal promoter of the trial and obtains the necessary trial insurance according to the legal requirements of the individual countries. The EORTC Data Center, which is specialized in the methodology of clinical trial design, conduct and analysis, is an essential ingredient in the conduct of EORTC phase II and phase III trials. The Data Center can also provide its expertise in new specialized areas of interest, such as in the fields of quality of life and health economics evaluations.

Previous chapters will have dealt with the need for carrying out randomized phase III trials when the goal is to compare the efficacy of two or more treatments. This chapter will emphasize the quality control, data monitoring, and reporting of results in the framework of multicenter, randomized phase III trials. The concepts presented in this chapter are based on the experience of the EORTC Data Center and are applicable to the conduct of phase III trials in general.

Quality Control and Data Monitoring of Clinical Trials

Inherent in the conduct of multicenter phase III clinical trials is the concept of a centralized data center whose task is to supply the necessary data management, computer, statistical and medical support for carrying out the trial. The various functions of such a data center are given in Table 1.

Quality control and data monitoring in a trial will be described in this chapter through a global overview of the tasks of the data manager, statistician, medical supervisor and study coordinator in such a multicenter setting, going from the design of a new trial to the publication of the final results.

Study Coordinator

The study coordinator is the clinician responsible for the overall conduct of the study. His tasks include: writing the protocol, helping to prepare the case

Table 1. Functions of a data center

1. Prior to study activation
   - Trial design and endpoints (including quality of life, health economics)
   - Statistical aspects: sample size, statistical analysis
   - Review of protocol prior to submission to a protocol review committee
   - Preparation and review of the case report forms
2. Trial execution
   - Central registration and randomization of patients
   - Collection, monitoring and quality control of data on the case report forms
   - Review of patient files by the medical supervisor and study coordinator (patient eligibility, response to treatment, side effects, mortality)
   - Computerization of patient data
3. Trial analysis
   - Preparation of interim administrative and statistical reports
   - Final statistical analysis
4. Participate in the publication of results

report forms (CRF), supervising the monitoring of the study, evaluating individual patient files, and presenting and publishing results. This is done in close collaboration with the personnel of the data center.

Medical Supervisor

The medical supervisor is responsible for insuring compliance of data center procedures with good clinical practice guidelines and to supervise all medical aspects related to the trials (protocol, CRF, trial monitoring, site visits, standard operating procedures, etc.).

Data Manager and Statistician

In conjunction with the medical supervisor, the data center statistician and data manager are involved with the following tasks:

Review of a New Protocol: At the design state, the statistician will review and amend the draft protocol which has been prepared by the study coordinator with respect to its methodology: the trial's design, objectives and endpoints, patient selection criteria, prognostic factors, criteria of evaluation, definition of endpoints, patient registration and randomization procedures, appropriate stratification factors, and the statistical considerations: sample size, trial duration and feasibility, statistical methods, interim analyses and early stopping rules.

The data manager will also review the draft protocol and write the sections dealing with the randomization checklist (questions asked at the time of the randomization) and the CRF: types of forms to be used and the form submission schedule.

All EORTC protocols must be written in a standardized format [1, 17] and then be approved by the EORTC protocol review committee prior to their activation.

Design of Case Report Forms: The first draft of the CRF is prepared by the data manager based on the protocol, input from the study coordinator and the medical supervisor, and experience from prior studies. They are then reviewed by the statistician, the medical supervisor, the study coordinator, other selected trial participants, and by various institutional data managers. The forms are then reviewed by the EORTC form review committee to assess their adequacy. Finally the forms will go through a pilot stage at the start of the trial so that they may be adapted if necessary prior to their final adoption.

Creation of the Registration/Randomization Procedure on Computer: A central registration/randomization is to be preferred to a system of envelopes in order to ensure that the randomization is correctly carried out without bias, that there is a uniform verification of the patient eligibility criteria, and that there has been a stratification for the most important prognostic factors [18]. In multicenter studies, it is recommended to stratify for the institution and for a small number of the most important prognostic factors using the minimization technique [18, 19]. A central randomization also permits the data center to know exactly how many patients have been entered in a trial at all times and their identity, thus allowing missing forms to be requested from the investigators.

Based on a general procedure for defining the questions to be asked at the time of randomization, the actual computer randomization is tailor made for each study. It involves inbuilt eligibility checks and warning messages, stratification for prognostic factors, takes into account lists of authorized/unauthorized investigators and provides the treatment assignment only once the required information has been furnished by the investigator.

The EORTC data center has implemented a centralized randomization via the EuroCODE (European Computerized Oncology Data Exchange) computer network whereby investigators can directly register and randomize patients 24 hours a day, 7 days a week. Such a system is highly desirable for sepsis trials where patients may need to be registered at any time of the day or night. EuroCODE also provides physician data query (PDQ), a database of cancer information and trials, to EORTC investigators.

Definition of the Database: The database is defined by content of the CRF. Each variable on a CRF is defined according to its type (date, categorical, integer or real), its name or index, its label or description, acceptable values or limits, coding of "unknown" values and whether the variable must be coded or may be left blank. The different types of forms may be filled out once for a given patient, for example the On Study form which provides patient characteristics prior to start of treatment, or they may be sequential forms and filled out more than once, Follow Up forms for example.

Computer Data Entry: Patient data received on the CRF are entered on computer by a keypuncher using a double entry technique to avoid typing errors. Alternatively, computer files containing the patient data defined on the CRF may be directly read into the computer.

Verification and Validation of Data on the Case Report Forms: All data entered on computer are initially read into a special "on hold" file until they are validated by the data manager. Data validation involves the following steps:

Data Validation by Computer: Data in the on hold file are subjected to a series of computer checks involving the range of permitted values, unknown values and missing values. Any data not within the specified limits are called to the attention of the data manager.

Review of the CRF and Protocol Compliance by the Data Manager: The CRF are reviewed with respect to the following aspects: patient eligibility, missing or inconsistent data, illegible data, protocol violations, misunderstandings of the protocol or of questions or codes on the CRF, the coding of comments, toxicity and serious adverse events. Whenever problems or questions arise, the medical supervisor and clinical investigators are contacted for clarification or for further information.

Computerized Cross-checks: Once the data manager is satisfied with the quality and correctness of the data, they are transferred to the master database where various computer cross-checks on the entire database for the trial can be carried out.

Data Modification: It should be emphasized that the data on the CRF are never modified without having obtained complementary explanations and the approval of the responsible physician. Any modifications that are made are done in accordance with the guidelines for good clinical practice (GCP) as explained below.

Review of Case Report Forms by the Study Coordinator: All patient files are reviewed by the study coordinator or by a special data review committee with respect to patient eligibility, protocol violations and response to treatment. This review forms part of a general quality control check on the participating institutions.

Implementation of Good Clinical Practice Requirements: In 1990, the European Community published a note for guidance concerning GCP for trials on medicinal products carried out in the European Community [20]. GCP is essentially a set of management tools designed to promote and maintain high quality data and to protect research subjects rights. This note covers the areas given in Table 2.

With respect to data monitoring these guidelines require that:

1. The data center establishes an internal quality control program and standard operating procedures.
2. The data center receives the original copy of the forms.
3. All corrections to the CRF must be initiated and they must not obscure the original entry.
4. All forms must be signed by the investigator.
5. The data center receives the curriculum vitae and bibliography of all investigators along with the normal laboratory values for their institution.

Reporting on the Progress and Conduct of the Trial: Feedback to the participants in the trial includes not only the reporting of problems pertaining to the patients they entered, but also 6 monthly status reports containing general administrative information about the trial: patient accrual rate by institution, patient ineligibility, protocol compliance, quality of the data, missing forms, patient characteristics, treatment side effects, and problems encountered in running the trial. In order not to bias the trial or to jeopardize future patient accrual, information concerning the relative treatment efficacy is not provided to the participants before the trial has been closed to patient entry.

Table 2. Areas covered by the EEC note for guidance on good clinical practice

1. Protection of trial subjects and consultation of ethics committees
   - Protection of trials subjects
   - Ethics committees
   - Informed consent
2. Responsibilities
   - Sponsor
   - Monitor
   - Investigator
3. Data handling
   - Investigator
   - Sponsor/monitor
   - Archiving of data
   - Language
4. Statistics
   - Experimental design
   - Randomization and blinding
   - Statistical analysis
5. Quality assurance

Interim Analyses and Interpretation of Efficacy Data: Interim statistical analyses of accumulating follow-up data are required in order to monitor the study with respect to efficacy, toxicity, and data quality, and to ensure that it is still ethical to continue patient entry in the trial [21, 22]. The frequency of such analyses depends on a number of factors such as the rate of patient entry in the trial and the event rate of the primary endpoint of interest.

Data Monitoring Committees: As previously mentioned, the presentation of interim results of treatment efficacy to trial participants while the study is still open to patient entry is not recommended since it may jeopardize further patient entry into trial, or may lead to investigators entering only very selected patients into the trial rather than all their eligible patients [23]. While in practice a data review or data monitoring committee composed at least of the study coordinator (who generally enters patients in the trial) and the trial statistician reviews the accumulating data, a completely independent data monitoring committee should be set up for this purpose in order to ensure a completely unbiased assessment of the data [22, 24–26].

Early Stopping Rules: A further problem in the monitoring and interpretation of accumulating data is related to the size of the type I and type II error rates α and β:
α = Prob(Reject the null hypothesis when the null hypothesis is true)
β = Prob(Accept the null hypothesis when the null hypothesis is false)

The more often accumulating data are analyzed, the greater the risk of rejecting the null hypothesis of no treatment difference just by chance unless special precautions are taken [27, 28].

Standard sequential designs call for the continuous monitoring and analysis of accumulating data. A truly sequential approach is not generally feasible due to the delay in observing the endpoint of interest. In practice, a small number of interim statistical analyses are carried out based either on the cumulative number of patients entered, the cumulative number of events observed, or on fixed calendar dates corresponding to meetings.

In the monitoring of data, one might be tempted to reject the null hypothesis of no treatment difference whenever $P<0.05$ at any interim analysis. If in fact there is no difference in efficacy between two treatments, then Table 3 presents the overall probability of finding a significant difference (rejecting the null hypothesis) if a number of interim analyses are each carried out at the nominal 5% level. If only one analysis is carried out, then by definition $\alpha = 0.05$. If on the other hand, 5 analyses are each carried out at the 5% level, then the size of the overall type I error is no longer 5%, but it is approximately 14%. Thus, even if there is no difference in efficacy between the two treatments to be compared, the probability of rejecting the null hypothesis of no treatment difference is approximately 14% if 5 different analyses are each carried out at the 5% level. As the number of analyses at the 5% level increases, so does the probability of incorrectly rejecting the null hypothesis of no treatment difference. This implies that one cannot declare a dif-

Table 3. Overall probability of finding a significant difference (rejecting the null hypothesis) if each analysis is carried out at the 5% level and there is no difference in treatment effect

Number of analyses	Overall significance level
1	0.050
2	0.083
3	0.107
4	0.126
5	0.142
10	0.193

Nominal Significance Level = 0.05

ference to be statistically significant as soon as the P value falls below the 5% level in a given analysis. Based on the number of analyses to be carried out, Table 4 presents the nominal significance levels to be used at each analysis in order to ensure an overall experiment wise error rate of 5%. If 5 analyses are to be carried out, then each analysis should be carried out at the 1.6% level in order for the overall level to be 5%.

This design is an example of what is more generally known as group sequential designs [29] whereby trial results are analyzed after each of K groups of observations become available. The advantage of group sequential designs is that they allow a trial to be stopped prior to the planned maximum sample size while controlling the size of the type I and type II errors.

There are 3 main types of group sequential early stopping rules which control the overall size of the type I error: those based on the Pocock design [30–31], the O'Brien-Fleming design [32], and the Peto design [29]. Examples of these designs are illustrated in Table 5 for the case of 2, 3 or 4 analyses.

Pocock Design

With the Pocock design, the same P value is used at each analysis. While this has the advantage that early interim analyses are carried out at less extreme P values than with the other two designs, it has the disadvantage that the final analysis must be carried out at a *more* extreme P value. There is thus less overall power to detect a given difference unless the sample size is increased by an inflation factor of between 10% and 30%.

Table 4. Significance level at which each analysis has to be carried out in order to maintain an overall significance level of 5%

Number of analyses	Nominal significance level
1	0.0500
2	0.0296
3	0.0221
4	0.0183
5	0.0159
10	0.0107

Table 5. Nominal significance levels at each analysis for early stopping in order to insure an overall level of $\alpha = 0.05$

Two Analyses			
Analysis	Pocock	O-F	Peto
1	0.029	0.005	0.001
2	0.029	0.048	0.05
Three Analyses			
Analysis	Pocock	O-F	Peto
1	0.022	0.0005	0.001
2	0.022	0.014	0.001
3	0.022	0.045	0.05
Four Analyses			
Analysis	Pocock	O-F	Peto
1	0.018	0.0001	0.001
2	0.018	0.004	0.001
3	0.018	0.019	0.001
4	0.018	0.043	0.049

O'Brien-Fleming Design
With the O'Brien-Fleming design, the nominal P value increases at each analysis. Early interim analyses are carried out using very extreme significance levels so that a trial is stopped very early on only for very small P values. It has the advantage that the final analysis can be carried out at *close* to the 5% level so that only a very small increase in the total sample size is required.

Peto Design
With the Peto design, each interim analysis is carried out at the 0.001 level which corresponds to 3 standard deviations. The final analysis is carried out at approximately the 0.049 level. Thus all interim analyses are very conservative, even the later ones. However it has the advantage that the final analysis can be carried out at approximately the 5% level so that no increase in sample size is required.

The disadvantage of all these designs is that it is necessary to pre-specify the maximum number of analyses to be done and that the analyses must be carried out at equal increments of information (patients or events). These conditions are not very practical, especially in the multicenter setting where analyses are timed to coincide with the meeting of cooperative groups or data monitoring committees.

Alpha Spending Functions: One solution to this problem is to use an alpha spending function which specifies how much alpha may be "spent" at each analysis according to the amount of information which is available [33]. With this technique, it is not necessary to prespecify the maximum number of analyses or to carry them out at equal increments of information. Thus one can test at arbitrary times, adjusting the nominal P value for the amount of information accrued.

There are many potential disadvantages to stopping a trial early [22]. In particular there may be a lack of credibility since small trials are not generally convincing due to their imprecision and the increased potential for bias. When an early stopping rule is used, there is no one rule which can be uniformly recommended. However an alpha spending function based on an O'Brien-Fleming design meets the practical requirements associated with many *long-term* clinical trials.

Reporting of Results of Clinical Trials

Simon [34] has stated that "the main purpose of clinical trials is to improve public health by generating and communicating knowledge about the presence or absence of treatment effectiveness". The confidence that a reader has in the validity of the reported findings is often influenced by the quality of the report. Clinicians need precise information to be able to judge whether the conclusions of the trial are relevant to their practice. The impact of clinical trials on medical practice is limited by difficulties in the communication of results, the interpretation of reports by practicing physicians and by the multiplicity of trials.

One particular problem in assessing the value of a given treatment is related to the concept of publication bias whereby studies with statistically significant findings are more likely to be published than those with non-significant results [35, 36]. This implies that literature reviews and even meta-analyses, both of which may have an important impact on general medical practice, may be biased if they are restricted to published trials. Temporary prominence may thus be given to treatments that are eventually found to be of no benefit. For this reason, it is important that the results of all trials be published. One step in this direction would be to establish a prospective register of all trials which are carried out in a given disease.

The quality of the reporting of results has been the subject of a number of surveys and publications [37–41]. The general conclusion is that there is still much room for improvement, not only with respect to the statistical content of the report, but also with respect to the format of the report itself. In 1985, George [39] published the results of a survey of the policies of medical journal editors with respect to statistical refereeing. Among 83 of 98 journals which responded, in 75% the decision about whether a statistical review was needed was taken by the editor and only 16% had a policy that guaranteed a statistical review. More recently in 1991, Altman [40] concluded that the misuse of statistics in medical journals was still far too common. He found that

1. There has been an increase in the use of statistical techniques employed;
2. Too many analyses are carried out, many of them incorrectly; and
3. The medical literature is obsessed with significant P values.

It is obvious that the incorrect reporting of results has serious consequences with respect to the every day care and treatment of patients.

As mentioned above, the reporting of results of treatment efficacy comparisons while the trial is still open to patient entry may seriously bias further patient accrual, treatment, and data collection and should thus be avoided [23]. In addition, the preliminary nature of the results may change with time and may not be consistent with the final results. The decision to publish a trial's results should always be based on a reasonable expectation that the results will not change if more follow-up data are collected.

Despite the fact that a number of authors have published checklists or guidelines for the publication of the results of a clinical trial [6, 42–52], considerable heterogeneity still exists in the literature. A general proposal for the format and content of published reports is given in Table 6. Specific details should take into account the recently published guidelines for the evaluation of anti-infective drug products [15, 16].

With respect to the reporting of comparisons of treatment efficacy:

1. Include *all* eligible patients in the main statistical analysis. The exclusion of inadequately treated patients or patients with protocol violations may seriously bias the treatment comparisons. That is, patients should be analyzed according to the intent-to-treat principle: analyze all patients as randomized without exclusions [53–54].
2. The analysis should be focused on the main endpoints described in the protocol and should generally include information concerning the response to treatment, reason for failure, cause of death, and adverse reactions.
3. Estimate time to event curves using the Kaplan-Meier technique [55] and compare them using a (non-parametric) test that takes into account the entire survival experience, possibly giving more weight to early deaths [56].
4. In addition to providing P values, provide an estimate of the size of the treatment effect or difference, and its 95% confidence interval [57–58].
5. For non significant results, provide the conditional power of detecting a treatment difference of the size specified in the protocol.
6. Indicate variables and methods used (retrospective stratification, multivariate models) to adjust treatment comparisons for prognostic factors.
7. Any subset analyses should be based on *a priori* hypotheses and interpreted very carefully. Conclusions should not be based on exploratory data analyses or data dredging [59].
8. The number and frequency of interim analyses should be reported along with the rationale for stopping the trial and reporting the results.
9. The necessary statistics to allow a trial's inclusion in a meta-analysis [60] should also be provided: for example (O)bserved, (E)xpected, var(O-E), and the odds ratio.

Note: the comparison of the survival of responders versus non-responders is not an acceptable method for showing therapeutic efficacy.

Table 6. Format for the reporting of results

1. *Introduction*
   - Background
   - Current state of knowledge
   - Goal and rationale of the trial

2. *Material and methods*

   A. Trial design
   - Type of trial
   - Design
   - Treatment assignment method
   - Endpoints

   B. Patient population
   - Inclusion/exclusion criteria
   - Diagnostic procedures used

   C. Treatments
   - Description
   - Time sequence
   - Dose modifications

   D. Pre-treatment and follow-up examinations
   - Required examinations and their frequency

   E. Criteria of evaluation and definition of (objective) endpoints
   - Response to treatment (clinical, microbiological)
   - – Colonization and further infection
   - – Need for treatment change or modification
   - – Concomitant supportive care
   - Survival/Cause of death
   - Adverse reactions

   F. Quality control
   - Data management
   - Extramural review
   - Site visits
   - Independent data monitoring committee
   - Patient compliance

   G. Statistical methods
   - Randomization technique
   - Stratification factors
   - Sample size determination
   - Statistical analysis techniques
   - Frequency of interim analyses
   - Early stopping rules
   - Policy of reporting interim results

3. *Results (by treatment group)*

   A. Descriptive statistics
   - Number of patients entered
   - Number of institutions
   - Period of patient accrual
   - Median and maximum duration of follow-up
   - Number of ineligible or not evaluable patients and reasons

B. Patient characteristics
   - Demographic factors (age, sex, etc)
   - Prior disease history and treatment
   - Underlying disease
   - Signs of sepsis and septic shock
   - Site and severity of infection (APACHE, SAPS, MPM, etc)
   - Nature of the invading micro-organism
   - Organ failure

   Note: the use of P values to compare the distribution of patient characteristics across treatment groups is meaningless

C. Treatment results (see text)

D. Toxicity
   - Attitude towards reporting side effects (relation to treatment)
   - Standardized grading scale
   - Documentation of toxic deaths
   - Late toxic effects

4. *Discussion/Conclusion*
   - Interpretation of results: Subgroup analyses – Surrogate endpoints
   - Consistency of results with other trials
   - Generalization of results to clinical practice
   - Clinical impact
   - New questions, future research

5. *References*

6. *Tables and Figures*

7. *Summary, Abstract, Key Words, Acknowledgments, Source of Financial Support*

Conclusion

There are still many controversies which exist regarding both the treatment and the evaluation of treatment efficacy in patients with sepsis. Studies will be carried out in order to determine the precise role of new promising agents. However, the criteria of response to treatment may vary from one group of investigators to the next making it difficult to put the results of different studies into their proper perspective. Should any treatment modification imply treatment failure or should the patient's overall treatment management be assessed?

These difficulties stress the need for a high level of cooperation and professionalism between all parties involved in the conduct of clinical trials in order to produce scientifically convincing results and to minimize the overall delay between the first testing or discovery of an effective new agent and its adoption in routine practice. Only well-controlled, large scale clinical trials will produce results which are convincing enough to have the necessary impact on daily clinical practice. In this respect, the involvement and value of a centralized data center which is specialized in the science and conduct of clinical trials cannot be overemphasized.

References

1. Sylvester R (1984) Planning cancer clinical trials. In: Buyse M, Staquet M, Sylvester R (eds) Cancer Clinical Trials: Methods and Practice. Oxford Medical Publications, Oxford, pp 47–63
2. Norrby SR (1984) Quality of antibiotic trials. J Antimicrob Chemother 14:205–208
3. Norrby SR (1990) Challenges in the design of trials to evaluate antibacterial agents in serious infections. J Hosp Infect 15 (Suppl A):13–22
4. Norrby SR (1993) Clinical trials of antibiotics: Need for better investigators. Int J Antimicrob Agents 3:139–143
5. Klastersky J, Zinner S, Calandra T, et al (1988) Empiric antimicrobial therapy for febrile granulocytopenic cancer patients: Lessons from four EORTC trials. Eur J Cancer Clin Oncol 24 (Suppl 1):S35–S45
6. Donnelly JP (1991) For Debate: Assessment and reporting of clinical trials of empiric therapy in neutropenic patients. J Antimicrob Chemother 27:377–387
7. Pizzo PA, Hathorn JW, Hiemenz J, et al (1986) A randomized trial comparing ceftazidime alone with combination antibiotic therapy in cancer patients with fever and neutropenia. N Engl J Med 315:552–558
8. Sanders JW, Powe NR, Moore RD (1991) Ceftazidime monotherapy for empiric treatment of febrile neutropenic patients: A meta-analysis. J Infect Dis 164:907–916
9. Baumgartner JD, Eggimann P, Glauser MP (1992) Management of septic shock: New approaches. In: Remington J, Swartz M (eds) Current Clinical Topics in Infectious Diseases. Blackwell Scientific Publications, pp 165–187
10. Bone RC (1991) A critical evaluation of new agents for the treatment of sepsis. JAMA 266:1686–1691
11. Infectious Diseases Society of America (1987) Report from the Antimicrobial Agents Committee. J Infect Dis 156:700–705
12. Gilbert DN (1987) Guidelines for evaluating new antimicrobial agents. J Infect Dis 156:934–941
13. Finch RG, Norrby SR, Reeves DS, et al (1989) The clinical evaluation of antibacterial drugs. J Antimicrob Chemother 23 (Suppl B):1–35
14. Immunocompromised Host Society (1990) The design, analysis and reporting of clinical trials on the empirical antibiotic management of the neutropenic patient. J Infect Dis 161:397–401
15. Beam TR, Gilbert DN, Kunin CM (1992) Guidelines for the evaluation of anti-infective drug products. Clin Infect Dis 15 (Suppl 1):S1–S346
16. European Society of Clinical Microbiology and Infectious Diseases (1993) In: Beam TR, Gilbert DN, Kunin CM (eds) European guidelines for the clinical evaluation of anti-infective drug products, pp 1–354
17. EORTC Data Center Procedures Manual, Second edition, September 1992, Brussels, Belgium
18. Lagakos S, Pocock S (1984) Randomization and stratification in cancer clinical trials: An international survey. In: Buyse M, Staquet M, Sylvester R (eds) Cancer Clinical Trials: Methods and Practice. Oxford Medical Publications, Oxford, pp 276–286
19. Staquet M, Dalesio O (1984) Designs for phase III trials. In: Buyse M, Staquet M, Sylvester R (eds) Cancer Clinical Trials: Methods and Practice. Oxford Medical Publications, Oxford, pp 261–275
20. EEC Note for Guidance: Good clinical practice for trials on medicinal products in the European Community (1990) Pharmacol Toxicol 67:361–372
21. Machin D (1992) Interim analysis and ethical issues in the conduct of trials. In: Williams CJ (ed) Introducing new treatments for cancer. JW Wiley & Sons, Chichester, pp 203–215
22. Pocock S (1993) Statistical and ethical issues in monitoring clinical trials. Statistics Med 12:1459–1469

23. Green SJ, Fleming TR, O'Fallon JR (1987) Policies for study monitoring and interim reporting of results. J Clin Oncol 5:1477–1484
24. Fleming TR, DeMets DL (1993) Monitoring of Clinical Trials: Issues and Recommendations. Controlled Clin Trials 14:183–197
25. PMA Biostatistics and Medical Ad Hoc Committee on Interim Analysis (1993) Interim analysis in the pharmaceutical industry. Controlled Clin Trials 14:160–173
26. Proceedings of "Practical issues in data monitoring of clinical trials" (1993) Bethesda, Maryland, USA. Statistics Med 12:415–416
27. McPherson K (1984) Interim analysis and stopping rules. In: Buyse M, Staquet M, Sylvester R (eds) Cancer Clinical Trials: Methods and Practice. Oxford Medical Publications, Oxford, pp 407–422
28. Armitage P (1991) Interim analysis in clinical trials. Statistics Med 10:925–937
29. Geller NL, Pocock SJ (1987) Interim analyses in randomized clinical trials: Ramifications and guidelines for practitioners. Biometrics 43:213–223
30. Pocock SJ (1977) Group sequential methods in the design and analysis of clinical trials. Biometrika 64:191–199
31. Pocock SJ (1982) Interim analysis for randomized clinical trials: The group sequential approach. Biometrics 38:153–162
32. O'Brien PC, Fleming TR (1979) A multiple testing procedure for clinical trials. Biometrics 35:549–556
33. Lan KKG, DeMets DL (1983) Discrete sequential boundaries for clinical trials. Biometrika 70:659–663
34. Simon R (1991) A decade of progress in statistical methodology for clinical trials. Statistics Med 10:1789–1817
35. Begg CB, Berlin JA (1989) Publication bias and dissemination of clinical research. J Nat Cancer Inst 81:107–115. Also in: Williams CJ (ed) Introducing new treatments for cancer. J Wiley & Sons, Chichester, pp 367–382
36. Dickersin K, Chan S, Chalmers TC, Sacks HS, Smith H (1987) Publication bias and clinical trials. Controlled Clin Trials 8:343–353
37. Meinert C, Tonascia S, Higgins K (1984) Contents of reports on clinical trials. Controlled Clin Trials 5:328–347
38. Altman DG (1982) Statistics in medical journals. Statistics Med 1:59–71
39. George SL (1985) Statistics in medical journals: A survey of current policies and proposals for editors. Med Pediatr Oncol 13:109–112
40. Altman DG (1991) Statistics in medical journals: Developments in the 1980's. Statistics Med 10:1897–1913
41. Gotzsche P (1989) Methodology and overt and hidden bias in reports of 196 double blind trials of nonsteroidal antiinflammatory drugs in rheumatoid arthritis. Controlled Clin Trials 10:31–56
42. Zelen M (1983) Guidelines for publishing papers on cancer clinical trials: Responsibilities of editors and authors. J Clin Oncol 1:164–169
43. Altman DG, Gore SM, Gardner MJ, Pocock SJ (1983) Statistical guidelines for contributors to medical journals. Br Med J 286:1489–1493. Also in: Gardner M, Altman D (eds) (1989) Statistics with confidence: Confidence intervals and statistical guidelines. Br Med J, pp 83–100
44. Gardner MJ, Machin D, Campbell MJ (1986) Use of check lists in assessing the statistical content of medical studies. Br Med J 292:810–812. Also in: Gardner M, Altman D (eds) (1989) Statistics with confidence: Confidence intervals and statistical guidelines. Br Med J, pp 101–108
45. Simon R, Wittes R (1985) Methodologic guidelines for reports of clinical trials. Cancer Treat Rep 69:1–3
46. Bailar JC, Mosteller F (1988) Guidelines for statistical reporting in articles for medical journals: Amplifications and explanations. Ann Intern Med 108:266–273
47. Miller AB, Hoogstraten B, Staquet M, Winkler A (1981) Reporting results of cancer treatment. Cancer 47:207–214

48. Dalesio O, Barton B, Hisazumi H, et al (1986) Standardization of format of reporting results. In: Denis L, Niijima T, Prout G, Schröder F (eds) Developments in bladder cancer. Alan R Liss, New York, pp 15–31
49. Louis T, Bouffioux C, Tazaki H, et al (1986) Policy on monitoring and reporting results. In: Denis L, Niijima T, Prout G, Schröder F (eds) Developments in bladder cancer. Alan R Liss, New York, pp 33–48
50. Hoogstraten B (1984) Reporting treatment results in solid tumors. In: Buyse M, Staquet M, Sylvester R (eds) Cancer Clinical Trials: Methods and Practice. Oxford Medical Publications, Oxford, pp 139–156
51. Kisner D (1984) Reporting treatment toxicities. In: Buyse M, Staquet M, Sylvester R (eds) Cancer Clinical Trials: Methods and Practice. Oxford Medical Publications, Oxford, pp 178–190
52. Zeittoun R, Preisler H (1984) Reporting treatment results in non-solid tumors. In: Buyse M, Staquet M, Sylvester R (eds) Cancer Clinical Trials: Methods and Practice. Oxford Medical Publications, Oxford, pp 157–177
53. Gail MH (1985) Eligibility exclusions, losses to follow-up, removal of randomized patients, and uncounted events in cancer clinical trials. Cancer Treat Rep 69:1107–1112
54. Peto R, Pike M, Armitage P, et al (1976) Design and analysis of randomized clinical trials requiring prolonged observation of each patient. Br J Cancer 34:585–612
55. Peto J (1984) The calculation and interpretation of survival curves. In: Buyse M, Staquet M, Sylvester R (eds) Cancer Clinical Trials: Methods and Practice. Oxford Medical Publications, Oxford, pp 361–380
56. Breslow N (1984) Comparison of survival curves. In: Buyse M, Staquet M, Sylvester R (eds) Cancer Clinical Trials: Methods and Practice. Oxford Medical Publications, Oxford, pp 381–406
57. Gardner M, Altman DG (1986) Confidence intervals rather than P values: Estimation rather than hypothesis testing. Br Med J 292:746–750
58. Simon R (1986) Confidence intervals for reporting results of clinical trials. Ann Intern Med 105:429–435
59. Yusif S, Wittes J, Probstfield J, Tyroler H (1991) Analysis and interpretation of treatment effects in subgroups of patients in randomized clinical trials. JAMA 266:93–98
60. Gelber R, Goldhirsch A (1991) Meta-analysis: The fashion of summing up evidence. Ann Oncol 2:461–468

Economic Evaluation in the Critical Care Literature

D. J. Cook

Introduction

Two interwoven themes have emerged over the last decade which illustrate the compelling need for more rigorous economic evaluation in the future of critical care research. First, the current tension over spiralling health care costs has reached its pinnacle in discussions about scarce resource allocation to the intensive care unit (ICU). In this setting, critically ill patients consume a large proportion of hospital budgets, usually in the last few days of life [1]. Thus, the highly skilled personnel, and complex, expensive technology utilized in the ICU make it particularly vulnerable to increasing health care costs [2].

Second, the relatively nascent specialty of critical care medicine is continually confronted with new diagnostic and therapeutic technologies. The desire for intensivists to use all the tools at their disposal, regardless of the cost-effectiveness ratio, has been coined the "technologic imperative" by Fuchs [3]. Unfortunately, these diagnostic and therapeutic tools are inevitably introduced into the critical care arena with insufficient evaluation of their impact on clinically important outcomes [4], and their economic consequences.

While an increasing portion of the general medical literature has focused on categorizing and justifying the need for economic evaluations [5, 6], the critical care literature has been flooded with articles about the costs of intensive care. Ironically, there has not been a parallel growth in true economic evaluation of critical care [7]. Redressing this imbalance is long overdue.

To practice effective, compassionate and yet fiscally responsible medicine, ICU health workers need to be empowered with better information about the costs and consequences of their actions. These actions, in the biomedical paradigm, include, but are not limited to, decision-making about diagnosis, prognosis, therapies, and often withdrawing and withholding life support [8].

In this chapter, I will review the need for economic evaluation, define and describe the components of an economic evaluation, outline the prerequisites, present an organizational framework for categorizing these analyses, summarize the different types of economic evaluation, and provide some guidelines for critically appraising an economic evaluation. The latter exercise may demonstrate the complexity of an economic evaluation, and could be useful to readers interested in conducting their own economic evaluation in their field of interest. Throughout this chapter, I will use cogent examples taken from the critical care and other medical literature.

Why do we Need Economic Evaluations?

Those who plan, provide, receive, or pay for critical care health services face an incessant barrage of questions such as:

a) Should ICU physicians offer all patients with life-threatening community acquired pneumonia mechanical ventilation?
b) Should hospitals buy every new, apparently useful piece of life-sustaining or life-saving equipment?
c) Should all stable patients with central venous catheters have daily radiographs performed?
d) Should hospitals develop a triage system to decide on admission and discharge policies for the ICU?
e) Should nursing expertise be shifted from the ICU to other venues so that nurses can spend more time on preventative medicine?

These questions can be summarized as follows: Who should do what to whom? ... with what health care resources ... and with what relation to other health care resources?

The answers to the foregoing questions are most strongly influenced by our estimates of the relative merits of the alternative courses of action they pose. Economic evaluation is concerned with the strategies whereby these estimates of relative value can be ascertained and interpreted. Economic evaluation, more specifically is asking [9]:

1) Is this health procedure, service or program worth doing compared to other things we could be doing using the same resources?
2) Are we satisfied that the health care resources (required to make the procedure, service, or program available to those who could benefit from it) should be spent in this way rather than some other way?

Components of an Economic Evaluation

Two features characterize economic evaluations. First, they deal with both inputs and outputs, which are referred to as costs and consequences. For example, in an economic evaluation of an ICU health care program to decrease stress ulcer bleeding, the inputs, or costs, would be the resources consumed by the program, which would include direct costs (e.g. the drugs themselves, and personnel time to administer them), indirect costs (e.g. overhead costs of the ICU) and intangible costs (which vary considerably depending on the analysis). In this example, the outputs, or consequences of the program would be the effects on health. These effects can be measured in a number of ways, such as in natural units (bleeding events, pneumonia episodes, and death); in quality-adjusted life years gained or lost; or in the associated fiscal benefits such as net dollars saved or lost.

The second feature which characterizes economic evaluations is that they deal with choices. Unfortunately, resources (that is, personnel, time, ICU beds, and equipment) are not unlimited. Choices must be made concerning the use of our precious resources. Intensivists make many choices that have economic sequelae in their daily practice. The basis for many of these choices is the educated guess, evidence from the biomedical literature, gut feelings, established patterns of practice, etc. However, these choices are frequently not as informed as the structured consideration of factors involved in a decision to commit resources to one use instead of another (as would be found in an economic evaluation). Non-systematic decision making is limited for the following reasons:

Without Systematic Analysis, it is Difficult to Clearly Identify the Relevant Alternatives

For example, in deciding whether to purchase a set of home ventilators for patients with end-stage respiratory failure, often little or no effort is made to describe existing alternative programs (such as special "self-medication and self-mastery" clinics for severely disabled patients with chronic airflow limitation). If the objective is to reduce morbidity and delay mortality due to chronic airflow limitation, then preventative medicine initiatives such as smoking cessation programs may represent more efficient means to achieving this goal, and should be added to the set of alternative programs in an economic analysis.

The Viewpoint assumed in the Analysis is Important

A program which looks attractive from one view point may not look as attractive when other viewpoints are considered. For example, hospital subsidization of home ventilators may appear attractive to patients and their families, but from society's point of view, this may be less compelling because it may mean foregoing the purchase of sorely needed neonatal ventilators for hospitalized infants.

Without Some Attempt at Measurement, the Uncertainty Surrounding Orders of Magnitude can be Critical

For example, when the American Cancer Society endorsed a protocol of six sequential stool tests for cancer of the large bowel, the cost per case of colon cancer detected was predicted to increase considerably with each test. It is unlikely that society expected that it would reach $47 million dollars for the sixth test, as has now been demonstrated [10]. This example illustrates that the real cost of any program is not the number recorded on the budget, but it is the health outcomes achievable in some other program which have been forgone by committing the resources in question to the first program. It is this "opportunity cost" which economic evaluation seeks to estimate and to compare with program benefits.

The Definition and Goals of Economic Evaluations

In summary, economic evaluations attempt to identify and to make explicit one set of criteria which may be useful in deciding among different uses for scarce resources. Thus, an economic evaluation can be defined as the comparative analysis of alternative courses of action in terms of both their costs and consequences. The task of an economic analysis is therefore to identify, measure, value and compare the costs and consequences of the alternatives being considered.

Prerequisites of an Economic Evaluation

Although economic evaluation provides important information for decision makers, it addresses only one dimension of decision-making about health care programs. An economic evaluation is most appropriately conducted, and therefore most useful, when it is preceded by three other types of evaluation [11] which address a different but essential complementary question.

Can it Work?

Does the health procedure, service or program do more good than harm to people who fully comply with the associated recommendations or treatments? This type of evaluation is concerned with efficacy, and can best be addressed in the format of large double-blind, high quality randomized trial in which adherence to protocol and patient compliance is close to perfect, and co-intervention and contamination are minimal or non-existent [12].

Does it Work?

Does the procedure, service or program do more good than harm to those people to whom it is offered? This type of evaluation is called an effectiveness evaluation, and considers both the efficacy of a service and its acceptance to those to whom it is offered. Both an effectiveness analysis and an efficacy analysis are best addressed in a high quality randomized trial. An effectiveness approach dictates that the trial is conducted in such a way that it better approximates real life. So for example, in a randomized trial of carotid end-arterectomy versus aspirin for symptomatic carotid stenosis, some patients who are randomized to surgery may refuse, or be unfit for surgery and some patients randomized to medical management may cross over to the other treatment arm and subsequently undergo end-arterectomy. Some patients may not take their medications; some may receive ancillary interventions like antihypertensive medications, which may be unequally distributed across the two groups; other patients may be lost to follow-up. An effectiveness approach considers all of these possibilities in the analysis, and considers them in interpreting the results of the trial. Note the contrast with a strict efficacy analysis described in the foregoing section, which is concerned with patients who fully comply with the program.

Is it Reaching those Who Need it?

Is the procedure, service or program accessible to all people who could benefit from it? Evaluation of this type is concerned with availability. There are relatively few studies published whose goal it is to evaluate the availability of programs to all sectors of the population.

Economic evaluations may make assumptions about the certainty that interventions or programs being analyzed are of proven efficacy, effectiveness or availability.

Studies Evaluating Costs and Consequences – The Conceptual Framework

Many different types of studies are published in the literature, some of which evaluate costs and some of which evaluate consequences. Only economic evaluation requires consideration of both costs and consequences. Let us now put these different studies into a conceptual framework.

Readers will be most familiar with studies evaluating consequences. For example, when the only consequences of a condition are described (without any comparisons), this may take the form of a natural history or prognosis study. An example would be a cohort study of potentially weanable patients receiving mechanical ventilation who underwent serial gastric intramural pH measurements to determine the sensitivity and specificity of pHi in predicting weaning success or failure [13]. When only the consequences of a condition are described (now with some comparison), this may take the form of a classic randomized trial of two types of interventions, which provides the highest form of evidence in evaluating the impact of different interventions.

On the other hand, when only the costs of a condition are reported (without any comparisons), this takes the form of a "cost description" study. When only the costs are described (with a comparison incorporated), this takes the form of a "cost analysis". An example of a cost analysis is the study by Lowson, Drummond and Bishop on the comparative costs of three methods of providing long-term home oxygen [14]. The authors argued that a cost analysis was sufficient since the relative effectiveness of the three methods was not a contentious issue.

One type of economic evaluation in which both costs and outcomes of a single service or program are being described is called a "cost outcome description". One example of a cost outcome study describes the costs of one coronary care unit and the estimated number of lives saved in that unit [15]. In this study, there was no attempt made to compare the costs and consequences of this coronary care unit with another alternative unit or ward. Such a study is only a partial economic analysis since, although both costs and outcomes are included, there is no comparison involved.

Let us now turn to studies evaluating both costs and consequences that include a relevant comparison among alternatives; these represent full economic evaluations.

Types of Economic Evaluations

The identification of costs and their valuation in currency is similar across most types of economic evaluations. However, the nature of the consequences of the alternatives being considered may vary considerably. In this section, we will consider four different economic analyses – a cost-minimization study, a cost-effectiveness study, a cost-benefit study, and a cost-utility study. The unique ways in which the consequences are valued in each of these four types are presented in Table 1.

Table 1. Comparison of different types of economic evaluation

Type of economic analysis	Identification of consequences	Measurement of consequences
Cost-minimization analysis	Identical in all respects	None
Cost-effectiveness analysis	Single effect of interest common to both alternatives	Natural units (e.g. strokes prevented, life years gained)
Cost-benefit analysis	Single or multiple effects, not necessarily common to both alternatives	Money
Cost-utility analysis	Single or multiple effects, not necessarily common to both alternatives	Quality adjusted life years

Popularization of the term "cost-effective" has resulted in an all-encompassing misuse of this term in the literature [16]. For example, the term cost-effectiveness has been used to describe effectiveness in the absence of considering monetary cost (bone scans were deemed the most cost-effective means of examining for metastases in patients with lung cancer, when in fact, fiscal consequences were not considered) [17]. Cost-effective does not equate with saving money; in a true cost-effectiveness study, the most cost-effective program is the one associated with the lowest cost. Thus, for only one type of economic analysis is the term cost-effectiveness analysis appropriate.

Cost-minimization Analysis

When we are searching for the least costly approach to a problem for which two equally viable options exist, we search for a cost-minimization study. For example, if tracheostomies for difficult to wean patients can be performed in the operating room or more conveniently in the patient's ICU bed, and we know that successful procedures can be achieved to the same degree using both approaches, a cost-minimization study would help us to decide on an appropriate policy for tracheostomies. In such an analysis, proof of the unimportant or non-existent differences in effectiveness of the two approaches would ideally be obtained in a randomized controlled trial, and the economic analysis would seek to determine the cost per surgical procedure, and thus, the least costly alternative. There are few cost-minimization studies published that are relevant to critical care clinicians.

Cost-effectiveness Analysis

Cost-effectiveness studies report the cost (e.g. dollars spent) in relation to a single outcome achieved (e.g. per unit of outcome obtained). Suppose that a group of intensivists were interested in prolonging life in patients with acute renal failure. They could compare the costs and consequences of CAVHD with intermittent hemodialysis. The outcome of interest would be common to both programs – life years gained. However, these two approaches may have different success in achieving life years gained, and they might incur different costs.

Using cost-effectiveness analyses allows for comparisons of many different programs. For example, we could compare the role of mandatory seatbelt legislation for the entire population with antihypertensive therapy for patients at least 50 years of age, with intermittent hemodialysis in acute renal failure, as long as a common outcome (life years gained) was used.

There are many examples of cost-effectiveness analyses in the literature. In a study examining the cost-effectiveness of thrombolytic therapy with streptokinase in elderly patients with suspected myocardial infarction [18], the authors found that for every 33 patients over age 75 treated with streptokinase, one life would be saved. For every 56 patients treated who were less than 65 years of age, one life would be saved. In sensitivity analyses, treatment benefit persisted if the probability of infarct was >9% on admission, if the relative reduction in mortality was >1%, and if the risk of in-hospital mortality without streptokinase was >3%. When assumptions were varied widely, the cost of streptokinase remained <$55000 per year of life saved. This cost-effectiveness ratio compares favorably with those associated with other effective health interventions such as secondary prevention of heart disease in hypertensive patients. This study reminds us of the reluctance of clinicians to deliver therapies such as streptokinase and warfarin to elderly patients, perhaps because of their fear of increased side effects such as serious bleeding. However, clinicians often fail to consider that benefits may be greater for elderly patients.

The recent profusion of research on immunotherapy in sepsis, and the great cost of these agents has prompted timely pieces on the cost-effectiveness of synthetic antibodies [19, 20].

Cost-benefit Analysis

In a cost-benefit study, all outcomes are valued in dollars to facilitate direct comparison of programs with different objectives. If we were interested in the effect of two different ICU programs, for example, an early enteral nutrition program, and bedside laboratory testing machinery, it would be challenging to directly compare them, given that their consequences are different. For the first alternative, nutritional status and aspiration pneumonias would be considered consequences; in the second, the benefits of detecting aberrant but important laboratory results and iatrogenic anemia would be considered. This common denominator of dollars is one of the attractive features, and challenges of a cost-benefit analysis; very few studies lend themselves to a comparison of those costs and benefits that can easily be expressed in monetary terms. One example of a cost-benefit study which did attempt to quantify and value a wide range of costs was a community-based versus hospital-based program for mental illness; although the community-based program was more costly, this was offset by its extra value in terms of patients being able to maintain employment [21].

Cost-utility Analysis

Even though the outcome of an ICU stay might be technically the same for two patients (living in an institution, able to conduct self-care and conversation, but needing help with mobilization and medication administration), these two people might value this health state differently. Utility refers to the value or worth of a specific level of health (or improvement in health) and can be measured by the preferences of individuals or society for any particular set of health outcomes. Cost-utility analyses are a relatively new type of economic evaluation that allow for an outcome to be adjusted for quality of life. They also provide a common denominator for the comparison of costs and outcomes for different programs. Thus, the outcome of quality-adjusted life years is determined by adjusting the length of time affected throughout the health state by adjusting this length of time by the utility value (on a scale of zero to one) of the resulting level of health.

Cost-benefit analyses should be conducted when quality of life is the primary, or one of the primary outcomes, or when it is desirable to combine both morbidity and mortality.

An example of a cost-utility study is provided in a paper examining the costs and outcomes of management of very low birthweight infants either by a regional program with a specialized neonatal ICU or by previously existing facilities within the region [22]. For newborns weighing 1000 to 1499 g, neonatal ICU increase both survival rates and costs. The cost in 1978 Canadian dollars was $3200 per quality adjusted life year gained; the corresponding figure for infants weighing 500 to 999 g was $22400 per quality adjusted life year gained.

Critical Appraisal of Economic Evaluations

Clinicians are likely to be reading relatively more synthetic research in the future (synthetic research includes systematic overviews, practice guidelines, and economic evaluations). As clinicians try to cope with the burgeoning medical literature, they are increasingly using guides for quick, reliable interpretation of publications in their field [23–28], some of which have been adapted to the critical care setting [29]. The questions that readers face each day are, in essence: are the results of this study valid? and if so, do they apply to my clinical setting?

Cost-benefit and cost-effectiveness studies are increasingly being integrated into the medical literature [30]. The following section addresses the validity of an economic analysis by posing a set of questions which examine the methods used to formulate the economic analysis (Table 2). While, like any clinical study, it is unlikely that any economic analysis will satisfy all validity criteria, addressing each of these questions will help readers to identify the strengths and weaknesses of the publication.

Was a Well-Defined Question posed in an Answerable Form?

A well-defined question for an economic analysis identifies the alternatives being compared and the viewpoint from which the comparison is to be made. For example "How much does it cost to operate our intensive care unit?" is not directly answerable in a full scale economic analysis because the alternative for comparison is not identified and the point of view is not specified.

Table 2. Guidelines for critical appraisal of an economic evaluation

1. Was a well-defined question posed in an answerable form?
2. Was a comprehensive description of competing alternatives given?
3. Was there evidence that the program's effectiveness had been established?
4. Were all the important and relevant costs and consequences for each alternative identified?
5. Were costs and consequences measured accurately in appropriate physical units?
6. Were costs and consequences measured credibly?
7. Were costs and consequences adjusted for differential timing?
8. Was an incremental analysis of costs and consequences of alternatives performed?
9. Was a sensitivity analysis performed?
10. Did the presentation and discussion of study results include all issues of concern to readers?

A better formulated question would read as follows: "From the societal point of view, is the development of more intermediate care units in community hospitals preferable to expanding the number of beds in existing ICUs?"

Was a Comprehensive Description of Competing Alternatives given?

Just as the methods section of any primary research paper is crucial for the interpretation of results, specific details about the primary objective of each alternative program, treatment or service is crucial in an economic analysis. Readers need this information to judge themselves whether any costs or consequences have been omitted, and they need to assess the applicability of these programs to their own settings.

Was there Evidence that the Program's Effectiveness had been Established?

We are most interested in the efficient provision of services which have been shown to do more good than harm, and all economic evaluations should make the effectiveness of the program(s) explicit (whether through previous or simultaneous evidence). Most economic evaluations assume that effectiveness has been established (often this is established by previously conducted randomized clinical trials). Sometimes, however, effectiveness is established simultaneously with the economic evaluation; that is, some randomized trials also include a comparison of costs of the experimental and control programs. This was the case in a report describing the effectiveness of an air suspension bed for the prevention of pressure ulcers [31]. This study demonstrated that significantly fewer patients on the air suspension bed as compared with the standard bed developed pressure ulcers, and data suggesting that these beds are cost-effective were presented.

Were all the Important and Relevant Costs and Consequences for each Alternative Identified?

A full identification of the relevant costs and consequences of the alternatives under comparison is necessary. Examples of the types of costs which should be accounted for include the costs of organizing and delivering the intervention or program: direct costs (variable costs such as supplies, equipment, personnel costs and fixed costs such as overhead, light, heat, rent and capital costs). Other costs borne to the patient or family include direct costs (such as pain, costs incurred by relatives paying for gas and parking), and indirect costs (such as psychological stress and production losses when patients or families do not go to work on account of illness).

There are several categories of consequences to consider in an economic evaluation. The first is simply the effects, or therapeutic outcomes, of the alternatives in question, such as the change in physical, emotional or social status of patients after they leave the ICU. While these effects are consequences of an economic analysis on their own, they can also give rise to another extremely important category of consequences which attach value to these outcomes – that is, the changes in quality of life as perceived by patients and their families. Finally, in reading an economic evaluation, readers should consider whether the consequences of primary interest are the therapeutic effects themselves (thus implying that a cost-effectiveness analysis is appropriate); or whether the primary interest is quality of life of patients and their families (implying that a cost-utility analysis is appropriate); or whether the primary interest is net change in resources (implying that a cost-benefit analysis is appropriate).

Were Costs and Consequences measured Accurately in Appropriate Physical Units?

Once the important and relevant costs and consequences have been identified, they must be measured in appropriate physical and natural units (i.e. charge for drug acquisition, 24 h shift of one-to-one nursing, etc.). It is a particular challenge to economists to accurately measure resources when they are used jointly by one or more programs. The complexities of evaluating costs should not be underestimated; recommendations exist to aid analysts in handling the challenges of cost estimation [32].

Were Costs and Consequences measured Credibly?

The valuation of costs, benefits and utilities should be clearly stated in an economic evaluation. Costs are usually valued in local currency, based on a certain year, to account for inflation. Valuation is most difficult in cost-benefit studies, in which not only the costs, but also the outcomes of medical care are measured in monetary terms (e.g. the dollar value of the benefits obtained). Valuation is simplest for cost-minimization studies, in which the programs or services being compared are of equal efficacy. The valuation of utilities or preferences attempts to ascertain how much better the quality of life is in one health state as a consequence of one of the alternatives compared with the health state as a consequence of another alternative. The results of utility analyses are often expressed as quality-adjusted life years gained or lost [33], determined either through population interviews of patients, or a consensus forming exercise. Measuring quality of life and establishing utilities is a relatively new field in health economics, and readers are referred to a comprehensive review for further details [34]. Economic evaluations should be sure to specify whose values were used to develop the utility; patients, a general population, health care providers, or administrators. Readers will want to be satisfied that the persons whose values were used fully understood the health state, through either experience or realistic case scenarios.

Were Costs and Consequences adjusted for Differential Timing?

In preparing an economic analysis, comparisons of programs or services must be done at one point in time (usually the present). The timing of program costs not occurring in the present need's to be accounted for, so often future dollar costs and benefits are discounted to reflect that dollars spent or saved in the future do not weigh as heavily in program decisions as dollars spent and saved in the present. The reasons for this process of discounting is that people tend to value positive outcomes more highly when offered in the present than in the future. Moreover, there is always uncertainty about the future – if the consumption of a service is deferred, it may never be enjoyed at all, because individual tastes and values may change over time (i.e. elderly patients may attach greater or lesser value to a hospital's provision of widely available intensive care than they would when they were middle aged); alternatively, patients may die during the period of deferment. Another reason for discounting is the law of diminishing marginal utility; additional consumption of a benefit at a later date may add less to patient well being than consumption now.

Was an Incremental Analysis of Costs and Consequences of Alternatives Performed?

It is often necessary to examine additional costs that one program imposes over another, compared with the additional effects or benefits that it delivers. This incremental approach to economic analysis can be described by referring back to the colon cancer screening example used earlier; there was a big difference between the average cost per case detected of colon cancer after six sequential tests, and the incremental cost of performing a sixth test.

Was a Sensitivity Analysis Performed?

Economic evaluations, like clinical trials, always contain some degree of uncertainty, methodologic controversy or imprecision. After identifying these areas of uncertainty, economists often rework the analysis employing different assumptions or estimates in order to test the sensitivity of the results and conclusions to such changing assumptions. If the conclusion is not altered by varying the estimates or measurements that are used, then the reader can feel more comfortable in letting the economic analysis guide decision-making.

Did the Presentation and Discussion of Study Results include all Issues of Concern to Readers?

A sound economic evaluation will help the reader interpret results by making the viewpoint of the analysis clear, and indicating exactly how the judgements were made about the costs and consequences of the study. Statements about the generalizability of the findings is also helpful.

Limitations of Economic Evaluations

Like all information at the disposition of a health care provider, economic analyses have some limitations. First, they assume, rather than establish or challenge, program effectiveness. In fact, some economic evaluations are predicated on the conduct of methodologically rigorous trials of program effectiveness. Second, economic analyses assume that resources saved by preferred programs will not be wasted, but will be used in alternative worthwhile programs. This may not be the case; if resources saved are consumed for other ineffective or unproven programs, then there may be no net savings, or a net loss of resources. Third, economic analyses will not themselves control health expenditures; forward-looking financial and organizational mechanisms are needed to facilitate that process. Fourth, there are some situations in which economic analyses are not desirable; sometimes their production uses up scarce research resources, and the end product is not worth the expense. Their impact may be greatest in situations in which program objectives need clarification, when the competing alternatives are very different in nature, or when large resources are under consideration. Finally, some physicians have not yet accepted their dual role as agent of the patient, and responsible member of the broader health economic mosaic. The natural extension of denying this dual role is that physicians have no responsibility whatsoever for the appropriate use of health care resources – a position that is untenable and retrogressive! Fortunately, clinicians appear to be rising to meet this challenge [35].

Conclusions

It is universally realized that the resources available to meet the demands for health care are limited. Decisions about allocative efficiency have been made for decades, implicitly, or more rarely, explicitly. To better inform these difficult allocative decisions, the best current evidence about the efficacy of medical practices and their costs must be made available to decision makers, so that useful comparisons among alternative uses of resources can be made.

Physicians potentially have a great deal to contribute to the development of economic analyses. Indeed, it is a heavy focus on the macro-economic level that has tended to obscure the crucial importance of decisions made every day by physicians at the micro level [36]. However, physicians cannot always be aware of the costs and benefits of their decisions. Increasingly, physicians are called upon to balance their role as agent of the patient and resource manager for society; this role conflict generally comes without much support [37]. Nevertheless, it is likely that improvements in allocative efficiency will occur when physicians demonstrate an increased commitment to their dual roles.

Although it is not necessary for every clinician to know how to perform a cost-benefit or cost-effectiveness analysis, it is essential that we all understand the underpinning principles, and why such analyses are necessary. If economic analyses were to become more widely understood and accepted by key decision makers in the health care sector, including physicians, important health benefits or cost savings might be realized.

References

1. Detsky AS, Stricker SC, Mulley AG, Thibault GE (1981) Prognosis, survival and the expenditure of hospital resources for patients in an intensive care unit. N Engl J Med 305:667–672
2. Jacobs P, Noseworthy TW (1990) National estimates of intensive care utilization and costs: Canada and United States. Crit Care Med 18:1282–1286
3. Fuchs VH (1979) Who shall live? Basic Books, New York, New York, p 60
4. Cook DJ, Brun-Buisson C, Guyatt GH, Sibbald WJ (1994) Evaluation of new technology: The bronchoalveolar lavage for diagnosing ventilator-associated pneumonia. Crit Care Med (in press)
5. Weinstein MC, Stason WB (1977) Foundations of cost-effectiveness analysis for health and medical practices. N Engl J Med 296:716–721
6. Warner KE, Hutton RC (1980) Cost-benefit and cost-effectiveness analysis in health care: Growth and composition of the literature. Med Care 11:1069–1084

7. Gill RS, Inman KJ, Eberhard JA, Sibbald WJ (1993) An evaluation of the health economic literature in the intensive care setting. Chest 104:98S (Abst)
8. Campbell ML, Field BE (1991) Management of the patient with do not resuscitate status. Heart Lung 20:345–348
9. Drummond MF, Stoddart GL, Torrance GW (1986) Basic types of economic evaluation. In: Drummond MF, Stoddart GL, Torrance GW (eds) Methods for the economic evaluation of health care programs. Oxford Medical Publications, Oxford, pp 5–17
10. Neuhauser D, Lewicki AM (1975) What do we gain from the sixth stool guaiac? N Engl J Med 293:226–228
11. Department of Clinical Epidemiology & Biostatistics (1981) How to read clinical journals: To understand an economic evaluation. Can Med Assoc J 130:1428–1433
12. Department of Clinical Epidemiology & Biostatistics (1981) How to read clinical journals: To distinguish useful from useless or even harmful therapy. Can Med Assoc J 124:1156–1162
13. Mohsenifar Z, Hay A, Hay J, Lewis MI, Koerner SK (1993) Gastric intramural pH as a predictor of success or failure in weaning patients from mechanical ventilation. Ann Intern Med 119:794–798
14. Lowson KV, Drummond MF, Bishop JM (1981) Costing new services: Long-term domiciliary oxygen therapy. Lancet 2:1146–1149
15. Reynell PC, Reynell MC (1972) The cost-benefit analysis of a coronary care unit. Br Heart J 34:897–900
16. Doubilet P, Weinstein MC, McNeil BJ (1986) Use and misuse of the term "cost-effective" in medicine. N Engl J Med 314:253–256
17. Kelly RJ, Cowan RJ, Feree CB, Raban M, Maynard CD (1979) Efficacy of radionuclide scanning in patients with lung cancer. JAMA 242:2855–2857
18. Krumholz HM, Pasternak RC, Weinstein MC, et al (1992) Cost-effectiveness of thrombolytic therapy with streptokinase in elderly patients with suspected acute myocardial infarction. N Engl J Med 327:7–13
19. Schulman KA, Glick HA, Rubin H, Eisenberg JM (1991) Cost-effectiveness of HA-1A therapy for gram-negative sepsis. JAMA 266:3466–3471
20. Chalfin DB, Holbein MEB, Fein AM, Carlon C (1993) Cost-effectiveness of monoclonal antibodies to gram-negative endotoxin in the treatment of gram-negative sepsis in ICU patients. JAMA 269:249–254
21. Weisbrod BA, Test MA, Stein LI (1980) Alternatives to mental hospital treatment: Economic cost-benefit analysis. Arch Gen Psych 37:400–405
22. Boyle MH, Torrance GW, Sinclair JC, Horwood SP (1983) Economic evaluation of neonatal intensive care of very low birth weight infants. N Engl J Med 308:1330–1337
23. Sackett DL (1981) How to read clinical journals: Why to read them and how to start reading them critically. Can Med Assoc J 124:555–558
24. Tugwell PX (1981) How to read clinical journals: To learn the clinical course and prognosis of disease. Can Med Assoc J 124:869–872
25. Haynes RB (1981) How to read clinical journals: To learn about a diagnostic test. Can Med Assoc J 124:703–710
26. Guyatt GH, Sackett DL, Cook DJ and the Evidence-Based Medicine Working Group (1993) Users' guides to the medical literature: Part I: How to use an article about therapy. JAMA 270:2093–2095
27. Guyatt GH, Sackett DL, Cook DJ and the Evidence-Based Medicine Working Group (1993) Users' guides to the medical literature: Part II: How to use an article about therapy or prevention. JAMA 270:2598–2601
28. Oxman AD, Cook DJ, Guyatt GH and the Evidence-Based Medicine Working Group (1994) Users' guides to the medical literature: How to use an overview. JAMA (in press)
29. Cook DJ, Jaeschke R, Guyatt GH (1992) Critical appraisal of therapeutic interventions

in the intensive care unit: Human monoclonal antibody treatment in sepsis. J Intensive Care Med 7:275–282
30. Fuchs VR (1980) What is CBA/CEA and why are they doing this to us? N Engl J Med 303:937–938
31. Inman KJ, Sibbald WJ, Rutledge FS, Clark BJ (1993) Clinical utility and cost-effectiveness of an air suspension bed in the prevention of pressure ulcers. JAMA 269:1139–1143
32. Luce BR, Elixhauser A (1990) Estimating costs in the economic evaluation of health services. Int J Tech Assess Health Care 6:57–75
33. Torrance GW, Feeny DH (1989) Utilities and quality-adjusted life years. Int J Tech Assess Health Care 5:559–575
34. Guyatt GH, Feeny DH, Patrick DL (1993) Measuring health-related quality of life. Ann Intern Med 118:622–629
35. Naylor D, Lington AL (1986) Allocation of health care resources: A challenge for the medical profession. Can Med Assoc J 134:333–340
36. Stoddart GL, Barer ML (1992) Toward integrated medical resource policies for Canada: Analytic framework for policy development. Can Med Assoc J 146:1169–1174
37. Stoddart GL, Barer ML (1992) Toward integrated medical resource policies for Canada: Improving effectiveness and efficiency. Can Med Assoc J 147:1653–1660

Ethical Issues in Clinical Trials

C.L. Sprung, L.A. Eidelman, and D.J. Nyman

Introduction

Research on human beings is important and necessary for the common good of society. Human experimentation is essential for the expansion of scientific knowledge in order to prevent, treat and cure disease. Despite the value of medical research in saving lives and relieving pain, the use of humans for experimental purposes often meets with opposition [1]. Medical progress requires clinical trials to introduce beneficial treatments and prevent the introduction of non-useful or harmful therapies. It would be helpful if the lay public became aware of the importance of clinical trials and became more knowledgeable about them before they were asked to participate in them. In 1747, one of the earliest reported clinical trials was performed by Sir James Lind in sailors with scurvy [2]. The first randomized controlled trial in modern times which occurred after World War II was the treatment of pulmonary tuberculosis with streptomycin [3]. There are those who believe that experimentation on human beings takes place continually in every doctor's office and that deliberate experimentation on a group of patients is merely an efficient way to collect and interpret data that would otherwise be lost [1]. Some physicians believe all therapies should be given as part of clinical trials. Clearly, modern clinical investigations are different than research done in the past.

Many medical procedures and therapies given by physicians to patients on a daily basis have not been proven to be effective by clinical studies. Widely recognized safe and effective therapies such as penicillin, aspirin, and many surgical procedures have never been studied with randomized trials. The history of medicine is replete with instances of "effective" therapies that were widely used and subsequently shown to be ineffective or even harmful. Therapies adopted by consensus based on observational studies and physiological mechanisms, but without randomized studies, may be classified by future physicians as useless or even toxic [4]. Interventional trials of the greatest benefit demonstrate validity, generalizability, and efficiency, and since validity has become a non-negotiable demand [5], the randomized trial has become the gold standard of assessing new drugs and treatments. The randomized, controlled, double-blind clinical trial reduces error, bias, and uncertainty of results, and increasingly refines approximations of the truth [6]. Unfortunately, these trials are not perfect and other types of studies may also be useful [4, 6–8].

When making ethical decisions in medicine and in clinical trials, it is most important to have accurate medical information. One cannot make good ethical decisions without good science. All the necessary components for a properly designed and executed trial must be present [4, 9]. These include justification, methodology, conduct, monitoring of the trial, and interpretation of the data. The justification to begin a phase III clinical trial is based on an understanding of the pathophysiology of the disease and the proposed physiologic effects of the intervention, sufficient animal studies in several species and models inferring benefit and no increased risk in humans and human pilot and/or phase II studies [4, 9, 10]. Performing a poorly designed and conducted trial in patients is unethical. Patients participating in such studies may incur risks without benefit to them or others.

Abuses in Research

Despite the great advances and breakthroughs obtained because of human experimentation, there have been instances of abuse by physicians involved in human research. The "experiments" conducted in concentration camps in Nazi Germany attest to the potential of physicians for cruelty and inhumanity. Since that time, there have been many examples of research subjects that were exploited, manipulated and deceived. Investigators risked the health or life of their subjects not so much out of a willful disregard of their patient's rights but rather from thoughtlessness and carelessness [11]. Some examples include the withholding of penicillin from patients in the Tuskegee syphilis study [12], the administration of hepatitis virus to retarded children, and the injection of live cancer cells into unknowing subjects [11]. The previous misconduct and abuse in human research together with increasing numbers of experiments on humans has led to the development of several codes, declarations and regulations for the protection of human beings in research.

Research Codes and Regulations

Codes, declarations, and regulations have built safeguards into the performance of clinical trials. The Nuremberg Code of 1947 [13] and the World Medical Association Declaration of Helsinki, revised in 1975 [14] are the most well known. In the United States, there have been many regulations enacted to protect research subjects. One example, the National Research Act of 1974 [15], required prior peer review of human research projects by an investigational review board (IRB) at all federal grantee institutions. Several of the fundamental principles of the codes on biomedical research on human subjects are noted in Table 1 [13, 14].

Table 1. Several fundamental principles in the Nuremberg Code and the World Medical Association Declaration of Helsinki [13, 14]

1. Concern for the interests of the subject must always prevail over the interests of science and society [4].
2. Biomedical research involving human subjects must conform to generally accepted scientific principles and should be based on the results of adequately performed laboratory and animal experimentation and a knowledge of the natural history of the disease and scientific literature [13, 14].
3. The experiment should yield fruitful results for the good of society, unprocurable by other methods or means of study [13].
4. The voluntary informed consent of the subject should be obtained, preferably in writing. Where physical or mental incapacity makes it impossible to obtain informed consent, permission from the responsible relative replaces that of the subject in accordance with national legislation. Each potential subject should be informed that he can abstain from participating in the study. During the course of the study the subject should be at liberty to bring the experiment to an end at any time [14].
5. The design and performance of each experimental procedure should be clearly formulated in an experimental protocol which should be submitted to an independent committee for consideration, comment and guidance [14] (currently the IRB or Helsinki committee).
6. Every project should be carefully assessed for predictable risks in comparison with foreseeable benefits to the subject or others. The degree of risk to be taken should never exceed that determined by the humanitarian importance of the problem to be solved by the study [13, 14].
7. Research should be conducted only by scientifically qualified persons [13].
8. Studies should be performed in proper facilities to protect the subject against even remote possibilities of injury, disability or death [13].
9. During the course of the experiment, the scientist must be prepared to terminate the experiment at any stage, if he has probable cause to believe that a continuation of the experiment is likely to result in injury, disability or death to the subject [13].
10. Reports of experimentation not in accordance with ethical principles should not be accepted for publication [14].

Ethical Considerations in Clinical Trials

The bioethical principles that are important with regard to the use of human subjects in research are autonomy, beneficence, non-maleficence and justice [16]. Autonomy is a term derived from the Greek *autos* ("self") and *nomos* ("rule"). An individual has self-determination and determines his own course of action without constraints from another's actions or from physical or psychological limitations [16]. The patient is the one who experiences the benefits or complications of treatment and feels the pain. Participation in research should be based on freedom of the individual to choose without coercion and with sufficient understanding to make a decision. In contradistinction to the principle of autonomy is paternalism wherein an individual's liberty is restricted to achieve his best interests irrespective of his consent. Physicians believe they are in a better position than their patients to make medical decisions and have an ethical responsibility to help make decisions in the best interests of their patients. Non-maleficence is associated with the famous dictum *primum non nocere* or "above all, or first, do no harm [16]." Beneficence requires not only that one refrain from harming people but that one also confer benefits and actively prevent and remove harms [16]. Therefore, the research subject's well being always takes precedence over the interests of science and society, and the benefits of the research should outweigh the risks. Finally, justice is "giving to each his right or due [16]." Neither the benefits nor the risks of research should be unjustly distributed [16]. Research subjects should be chosen based on scientific issues and not because of their easy availability, their compromised position or their tendency to be manipulated [17].

If there are procedures or therapies which may help or harm patients, should patients be enrolled into randomized trials to evaluate these modalities? A major concern in human experimentation is that a person included in a study may be treated differently and exposed to risks which he would not ordinarily encounter if he did not participate in the study. In a randomized clinical trial, the various procedures performed are not all necessary for the treatment of the individual patient. As a subject in a clinical trial, the patient may be exposed to added hazards, discomforts, and inconveniences. Treatment may not be able to be tailored to the patient's specific needs. Patients may not benefit from advances that occur during the trial's duration. Towards the end of a several year trial, new treatments or technologies may become available that may be superior to those available to patients in the trial. On the other hand, there are benefits for the patient who becomes a research subject. The patient may have access to a new drug that would otherwise not be available. The patient may be positively affected by the Hawthorne effect because the patient is part of a research activity with more attention from specialists who would not be as involved if the patient were not in the trial [18]. In fact, outcomes in research trials tend to be better than treatment outside the trials irrespective of the treatment group [19]. Patients may also be gratified that they have done everything possible including extraordinary measures to overcome their illness.

Physicians have an ethical obligation to use the best available treatment for their patient. If a clinician has good reasons to believe that one therapy is better than another, it would be unethical to participate in a trial comparing the better therapy to an inferior one. If the physician has doubts as to which therapy is better and believes either is acceptable, he could ethically randomize patients into a clinical trial. Clinical equipoise must exist. Clinical equipoise occurs when competent physicians are content to have their patients receive any of the treatment groups in a randomized trial because based on available data, none has been proven preferable [20]. If two agents to be tested are known to be beneficial, the inclusion of a placebo group would be unethical. If doubt existed as to whether any of the agents is better, an experimental and a placebo group would be desirable and ethical [21]. There are differences between established therapies and promising but unproven treatments. Even if a new therapy is unproven, if the doctor believes it has promise, how can he allow his patient to be randomized into a placebo group if he is supposed to act in the patient's best interest? A physician may randomize patients into treatment and placebo arms because a new therapy might be beneficial but it also might be harmful. Several studies have documented accepted therapies to be not only not superior but more harmful than the placebo [22, 23]. Recruiting patients as research subjects into randomized clinical trials is believed to be morally permissible because at the time of the trial it is not clear what the best treatment is and the randomized clinical trial is not inconsistent with the physician's duty to provide the best possible treatment for his patient [24]. In fact, there are those who argue that it is more ethical to use patients as research subjects in a randomized clinical trial than to use treatments that are unproven. Most of the recent clinical trials for sepsis have compared a new therapeutic agent to a placebo whereas all other therapies were standard treatments.

Most physicians will have a treatment preference, a bias or a hunch and are not truly indifferent to the alternatives being tested [24]. Patients ask their doctors for a recommendation based upon the physician's knowledge, judgement, and experience. If a physician does have a strong preference even based on unscientific data, he should probably not participate in the trial. If the physician has a preference but not a strong one and is not certain what is best, then he may advise the patient to participate in the trial. Even if one has no opinion prior to a study, during the course of a trial, one may form an opinion especially if it is impossible to remain blinded to the therapies being given. Moreover, a single trial is often not sufficient for licensing of a drug and a second, confirmatory study must be performed. It may be difficult for a physician to participate in a second, confirmatory study unless there were problems with the first trial. The physician should inform the patient of his preferences and the previous studies even if this may cause the patient to decide not to participate in the trial because withholding this information would violate the physician's duty to his patient [24].

Should large, controlled, blinded randomized trials be performed initially or should pilot, open, uncontrolled, unblinded trials of a new therapy be performed first? Some argue that initial, uncontrolled studies should not be performed because without controls, the results lack validity, they may seriously mislead investigators and patients about the effectiveness of a new drug, and once physicians are persuaded by unscientific grounds that the drug is efficacious, they may mistakenly consider themselves ethically bound to use the drug and unable to randomize patients into a properly conducted trial [24, 25]. Others reject these assertions and state that randomized trials should not be performed for all therapeutic research. They state that it is unethical to undertake the enormous costs and demands of a large trial until there is some preliminary evidence of efficacy; at the time that there is dramatic evidence of benefit, appropriate patients can be enrolled into large, controlled trials [23, 25]. We believe it is extremely important to perform pilot studies in patients to show efficacy before large, multicenter trials are begun. For instance, initial studies of corticosteroids and prostaglandin E1 in single centers demonstrated benefit and led to large, multicenter trials which did not confirm the effectiveness [22, 27, 28].

Informed Consent

Conducting clinical trials in sepsis presents particular difficulties as patients may be extremely ill, unconscious, and have many other underlying diseases. In the United States, federal regulations concerning informed consent for research are more stringent than informed consent for therapeutic indications. The issue of informed consent has caused problems in performing research in critically ill patients in the United States [29]. Investigators are either avoiding the issue, not performing the research or doing the best they can with the present difficulties.

The obtaining of truly informed consent can be a major problem. It has been said that true informed consent may never be obtainable [11]. Informed consent for research presents additional ethical problems than informed consent for clinical situations. The elements of informed consent include disclosure of information, competency, understanding, voluntariness and decision making. The physician provides information to a competent patient who understands this information and who voluntarily makes a decision to accept or refuse the recommended procedure or treatment [30]. In some cultures, community leaders may have to be approached for consent before attempting to obtain consent from individuals [31]. Informed consent is based on the fundamental right of self-determinism which some believe should be honored universally no matter what the local custom [32].

The doctrine of informed consent is also designed to promote patient health [33, 34]. Society has an important interest in the well-being of its members. This societal interest in preserving health may at times outweigh the interest in protecting individual autonomy. The exceptions to informed consent such as emergency and incompetency illustrate this balancing process [33, 34]. Ultimate decision making authority usually rests with the individual. Since the critically ill patient may be unable to be informed or to consent, however, the interests of society in promoting health and in acting in the best interest of patients unable to make health care decisions for themselves are reflected in the exceptions to the informed consent doctrine.

The issue of informed consent is relevant not only to ethics but also to science. In the VA Cooperative trial of corticosteroids in sepsis [27], the central VA committee responsible for informed consent would not allow the trial to proceed without the actual informed consent of the subject. The investigators requested that patients with altered sensorium and more serious illness be included with surrogate consent because they believed that the drug would be more effective in these patients. At this same time, patients were being enrolled into trials with informed consent given by their next-of-kin and approved by local IRBs in VA hospitals throughout the United States. Despite these facts, surrogates were not allowed to give consent and only patients who gave informed consent were enrolled into the VA Co-operative trial. Because of this ethical decision related to informed consent, the overall mortality in the study was lower than other studies and as the investigators predicted, screened, non-enrolled septic patients with an altered sensorium had a higher mortality than septic patients with normal sensorium [35].

In general, the patient should be informed as to the nature of the medical problem, the nature, duration, and purpose of the proposed study treatment with its risks and benefits, alternatives, the method and means by which the study is to be conducted, all inconveniences and hazards reasonably to be expected, the effects on the subject's health which may occur because of participation in the study, and rights to compensation and treatment as a result of participation in the study. The patient should also be informed that he does not have to participate in the trial and that he can withdraw from the trial at any time. When accepted standard treatments are being given or compared, there is controversy whether a patient should be informed of the fact that he is participating in a trial or that the therapy to be given will be determined by randomization [24, 36, 37]. Today many authorities believe that the patient should be informed of these facts.

Most septic and/or critically ill patients will not have the decision making capacity to decide for themselves. A patient's lack of decision making capacity may be complete, limited or intermittent. Medications given for sedation, anxiety or analgesia may impair a patient's mental functioning as can a patient's fear, depression or denial. The patient is normally considered competent unless he has been formally judged to be incompetent [33]. Incompetency may be general or specific [33]. General incompetency refers to those patients who are unconscious, encephalopathic, intoxicated, grossly psychotic or senile. The term "specific incompetency" is applied to those who are incompetent to make certain decisions, but competent to make others [33]. Incompetent patients have the same rights as competent patients. The manner, however, in which these rights are exercised differs in that another person, a surrogate, exercises those rights for the incompetent patient [38, 39].

Questions arise whether surrogates can give informed consent for research purpose. The Nuremberg Code states that "the voluntary consent of the human subject is absolutely essential [13]." No exceptions are made. This would effectively forbid research in all seriously ill patients with an altered mental status and deny potential benefits to future patients. Federal regulations in the Unites States believed this to be inequitable [40]. The Declaration of Helsinki [14] approved of consent by proxy with the use of a responsible relative as noted in the research codes and regulations section above. Some countries and states in the United States specify that the surrogate must be "an authorized legal representative." Some attorneys take this to mean a court-appointed individual, a requirement that is quite impossible in an emergency treatment protocol. Although family members have no legal authority to make most medical decisions for incapacitated patients, relatives routinely participate with physicians in life and death diagnostic, therapeutic and experimental decisions [39].

Once a surrogate has been identified, respect for the patient's autonomy and the promotion of the patient's health are the two concerns that guide decision making [39, 41]. Although patient autonomy is respected through the surrogate, there are differences between what patients want and what their surrogates think they want [39]. The two main standards advocated for use by surrogate decision makers are substituted judgement and best interests [38, 39]. Substituted judgement occurs when a surrogate attempts to determine what the incompetent patient would have decided had the patient been able to choose. The best interests standard attempts to promote the good of the individual as viewed by the shared values of society [38, 39]. The course that will offer the greatest net benefit to the patient, as would be determined by a reasonable person in the patient's circumstances is followed. Most ethical and legal authorities have recommended the use of substituted judgement but if the patient's views are not known then the best interests standard is used [39, 41].

One of the issues with informed consent in clinical trials is whether the consent is truly voluntary. The patient may be dependent and submissive towards the physician who is responsible for his care. The burden of more detailed information and decisions as to the patient's medical condition and the trial which would not be disclosed if the patient were not a potential research candidate adds to the extreme stress and anxiousness of the patient and/or family. They probably wonder how the patient's care will be negatively affected if they refuse or how it will be positively affected if they agree. The investigator should explain that the patient will receive the best possible care by the treating physicians whether the patient participates in the trial or not but the patient or family may not be entirely convinced.

There also exists the concept of "deferred" consent for critically ill patients who must be given therapy immediately and when prior informed consent is impossible to obtain [42]. This typically occurs under the emergency exception to informed consent when there is an immediate threat to life or limb [33] and usually applies to standard, recognized medical therapies. Because the reasonable man and average patient wants to be treated in a life-threatening situation without informed consent, and society is interested in the health of its members, physicians may treat patients in an emergency situation without informed consent. Whether this includes experimental therapies in trials in emergency situations is unclear. Deferred consent in research involves the random assignment of patients who meet the medical criteria of the research protocol to either the standard or experimental therapy group without obtaining informed consent from either the patient (who lacks decision making capacity) or their families (who are not available in the short, critical time period during which treatment must be initiated) [42]. Once family members become available, however, an explanation of the research protocol is provided and they can withdraw the patient from the study or continue the patient in the study [42]. Deferred consent may conflict with the principle of autonomy. Patients are not required to accept an accepted or experimental treatment that is "best" for them. They may want to be free to make the "wrong" choice and decide for themselves.

In the United States, the Department of Health and Human Services (DHHS) requires that for biomedical research supported by federal funds "informed consent will be sought from each respective subject or the subject's legally authorized representative" [43] but also permits a waiver of informed consent under certain circumstances. These circumstances are that the IRB finds and documents that:

1) the research could not be carried out without the waiver;
2) the subjects will be provided with additional pertinent information after participation;
3) the research involves no more than minimal risk to the subjects; and
4) the waiver will not adversely affect the rights and welfare of the subjects [44].

It could be argued that the risks of research might be less than minimal if two available, yet to be proven therapies that were being used clinically were studied. This might not hold true for a new, experimental therapy. In addition, the randomization of treatment assignment and using an experimental therapy without consent might affect the patient's rights. The FDA also has regulations permitting the use of an investigational drug without informed consent under certain circumstances. These circumstances are:

1) the subject is confronted by a life-threatening situation necessitating the use of the drug;
2) informed consent cannot be obtained from the subject because of an inability to communicate with the subject;
3) time is not sufficient to obtain consent from the subject's legal representative; and
4) there is no alternative method of approved therapy that provides an equal or greater likelihood of saving the life of the subject [45].

Whether the use of an experimental drug is necessary or whether no other alternative therapy that provides equal or greater likelihood of saving the patient in resuscitation or sepsis trials could be debated. In evaluating the question of deferred consent for clinical trials, a study testing two standard therapies or experimental therapies which a reasonable physician and lay persons would consider in the best interests of the patient should be less problematic. An NIH-funded, international randomized clinical trial of cardiopulmonary-cerebral resuscitation after cardiac arrest, the Brain Resuscitation Clinical Trial (BRCT II), used deferred consent in 15 American and 8 European hospitals [42]. It could be argued that deferred consent might also be appropriate for studies in certain groups of septic patients such as severe septic shock which requires prompt treatment.

The regulations and practices in various countries around the world differ. Under British law, consent can only be granted by the patient or a legally authorized representative [46]. It is unusual for legal steps to be taken to appoint a legal guardian for a critically ill patient and permission is usually obtained from relatives [46]. Several countries are considering adhering to regulations formulated by the CPMP Working Party on Efficacy of Medicinal Products of the Commission of the European Communities which include consent to clinical studies (L.G.Thijs, personal communication). The regulations include a section stating that if a subject is incapable of giving consent, the inclusion of such subjects may be acceptable if the Ethics Committee is in agreement and the investigator believes participation will promote the welfare and interest of the subject. The agreement of a legally valid representative that participation will promote the welfare and interest of the subject should also be recorded by a dated signature. If neither signed informed consent nor witnessed signed verbal consent are possible, this fact must be documented with reasons by the investigator. In Switzerland, when consent for clinical research cannot be obtained from the patient or legal representative in due time because of an emergency situation, consent of an independent physician not participating in the study and selected for that purpose by the ethical research committee is obtained (M.Glauser, personal communication).

Conflicts of Interest

It is generally accepted that the physician's primary responsibility is to provide the best possible treatment to his patient and that this obligation overrides other competing goals such as the promotion of scientific knowledge [24]. There is a potential conflict of interest for the physician who is responsible or involved in the medical treatment of the patient and who is also the principal investigator of the research study [24]. In many clinical trials, the investigator is also the patient's physician. As the primary care physician, the doctor's commitment is exclusively to his patient. He may neglect the requirements of a trial which he fears are too burdensome for his patient. Because physicians believe in the potential usefulness of the agent being studied, some may enroll their patients into the trial (usually giving the patient at least at 50% chance of receiving the study drug in most randomized sepsis trials) despite the fact that the patients do not meet the entry criteria or have exclusion criteria. As a scientist, the principal investigator's obligation is to the proper running of the trial and scientific knowledge. His commitment is no longer exclusively and unequivocally to promote the interests of his patient [24]. He may lose sight of what is best for the patient when enthusiastically recruiting patients and performing the study. The physician may do what is best for the study and not advocate strongly to individualize therapy for the patient. Investigators may have a conflict of interest if they have financial ties as stockholders or as paid consultants to a company whose products they are investigating [47]. In addition, investigators in most industry-sponsored studies receive a payment and authorship based on patients enrolled and therefore have incentives to enroll patients. This may work to the disadvantage of the patient and the study. In most circumstances the priorities of the primary care physician and the investigator coincide, occasionally, however, they may conflict. Therefore, it may be better to separate these two roles entirely. The primary care physician can manage the medical care of the patient on a daily basis and be the patient's advocate, and another individual can be the principal investigator whose primary obligation is to the proper running of the study. Some investigators in multicenter trials have developed guidelines for disclosure and against buying, selling, or holding stock or serving as paid consultants to companies whose therapies they are investigating so there is no real or perceived conflict of interest [48].

There are other ethical issues that arise with industry-sponsored trials. There is great importance in the collaboration between industry and the scientific community in clinical trials. Both industry and physicians in academia are interested in the development of safe and effective therapies for patients. Unfortunately, there also may be a conflict of interest between the company and the investigator. Their goals and priorities may differ. Pharmaceutical corporations have a primary fiduciary responsibility to their shareholders. Because of the extreme competition to develop a new therapy for sepsis, there is great pressure on industry to quickly bring a successful product to market. This may not always be in the best interests of the patients or the study. There are also pressures on investigators to participate in corporate-sponsored research so they can acquire professional recognition and fund there own research activities as funding sources diminish. Because of these pressures on industry and investigators, some have questioned whether adequate numbers and ample types of animal studies and sufficient non-randomized human studies have been performed before large clinical trials [10]. In addition, as investigators have become more involved in industry-sponsored clinical trials, they have noted the differing goals of the investigator and the corporation [10]. Investigators want easy and quick access to study data and early publication of results whereas companies want control of the data they have contracted for and developed, and may set greater priorities for items other than publishing manuscripts. Who owns the data? The company, the investigators, or the patients? This will usually depend on the arrangements agreed upon before the study commences. Many investigators when signing contracts with companies agree that data are the property of the company and that data will not be disclosed or published without the prior written permission of the company.

Monitoring Clinical Sepsis Trials

Ethical issues which affect science also arise in monitoring a clinical trial. Who is to be responsible and how should they proceed? Some entity must be responsible for the development, implementation and monitoring of the randomization, the monitoring of compliance with the protocol, efficiency of data collection and processing, safety and efficacy, stopping the trial, and the analysis, interpretation and reporting of the results at interim analyses and at study end [10]. The primary purpose of a monitoring committee is to stop the trial if the accumulating data destroy the state of equipoise indicating efficacy or toxicity [4]. Because of the pressure to enroll patients quickly and because of the multiple centers enrolling patients into some large trials, patients may be enrolled too quickly for the adequate monitoring of safety and efficacy. IRBs typically review research protocols and informed consent issues prior to a trial and make perfunctory yearly reviews of enrolled patients. Most IRBs, however, do not prospectively monitor the informed consent process, the performance of the research, the complications, or the protocol violations.

Over the last decade, corporations have been responsible for most of the large, multicenter sepsis trials. Industry may choose to perform all, some or none of the above functions. Although there may be nothing wrong with a company performing these activities, they may be best performed by an independent entity so there is no potential for the introduction of bias [49]. Difficulties have occurred when a corporate representative had access to interim analysis data and changes were made in the analytic plan [50]. An example can be taken from the SOLVD trial which evaluated an angiotensin-converting-enzyme inhibitor in patients with congestive heart failure and low ejection fractions [51]. The investigators through the National Heart, Lung and Blood Institute designed, conducted and monitored the study, and analyzed, interpreted and reported the results of the study without company input [51].

In summary, we have reviewed the ethical considerations involved in clinical trials of sepsis. Ethical issues by their nature do not lend themselves to an evidence-based approach. We have specifically discussed bioethical principles, issues related to research codes and regulations, whether and when trials are ethical, informed consent, conflicts of interest, and the monitoring of trials. The most dependable safeguard for the research subject more than informed consent, an IRB, or a set of regulations is the presence of a competent, conscientious, compassionate, responsible and caring physician and investigator.

Conclusions

1. Human experimentation is essential for the expansion of scientific knowledge.
2. Ethical decision making in medicine and clinical trials requires accurate medical information.
3. The components for a properly designed and executed trial include justification, methodology, conduct and monitoring of a trial and the interpretation of the data.

4. The justification to begin a randomized controlled trial (RCT) is based on an understanding of the pathophysiology of the disease and the proposed physiologic effects of the intervention, sufficient animal studies in several species and models inferring benefit and no increased risk in humans, and human pilot and/or phase II studies.
5. Abuses in research have occurred in the past and could occur in the future.
6. Various codes, declarations and regulations on biomedical research have been developed to protect human subjects (Table 1).
7. The randomization of patients into a clinical trial is not inconsistent with the physician's duty to provide the best possible therapy if there is clinical equipoise.
8. Informed consent from the patient or a surrogate must be obtained prior to the randomization of a patient into a clinical trial.
9. Deferred consent or waiver of informed consent are mechanisms to enroll patients with life-threatening illnesses into clinical trials when therapy must be given immediately and prior informed consent is impossible.
10. Participation in a trial can influence the behavior of physicians and patients.
11. Conflicts of interest may occur between the physician's primary responsibility to the patient and the investigator's responsibility to the trial.
12. Conflicts of interest may occur between investigators and research sponsors. These conflicts can potentially lead to differences of opinion in many areas including the randomization, design of trials, monitoring compliance with the protocol, monitoring data collection and processing, monitoring safety and efficacy, stopping the trial, and analysis, interpretation, and reporting of the data in trials.
13. Research sponsors control and/or involvement in the above activities may lead to a potential for the introduction of bias and unfortunate results in trial outcomes.
14. Ethical issues and decisions in clinical trials can affect the scientific results of the trials and the use of new therapies.

Recommendations

1. The components for a properly designed and executed trial must be present.
2. RCTs should commence only after there is an understanding of the pathophysiology of the disease and the proposed physiologic effects of the intervention, there are sufficient animal studies in several species and models inferring benefit and no increased risk in humans, and there are sufficient pilot and/or phase II studies inferring the possibility of beneficial and not harmful effects.

3. Clinical trials should be performed in accordance with the various codes, declarations and regulations on biomedical research to protect human subjects.
4. Experimental and placebo groups are desirable if doubt exists as to which agent is best. When two proven beneficial agents are to be tested, a placebo group should not be included. Physicians with a strong preference for one treatment should not participate in these trials.
5. Informed consent from the patient or a surrogate must be obtained prior to the randomization of a patient into a clinical trial.
6. Deferred consent or waiver of informed consent after appropriate approval may allow the enrollment of patients with life-threatening illnesses into clinical trials when therapy must be given immediately and when prior informed consent is impossible.
7. The investigator should be someone other than the primary care physician to avoid a conflict of interest or a potential conflict of interest.
8. Investigators should disclose their financial interests in a therapy they are studying and should avoid buying, selling or holding stock or serving as paid consultants to companies whose therapies they are investigating to avoid a real or perceived conflict of interest.
9. Responsibilities for randomization, monitoring compliance with the protocol, data collection and processing, safety and efficacy, stopping the trial and data analysis should be performed by an independent, external group. Responsibilities for interpretation and reporting of the results of the trial should also be considered given to an independent, external group.
10. Data collection and processing should occur quickly enough to allow for adequate safety and efficacy monitoring.
11. Investigators should have ready access to data and have a copy of the trial data to allow for early interpretation and reporting of results.

References

1. Shinkin MB (1953) The problem of experimentation on human beings. 1. The research worker's point of view. Science 117:205–207
2. Thomas DP (1969) Experiment versus authority: James Lind and Benjamin Rush. N Engl J Med 281:932–935
3. Medical Research Council (1948) Streptomycin treatment of pulmonary tuberculosis. Br J Med 2:769–782
4. Passamani E (1991) Clinical trials – Are they ethical? N Engl J Med 324:1589–1592
5. Sackett DL (1982) The competing objectives of randomized trials. N Engl J Med 303:1059–1069
6. Hellman S, Hellman DS (1991) Of mice but not men. Problems of the randomized clinical trial. N Engl J Med 324:1585–1589
7. Gehan EA, Freireich EJ (1974) Non-randomized controls in cancer clinical trials. N Engl J Med 290:198–203
8. Byar DP, Schoenfeld DA, Green SB, et al (1990) Design considerations for AIDS trials. N Engl J Med 323:1343–1347

9. Inman KJ, Martin CM, Sibbald WJ (1992) Design and conduct of clinical trials in critical care. J Crit Care 7:118–128
10. Eidelman LA, Sprung CL (1994) Why have new effective therapies for sepsis not been developed? Crit Care Med 22 (in press)
11. Beecher H (1966) Ethics and clinical research. N Engl J Med 274:1354–1360
12. Brandt AM (1978) Racism and research: The case of the Tuskegee syphilis study. Hast Ctr Rep 8:21–29
13. Beauchamp TL, Childress JF (eds) (1983) Principles of biomedical ethics. 2nd ed. Oxford University Press, Oxford, pp 338–339
14. Beauchamp TL, Childress JF (eds) (1983) Principles of biomedical ethics. 2nd ed. Oxford University Press, Oxford, pp 339–343
15. National Research Act (1974) Pub Law 93-348, 42 USC 289L-3(a)
16. Beauchamp TL, Childress JF (eds) (1983) Principles of biomedical ethics. 2nd ed. Oxford University Press, Oxford, pp 59–220
17. National Commission for the protection of human subjects of biomedical and behavioral research (1979) The Belmont Report: Ethical principles and guidelines for the protection of human subjects of research. Department of Health, Education and Welfare, Washington D.C., 5. DHEW publication no (05) 9-12065
18. Levine RJ, Cohen ED (1974) The Hawthorne effect. Clin Res 22:111–112
19. Stiller C (1992) Survival of patients in clinical trials and at specialist centres. In: Williams CJ (ed) Introducing new treatments for cancer: Practical, ethical and legal problems. Wiley, Chichester, pp 119–136
20. Freedman B (1987) Equipoise and the ethics of clinical research. N Engl J Med 317:141–145
21. Shaw LW, Chalmers TC (1970) Ethics in cooperative clinical trials. Ann NY Acad Sci 169:487–494
22. Bone RC, Fisher CJ, Clemmer TP, et al (1987) A controlled clinical trial of high-dose methylprednisolone in the treatment of severe sepsis and septic shock. N Engl J Med 317:653–658
23. The Cardiac Arrhythmias Suppression Trial (CAST) Investigators (1989) Preliminary report: Effect of encainide and flecainide on mortality in a randomized trial of arrhythmia suppression after myocardial infarction. N Engl J Med 321:406–412
24. Schafer A (1982) The ethics of the randomized clinical trial. N Engl J Med 307:719–724
25. Sacks H, Kupfer S, Chalmers TC (1980) Are uncontrolled clinical studies ever justified? N Engl J Med 303:1067 (Lett)
26. Hollenberg NK, Dzau VJ, Williams GH (1980) Are uncontrolled clinical studies ever justified? N Engl J Med 303:1067 (Lett)
27. The Veterans Administration Systemic Sepsis Cooperative Study Group (1987) Effect of high-dose glucocorticoid therapy on mortality in patients with clinical signs of systemic sepsis. N Engl J Med 317:659–665
28. Bone RC, Slotman G, Maunder R, et al (1989) Randomized double-blind, multicenter study of prostaglandin E1 in patients with the adult respiratory distress syndrome. Chest 96:114–119
29. Sprung CL, Schein RMH (1986) Consent: Informed, implied or deferred. JAMA 256:1891–1892
30. Meisel A, Roth LH (1981) What we do and do not know about informed consent. JAMA 246:2473–2477
31. Barry M (1988) Ethical considerations of human investigation in developing countries. N Engl J Med 319:1083–1086
32. Angell M (1988) Ethical imperialism? Ethics in international collaborative clinical research. N Engl J Med 319:1081–1083
33. Sprung CL, Winick BJ (1989) Informed consent in theory and practice: Legal and medical perspectives on the informed consent doctrine and a proposed reconceptualization. Crit Care Med 17:1346–1354
34. Meisel A (1979) The exceptions to the informed consent doctrine: Striking a balance between competing values in medical decision-making. Wisc Law Rev 1979:413–488

35. Sprung CL, Peduzzi PN, Shatney CH, et al (1990) Impact of encephalopathy on mortality in the sepsis syndrome. Crit Care Med 18:801–806
36. Zelen M (1979) A new design for randomized clinical trials. N Engl J Med 300:1242–1245
37. Brewin TB (1982) Consent to randomised treatment. Lancet 2:919–921
38. Nyman DJ, Sprung CL (1991) Ensuring informed consent: Essentials and specific exceptions. J Crit Illness 6:89–96
39. Sprung CL (1990) Surrogate decision-making in critical care medicine. In: Lumb PD, Shoemaker WC (eds) Critical Care. State of the art 1990. Society of Critical Care Medicine, Fullerton, pp 367–377
40. Protection of human subjects (1973) 38 Fed Reg 31,739
41. President's Commission for the Study of Ethical Problems in Medicine and Biomedical and Behavioral Research (1983) Patients who lack decision making capacity. In: Deciding to forego life-sustaining treatment: Ethical, medical and legal issues in treatment decisions. Government Printing Office, Washington, D.C., pp 121–170
42. Abramson NS, Meisel A, Safar P (1986) Deferred consent. A new approach for resuscitation research on comatose patients. JAMA 255:2466–2471
43. Protection of human subjects (1983) 45 CFR §46.111(a)
44. Protection of human subjects (1983) 45 CFR §46.116(d)
45. Food and Drug Administration (1981) Protection of human subjects. 46 Fed Reg 8,951
46. Park GR (1989) Ethical and moral difficulties with trials in critically ill patients. Intensive Care World 6:11–12
47. Relman AS (1989) Economic incentives in clinical investigation. N Engl J Med 320:933–934
48. Healy B, Campeau L, Gray R, et al (1989) Conflict-of-interest guidelines for a multicenter clinical trial of treatment after coronary-artery bypass-graft surgery. N Engl J Med 320:949–951
49. O'Neill RT (1993) Some FDA perspectives on data monitoring in clinical trials in drug development. Statistics Med 12:601–608
50. Siegel JP, Stein KE, Zoon KC (1992) Anti-endotoxin monoclonal antibodies. N Engl J Med 327:890–891
51. The SOLVD Investigators (1991) Effect of enalapril on survival in patients with reduced left ventricular ejection fractions and congestive heart failure. N Engl J Med 325:293–302

Subject Index

Springer-Verlag and the Environment

We at Springer-Verlag firmly believe that an international science publisher has a special obligation to the environment, and our corporate policies consistently reflect this conviction.

We also expect our business partners – paper mills, printers, packaging manufacturers, etc. – to commit themselves to using environmentally friendly materials and production processes.

The paper in this book is made from low- or no-chlorine pulp and is acid free, in conformance with international standards for paper permanency.

MIX
Papier aus verantwortungsvollen Quellen
Paper from responsible sources
FSC® C105338

If you have any concerns about our products,
you can contact us on
ProductSafety@springernature.com

In case Publisher is established outside the EU,
the EU authorized representative is:
Springer Nature Customer Service Center GmbH
Europaplatz 3, 69115 Heidelberg, Germany

Printed by Libri Plureos GmbH
in Hamburg, Germany